T0175641

Tintinalli's
Emergency Medicine
Examination and Board Review

SUSAN B. PROMES, MD, MBA, FACEP
Professor and Chair
Department of Emergency Medicine
Pennsylvania State University
Penn State Health—Milton Hershey Medical Center
Hershey, Pennsylvania

New York/Chicago/San Francisco/Athens/London/Madrid/Mexico City/
Milan/New Delhi/Singapore/Sydney/Toronto

McGraw Hill Specialty Board Review Tintinalli's Emergency Medicine Examination and Board Review

Copyright © 2023 by McGraw Hill LLC. All rights reserved. Printed in China. Except as permitted under the United States Copyright Act of 1976, no part of this publication may be reproduced or distributed in any form or by any means, or stored in a data base or retrieval system, without the prior written permission of the publisher.

1 2 3 4 5 6 7 8 9   DSS   27 26 25 24 23 22

ISBN 978-1-260-02594-1
MHID 1-260-02594-2

Notice

Medicine is an ever-changing science. As new research and clinical experience broaden our knowledge, changes in treatment and drug therapy are required. The authors and the publisher of this work have checked with sources believed to be reliable in their efforts to provide information that is complete and generally in accord with the standards accepted at the time of publication. However, in view of the possibility of human error or changes in medical sciences, neither the authors nor the publisher nor any other party who has been involved in the preparation or publication of this work warrants that the information contained herein is in every respect accurate or complete, and they disclaim all responsibility for any errors or omissions or for the results obtained from use of the information contained in this work. Readers are encouraged to confirm the information contained herein with other sources. For example and in particular, readers are advised to check the product information sheet included in the package of each drug they plan to administer to be certain that the information contained in this work is accurate and that changes have not been made in the recommended dose or in the contraindications for administration. This recommendation is of particular importance in connection with new or infrequently used drugs.

This book was set in Minion Pro by KnowledgeWorks Global Ltd.
The editor was Kay Conerly.
The production supervisor was Catherine Saggese.
Project management was provided by Revathi Viswanathan, KnowledgeWorks Global Ltd.

This book is printed on acid-free paper.

Library of Congress Control Number: 2022947273

*This book is dedicated to my family and colleagues at Penn State University
without which this book would not have come to fruition.*

*Special thanks to my husband, Mark, who is my biggest supporter and my two amazing sons,
Alex and Aaron. Did I tell you? I love you!*

Contents

Contributors

Section Editors

Erica Bates, MD
Assistant Professor of Emergency Medicine and
   Internal Medicine
Department of Emergency Medicine
Pennsylvania State University
Penn State Health—Milton S. Hershey Medical Center
Hershey, Pennsylvania

Avram Flamm, DO
Assistant Professor of Emergency Medicine and
   Public Health Sciences
Department of Emergency Medicine
Pennsylvania State University
Penn State Health—Milton S. Hershey Medical Center
Hershey, Pennsylvania

Kathryn M. McCans, MD, FAAP
Associate Professor of Emergency Medicine and Pediatrics
Departments of Emergency Medicine and Pediatrics
Pennsylvania State University
Penn State Health—Milton Hershey Medical Center
Hershey, Pennsylvania

Authors

Andrew Beck, MD, MS
Assistant Professor
Department of Emergency Medicine
Brown University
Providence, Rhode Island
Chapter 6 Thoracic-Respiratory Disorders

Amber Billet, MD, FACEP
Program Director
Emergency Medicine Residency Program
WellSpan York Hospital
York, Pennsylvania
Chapter 7 Abdominal and Gastrointestinal Disorders

Ryan P. Bodkin, MD, MBA
Associate Professor of Emergency Medicine
University of Rochester
Rochester, New York
Chapter 14 Environmental Injuries

E. Page Bridges, MD
Assistant Clinical Professor
Department of Emergency Medicine
Prisma Health/University of South Carolina School of
   Medicine—Greenville
Greenville, South Carolina
Chapter 7 Abdominal and Gastrointestinal Disorders

Esther H. Chen, MD
Professor
Department of Emergency Medicine
University of California, San Francisco
San Francisco, California
Chapter 9 Obstetrics and Gynecology

Eleanor Dunham, MD, FACEP
Assistant Professor of Emergency Medicine
Department of Emergency Medicine
Pennsylvania State University
Penn State Health—Milton S. Hershey Medical Center
Hershey, Pennsylvania
Chapter 22 Psychosocial Disorders

Paolo Grenga, MD
Clinical Instructor of Emergency Medicine
University of Rochester
Rochester, New York
Chapter 14 Environmental Injuries

Mariana Guerrero, MD
Emergency Medicine Physician
Denver Health and Hospital Authority
Denver, Colorado
Chapter 3 Analgesia, Anesthesia, and Procedural Sedation

Alison Hayward, MD, MPH
Assistant Professor of Emergency Medicine
Warren Alpert School of Medicine
Brown University
Providence, Rhode Island
Chapter 8 Renal and Genitourinary Disorders

Shanna C. Jones, MD, FACEP
Associate Professor
Department of Emergency Medicine
Beaumont Health System
Troy, Michigan
Chapter 11 Systemic Infectious Disorders

Nikita K. Joshi, MD
Medical Director, Alameda Hospital
Department of Emergency Medicine
Alameda Health System
Oakland, California
Chapter 18 Dermatology

Annahieta Kalantari, DO
Associate Professor
Department of Emergency Medicine
Pennsylvania State University
Penn State Health—Milton S. Hershey Medical Center
Hershey, Pennsylvania
Chapter 12 Nervous System Disorders

Linda E. Keyes, MD, FACEP, FAWM
Adjoint Associate Professor of Emergency Medicine
Anschutz Medical Campus
University of Colorado
Aurora, Colorado
Chapter 3 Analgesia, Anesthesia, and Procedural Sedation

James A. Krueger, MD, FACEP
Consultant, The Poison Control Center at Children's Hospital
    of Philadelphia
Assistant Professor, Division of Medical Toxicology
Assistant Professor, Department of Emergency Medicine
Einstein Healthcare Network
Philadelphia, Pennsylvania
Chapter 13 Toxicologic Disorders

Heather M. Kuntz, MD
Associate Professor
Departments of Emergency Medicine and Pediatrics
Loma Linda University Health
Loma Linda, California
Chapter 10 Pediatrics

Eric J. Lee, MD
Assistant Professor
Program Director
Department of Emergency Medicine
University of Oklahoma
Tulsa, Oklahoma
Chapter 8 Renal and Genitourinary Disorders

Jordan Lull, MD
Pediatric Critical Care Fellow
Nationwide Children's Hospital
Columbus, Ohio
Chapter 10 Pediatrics

Nicholas Macklin, MD
Clinical Assistant Professor
Department of Emergency Medicine
Atrium Health Wake Forest Baptist
Winston-Salem, North Carolina
*Chapter 25 Point-of-Care Ultrasound in the Emergency
    Department*

Jade Malcho, MD
Clinical Instructor
Department of Emergency Medicine
University of Rochester Medical Center
Rochester, New York
Chapter 24 Special Situations

Kathryn McCabe, MD
Staff Physician Denver Health Medical Center
Clinical Instructor, Emergency Medicine
University of Colorado School of Medicine
Aurora, Colorado
Chapter 17 Eye, Ear, Nose, Throat, and Oral Disorders

Mary P. Mercer, MD, MPH, FAEMS
Professor of Emergency Medicine
University of California, San Francisco
San Francisco, California
Chapter 1 Prehospital Care and Disaster Management

Cathy Nelson-Horan, MD
Assistant Professor
Department of Emergency Medicine
Pennsylvania State University
Penn State Health—Milton S. Hershey Medical Center
Hershey, Pennsylvania
Chapter 16 Hematologic Disorders

J. Elizabeth Neuman, DO, FACEP
Assistant Professor of Emergency Medicine
Department of Emergency Medicine
Pennsylvania State University
Penn State Health—Milton S. Hershey Medical Center
Hershey, Pennsylvania
Chapter 19 Traumatic Disorders

Flavia Nobay, MD
Associate Dean of Student Affairs
Professor of Emergency Medicine
University of Rochester School of Medicine
Rochester, New York
Chapter 24 Special Situations

Robert P. Olympia, MD
Professor
Departments of Emergency Medicine and Pediatrics
Pennsylvania State University
Penn State Health—Milton S. Hershey Medical Center
Hershey, Pennsylvania
Chapter 10 Pediatrics

David M. Painter, MD
Department of Emergency Medicine
Duke University
Durham, North Carolina
Chapter 20 Injuries to Bones and Joints

Berenice Perez, MD
Clinical Instructor of Emergency Medicine
UCSF School of Medicine
Emergency Department Medical Director
Alameda Health System Highland Campus
Oakland, California
Chapter 18 Dermatology

Jordan S. Richardson, DO
Emergency Medicine Physician
Timpanogos Regional Medical Center
Orem, Utah
Chapter 5 Cardiovascular Disorders

Ross Rodgers, MD
La Jolla Emergency Specialists
Scripps La Jolla
La Jolla, California
Chapter 5 Cardiovascular Disorders

Carlo L. Rosen, MD
Executive Vice Chair
Department of Emergency Medicine
Associate Director of Graduate Medical Education
Beth Israel Deaconess Medical Center
Associate Professor of Emergency Medicine,
    Harvard Medical School
Boston, Massachusetts
Chapter 19 Traumatic Disorders

Kim A. Rutherford, MD
Assistant Clinical Professor of Emergency Medicine
Long Island School of Medicine
New York University
Mineola, New York
Chapter 23 Abuse and Assault

Evan S. Schwarz, MD, FACEP, FACMT
Associate Professor of Emergency Medicine
Medical Toxicology Division Chief
Washington University
St. Louis, Missouri
Chapter 5 Cardiovascular Disorders

Krystle Shafer, MD
Director of EM-Critical Care
Departments of Emergency Medicine and
    Critical Care Medicine
Wellspan York Hospital
York, Pennsylvania
Chapter 2 Resuscitation

Bijal Shah, MD
Clinical Assistant Professor
Department of Emergency Medicine
Prisma Health/University of South Carolina
    School of Medicine
Greenville, South Carolina
Chapter 7 Abdominal and Gastrointestinal Disorders

Luz M. Silverio, MD
Assistant Program Director (Affiliate)
Department of Emergency Medicine
Stanford University
Stanford, California
Attending Physician
Department of Emergency Medicine
Kaiser Permanente Santa Clara
Santa Clara, California
Chapter 6 Thoracic-Respiratory Disorders

Jessica L. Smith, MD, FACEP
Professor, Clinician Educator
Department of Emergency Medicine
The Alpert Medical School Brown University
Rhode Island Hospital/The Miriam Hospital/Newport Hospital
Providence, Rhode Island
Chapter 6 Thoracic-Respiratory Disorders

Paul Sokoloski, MD
Penn State Holy Spirit Medical Center
Penn State Hampden Medical Center
Penn State Health
Camp Hill, Pennsylvania
Chapter 4 Wound Management

Joshua J. Solano, MD, FAAEM, FACEP
Associate Professor of Emergency Medicine
Medical Student Clerkship Director
Department of Emergency Medicine
Florida Atlantic University
Boynton Beach, Florida
Chapter 19 Traumatic Disorders

Molly E.W. Thiessen, MD
Emergency Medicine Physician
Denver Health Medical Center
Denver, Colorado
Associate Professor
Department of Emergency Medicine
University of Colorado School of Medicine
Aurora, Colorado
Chapter 17 Eye, Ear, Nose, Throat, and Oral Disorders

Traci Thoureen, MD, MMCi, FACEP
Associate Professor
Department of Emergency Medicine
Duke University Medical Center
Durham, North Carolina
Chapter 20 Injuries to Bones and Joints

Steven J. Walsh, MD
The Poison Control Center at Children's Hospital of
  Philadelphia
Division of Medical Toxicology
Department of Emergency Medicine
Einstein Healthcare Network
Philadelphia, Pennsylvania
Chapter 13 Toxicologic Disorders

Monica Kathleen Wattana, MD, FAAEM
Associate Professor of Emergency Medicine
University of Texas MD Anderson Cancer Center
Houston, Texas
Chapter 15 Endocrine, Metabolic, and Nutritional Disorders

Sumintra Wood, MD, MHPE
Attending Physician
Department of Emergency Medicine
Maimonides Medical Center
Brooklyn, New York
Chapter 21 Musculoskeletal Disorders (Non-Traumatic)

Preface

This book is designed as a study tool to complement the popular ninth edition of *Tintinalli's Emergency Medicine: A Comprehensive Study Guide*. To aid in the preparation for the ABEM and AOBEM written examination as well as the annual emergency medicine residency program in-training examination, this edition presents over 800 questions and answers enhanced with tables and visual images, which are in full color. We have also added a new, dedicated chapter on point-of-care ultrasound. The explanation of the correct answer for each question is referenced directly to a chapter in *Tintinalli's Emergency Medicine: A Comprehensive Study Guide, 9th edition*. I hope you find this resource helpful as you prepare for your examination.

Susan B. Promes, MD, MBA, FACEP

Prehospital Care and Disaster Management

QUESTIONS

1. According to the Emergency Medical Treatment and Active Labor Act (EMTALA) of 1986, hospitals wishing to transfer a patient to another facility for a higher level of care must do the following prior to transferring the patient?
   (A) Complete all diagnostic tests
   (B) Collect payment from the patient
   (C) Have an existing transfer contract with the receiving hospital
   (D) Perform a medical screening examination and stabilization of the patient

2. Using the Utstein template for cardiac arrest helps an EMS system do which of the following?
   (A) Collect complete data on cardiac arrest patients and compare outcomes to other EMS systems
   (B) Create a high-performance cardiopulmonary resuscitation (CPR) program
   (C) Determine the number of ambulances needed to treat cardiac arrests promptly
   (D) Transfer cardiac arrest patients to regional ST segment elevation myocardial infarction (STEMI) centers

3. An ambulance unit responds to the scene of a cardiac arrest patient. Describe the differences or similarities between a defibrillator used by advanced life support (ALS) personnel, such as a paramedic versus that used by basic life support (BLS) personnel, such as an emergency medical technician (EMT)-basic.
   (A) A defibrillator used by both ALS and BLS personnel does not display the heart rhythm that the patient is experiencing, in case the EMS provider should get confused and delay delivering the shock.

   (B) The defibrillator used by both ALS and BLS personnel displays the heart rhythm, but the ALS unit can select whether or not to shock, whereas the BLS unit will always deliver a shock.
   (C) The ALS unit uses an automatic external defibrillator (AED), whereas the BLS unit uses a manual defibrillator.
   (D) The ALS unit uses a defibrillator with a manual defibrillator option, whereas the BLS unit uses an AED.

4. A football player cannot get up off of the field after a big tackle and is reporting that he cannot feel or move his legs. He is moving his arms and is in no respiratory distress. As the paramedics are seeking to transfer him to an ambulance, the coach asks if they should remove his helmet. Which of the following is the BEST action of the paramedic?
   (A) The face mask and helmet should be removed from the patients, but the shoulder pads left in place prior to transport, in order to maintain neutral positioning of the spine.
   (B) The face mask and shoulder pads should be removed from the patient, but most of the helmet left in place prior to transport, in order to maintain neutral positioning of the spine.
   (C) The helmet and shoulder pads should both be removed prior to transport, in order to maintain neutral positioning of the spine.
   (D) The helmet and shoulder pads should not be removed until the patient arrives at the emergency department, as they help to maintain neutral positioning of the spine.

5. An EMS medical director is looking to introduce a supraglottic airway device to his/her system. What is a factor that may influence this decision?
   (A) A laryngeal mask airway (LMA) is considered a definitive airway.
   (B) Endotracheal intubation is a skill that is easily maintained in daily practice by emergency medical technicians (EMTs).
   (C) Increasing the number of advanced prehospital providers within a system may reduce opportunities for individuals to maintain skills.
   (D) Rapid-sequence induction (RSI) medications have a low risk profile in the prehospital setting.

6. A 10-day-old infant is diagnosed with septic shock and requires transfer from a community hospital to a tertiary care center that is 30 minutes by helicopter or 2 hours by ground ambulance. What factor will determine if the child will be transferred by helicopter?
   (A) The child cannot be transferred via helicopter EMS if he is placed on a vasopressor drip.
   (B) Should the child develop respiratory distress during transport, the emergency medical technicians (EMTs) aboard the flight will not have the training or skills to manage a pediatric airway.
   (C) The method of transportation is determined by the receiving physician (at the tertiary center).
   (D) The pilot of the helicopter will determine whether or not the flight is feasible based on weather and other flight conditions.

7. What is a problem of which a helicopter air medical team should be aware?
   (A) Chest tubes should not be left to suction during flight, or a pneumothorax may expand.
   (B) Endotracheal cuff pressure could lead to tracheal mucosal damage or necrosis.
   (C) Medications used for rapid sequence intubation (RSI) in the air, have a different dose-effect than on land.
   (D) While transporting a patient with decompression illness, the altitude may improve or resolve their symptoms.

8. You have been asked to be the medical director for an upcoming, outdoor, rock concert that is expected to draw a crowd of over 100,000 people. Part of your responsibility includes creating a medical plan in advance of the event to submit to the city EMS agency. As you work to create this plan, you should consider a number of issues. Select the statement that is TRUE from the following options:
   (A) Environmental factors including changes in weather, temperature, time of day, access to food, water and toileting can all play a factor in the volume and range of medical emergencies that develop over the course of an event.
   (B) Local law enforcement agencies routinely train in addressing mass casualty incidents (MCIs) and can be relied on to render medical care should an MCI occur.
   (C) Medical treatment protocols that are authorized under your supervision are considered independent of local EMS policies and protocols.
   (D) You can expect your volunteer medical responders to rely on their personal cellphones to communicate between each other and the local 911 services.

9. What is the role of the lead safety officer within the incident command system (ICS) structure?
   (A) Develop processes and accountability to ensure the health and safety of the paid and volunteer workers who are supporting the event
   (B) Monitor the crowd size and movement, and direct foot traffic in a safe manner
   (C) Plan for the upcoming operational period and distribute important bulletins, including safety information to team members
   (D) Set up and operate rest stations for event staff

10. You have been asked to represent the emergency department on your hospital's disaster planning committee. Before the group moves on to updating the hospital disaster plans and organizing simulation exercises for staff, the committee chair has asked that the group first assess how the national and local environment has changed and may affect the likelihood of certain types of natural or man-made disasters. For example, a large chemical plant has recently opened about 1 mile from the hospital, and nowhere in the existing disaster plan is there a strategy for addressing an active shooter scenario. This process of assessing local threats and prioritizing preparedness efforts specific to your hospital is called a(n):
    (A) Hazard vulnerability analysis
    (B) Incident command system
    (C) Surge plan
    (D) Table-top exercise

11. You are working in the emergency department when a fire breaks out in a nearby large skilled nursing facility, requiring evacuation of 75 medically complex patients, some with burns and fire-related injuries, directed to your hospital. As your team is triaging and treating the large influx of patients, you realize that most of them require at least short-term admission until longer-term care facilities can be identified. Your hospital's incident command system has been activated. The hospital administration is opening areas of the hospital, calling in extra staff, doubling up patients in in-patient rooms, and modifying a medical ward into an intensive care unit in order to accommodate this large number of admitted patients. This process of finding additional space and expanding treatment capacity is known as:
    (A) Alternate standards of care
    (B) Incident command system
    (C) Surge plan
    (D) Triage plan

12. One of the MOST common types of illnesses to affect victims and relief workers following an earthquake is:
    (A) Fractures
    (B) Hypertension
    (C) Myocardial infarction
    (D) Respiratory illnesses

13. The National Disaster Medical System (NDMS) is a government agency that coordinates deploying highly organized and experienced medical teams into disaster areas as part of the first response. Relief workers on these teams are expected to be ready to depart to a disaster area within 6 to 12 hours of being activated, and they are expected to be self-sufficient for at least:
    (A) 2 days (48 hours)
    (B) 3 days (72 hours)
    (C) 7 days (168 hours)
    (D) 14 days (336 hours)

14. The MOST common cause of primary fatality among blast victims is injury to the:
    (A) Abdomen
    (B) Head
    (C) Heart
    (D) Lung

15. A 30-year-old woman who is 27 weeks pregnant is brought to your emergency department after being found at the site of a bomb explosion at an appliance store. She had been a few yards away from the center of the blast. She initially had ringing in her ears, but now is asymptomatic with normal vital signs and a normal examination.
    (A) Discharge home
    (B) Give steroids and admit the patient to labor and delivery for an urgent C-section
    (C) If initial examination and testing is normal and if the patient remains asymptomatic, admit her to labor and delivery for observation and fetal monitoring
    (D) If initial examination and testing is normal, observe the patient in the emergency department for 6 hours and if patient remains asymptomatic, discharge her to home

16. A 28-year-old woman is the first of 10 patients brought to your emergency department from an office building where there was a suspected nerve agent release. The patient is seizing, has copious frothy sputum and nasal secretions, wheezing, and an episode of diarrhea. In addition to managing her airway, which medications should you administer?
    (A) Adenosine, pralidoxime, and midazolam
    (B) Adenosine, physostigmine, and phenytoin
    (C) Atropine, pralidoxime, and midazolam
    (D) Atropine, pralidoxime, and phenytoin

17. A congresswoman's office received a letter in the mail that contains a death threat and a powdery, white substance. At least 12 people have been exposed to that letter and present to your emergency department. None are currently experiencing symptoms. The sample is sent to the lab to test for *Bacillus anthracis* and other substances. At this time, the 12 patients should be given the following treatment:
    (A) Anthrax immunoglobulin
    (B) Anthrax vaccination
    (C) Intravenous penicillin
    (D) Oral ciprofloxacin

18. In helping to manage an outbreak of an infectious disease (such as an agent of potential bioterrorism), among other things, a public health system should provide which of the following to the public?
    - (A) A clear and concise case definition for diagnosis of "presumptive" or "suspect" cases
    - (B) Immediate public vaccination programs
    - (C) Mandatory quarantine orders for any infectious agent
    - (D) Specialized treatment centers for people with suspected infections

19. You are treating patients brought from an explosion at a nuclear reactor, all of whom are presumed to have been exposed to radiation. While providing medical stabilization and decontamination, which laboratory test will help you estimate the amount of radiation exposure and prognosticate survival?
    - (A) Creatinine
    - (B) Lymphocyte count
    - (C) Stool guaiac
    - (D) Urine pH

20. Your emergency department has been notified that it will receive 15 patients from the site of an explosion at a nuclear reactor. Many have serious traumatic injuries, and all have presumed radiation exposure. Your treatment team has established the appropriate decontamination, treatment, and post-decontamination areas, with sufficient staff having donned personal protective equipment. You are helping to establish the triage process for this mass casualty event. The first patient to arrive from the scene is a 25-year-old woman who was struck in the chest and abdomen with a metal pipe. She is pale, cool, and diaphoretic with a respiratory rate of 36, a thready pulse, and chest wall crepitus. What is the MOST appropriate initial treatment for her?
    - (A) Perform a chest radiograph to determine if she has a pneumothorax
    - (B) Send her to the wet decontamination shower to remove any external radiation before definitive treatment
    - (C) Stabilize her injuries in a "contaminated" treatment room before completing decontamination
    - (D) Triage her to the "Green" zone, as she can walk

ANSWERS

1. **The answer is D.** (Chapter 1) The Emergency Medical Treatment and Active Labor Act (EMTALA) was enacted to ensure that patients seeking emergency care were not turned away or transferred to another facility at an unsafe time in their treatment. It is common for patients to be transferred from one facility to another for a higher level of care (e.g., a patient with severe traumatic injuries who presents to a community hospital could be transferred to a regional trauma center). EMTALA lays out clear requirements for transferring facilities and physicians to follow in order to optimize safe transfer. The most basic requirement is that the first facility must perform a medical screening examination and basic measures of stabilization before transferring the patient. Liability for adverse events during transfer is borne by the transferring physician (at the sending hospital).

2. **The answer is A.** (Chapter 1) The Utstein template is a standardized format for collecting data on cardiac arrests that has been validated through research studies. Use of standardized definitions allows EMS systems to compare outcomes for equivalent patient groups (e.g., cardiac arrests due to ventricular fibrillation vs. nonshockable rhythms). High-performance cardiopulmonary resuscitation (CPR) is a specific method of performing cardiopulmonary resuscitation that delivers real-time feedback to providers. Regionalization of care to specialty centers has been shown to be beneficial to patient outcomes for time-sensitive conditions such as for ST-elevation myocardial infarction and stroke.

3. **The answer is D.** (Chapter 2) The advanced life support (ALS) unit is staffed by a paramedic who can interpret the rhythm displayed on the defibrillator monitor and decide when to deliver a shock (and with how many joules of energy), whereas the basic life support (BLS) unit uses an automatic external defibrillator, which internally records and automatically interprets the rhythm, and then is automatically programmed to deliver a shock if the rhythm is interpreted as ventricular tachycardia or ventricular fibrillation.

4. **The answer is D.** (Chapter 2) The helmet and shoulder pads should not be removed until the patient arrives at the emergency department, as they help to maintain neutral positioning of the spine. The helmet and shoulder pads of the patient help to maintain the spine in a neutral position and should not be removed until after transport to the hospital. In fact, the recommendation is to wait until after initial assessment and radiographs are completed. Removal of the helmet and shoulder pads requires several people in order to maintain spinal alignment. However, the face-mask of a helmet can and should be removed early on in evaluation in order to better access the patient's airway.

5. **The answer is C.** (Chapter 2) Airway and ventilatory management are important prehospital skills for addressing life-threating conditions, such as respiratory distress. Endotracheal intubation and cricothyrotomy are the only definitive airway management techniques. However, both are also high-risk procedures with opportunity for error and increased patient harm if not performed correctly. Both skills may be difficult to maintain due to infrequency of the procedure, and some EMS systems may elect to limit (or not include them) in local scope of practice for certain patient populations (such as pediatrics). A system that has a high number of paramedics performing a small number of infrequent procedures (such as intubation) may determine that they have insufficient volume or simulation time to maintain proficiency of the skills. Although not considered truly definitive airways, supraglottic devices such as the laryngeal mask airway (LMA) can provide an effective bridging intervention to maintain oxygenation and ventilation of critical patients in the prehospital setting. Rapid sequence induction medications have a high-risk profile in the prehospital setting.

6. **The answer is D.** (Chapter 3) Air medical transport is an important part of prehospital care, especially for EMS systems serving more rural communities. There can be many different configurations of the team members on an air medical transport unit. The most common is nurse-paramedic. Due to the higher-risk patient care needs and longer transport times, air medical crews undergo increased training and have expanded scope of practice (increased medications, drips, etc.). Flight safety is a key principle of air medical EMS in order to ensure the lowest risk of accidents. It is standard practice that a pilot will be blinded to the clinical details (including age and condition of the patient) to ensure that the decision to fly is being made exclusively based on the flight conditions and not due to emotional considerations for the patient in need.

7. **The answer is B.** (Chapter 3) Pressure-related problems can occur at altitude. This is described by Boyle's law: the volume of gas increases when pressure decreases at a constant temperature. Therefore, as the volume of an endotracheal tube (ETT) cuff cannot change at altitude, the pressure of the air inside the cuff could increase above the perfusion pressure of the tracheal mucosa and cause necrosis.

8. **The answer is A.** (Chapter 4). Planning for an appropriate medical response during a mass gathering is critical for maintaining the health and safety of participants and spectators, as well as for ensuring the maintenance of services for the surrounding community. Preparations should include an interdisciplinary team and all-hazards approach to planning. It is important for medical directors to understand the conditions that could be exacerbated by the crowd size, venue, and the nature of the event. Historical data about the event or similar events are important for preparation of the medical plan. Environmental factors including changes in weather, temperature, time of day, access to food, water, and toileting can all play a factor in the volume and range of medical emergencies that occur during a mass gathering. An appropriate plan should include resources and communication systems that do not jeopardize the local medical response system. Sometimes, additional EMS personnel may contract with an event organizer to provide care or transportation for medical emergencies. These providers must still work within the local scope of practice and EMS policies. Medical directors should also coordinate with local safety officials including law enforcement and fire to plan for potential response to different types of mass casualty incidents that could result due to crowd conditions or terrorism. While some law enforcement agencies understand the basics of medical care, the medical director should not assume that police or fire personnel will be assisting in rendering medical attention.

9. **The answer is A.** (Chapter 4) Within the incident command system (ICS), the safety officer is a member of the command staff and his or her role is to develop processes and accountability to ensure the health and safety of the paid and volunteer workers who are supporting the event (or disaster response). Members of the operations and logistics sections would be responsible for ensuring the health and safety of the event participants, as well as executing the plan and processes outlined by the safety officer (including setting up and operating rest stations). Members of the planning section are responsible for planning ahead for the next operational period.

10. **The answer is A.** (Chapter 5) A hazard vulnerability analysis (HVA) is an assessment performed by a local hospital or EMS agency that helps to categorize the different types of disasters that might affect their community (e.g., earthquake, flood, active shooter, etc.). By assessing which events are the most likely to occur and which would produce the significant strain on the response capabilities, a hospital can prioritize disaster planning efforts. The incident command system (ICS) is a standardized organizational system for the immediate response phase of a disaster. A surge plan is the specific plan of action that hospital will take in response to a sudden large increase (or "surge") in patient volume or critical care needs. A tabletop exercise is a written and verbal simulation exercise in which a group of key stakeholders will reason through a series of challenges that could occur in the setting of a disaster or mass casualty incident (MCI).

11. **The answer is C.** (Chapter 5) A surge plan is the specific plan of action that hospital will take in order to increase treatment capabilities in response to a sudden large increase (or "surge") in patient volume or critical care needs. Alternate standards of care denote a specific legal determination that can only be claimed when the governor of a state has requested a declaration of state of emergency, under the Stafford Act. The Incident Command System (ICS) is a standardized organizational system for the immediate response phase of a disaster. A triage plan describes the process for receiving and sorting a large volume of patients from a mass casualty incident (MCI).

12. **The answer is D.** (Chapter 6) Respiratory illnesses are the most common types of illnesses to occur among victims *and* relief workers following an earthquake. This phenomenon is thought to be due to the large amount of particulate matter from collapsed buildings and roads and which can cause reactive airway disease in victims and relief workers. Additionally, in the weeks to months that follow large groups of victims and volunteers may still be living in crowded shelters and other enclosed spaces, with opportunity to spread infectious respiratory illnesses. Acute conditions including fractures and myocardial infractions are more common (than at baseline) during or immediately following an earthquake. And chronic conditions such as hypertension can become exacerbated among survivors due to lack of access to medications.

13. **The answer is B.** (Chapter 6) Relief workers who respond with the National Disaster Medical System (NDMS) are expected to be self-sufficient (with supplies for their personal care and for basic team operations for delivery of medical care) for at least 72 hours (3 days) after deployment to a disaster area.

14. **The answer is D.** (Chapter 7) Pulmonary barotrauma is the most common cause of fatal primary blast injury. The lung is particularly susceptible to blast injuries because of the number of air-filled spaces and vasculature, which allow for significant pressure differentials to be generated across tissue barriers (thereby damaging them). Such pressure differentials can lead to hemorrhage, contusions, pneumothorax, hemothorax, and pneumomediastinum.

15. **The answer is C**. (Chapter 7). Direct injuries to the fetus are uncommon in pregnant women who are victims of a blast event, as the fetus is surrounded by amniotic fluid. However, direct injuries to the placenta are common. After life-threatening conditions have been stabilized or ruled out, any woman in the second or third trimester of pregnancy should be admitted to the labor and delivery floor for continuous fetal monitoring and obstetric evaluation.

16. **The answer is C**. (Chapter 8) The syndrome being described is consistent with an anticholinergic toxidrome which could be caused by organophosphate poisoning (OP) including intentional OP poisoning such as from sarin gas (an acetylcholinesterase inhibitor). Treatment includes atropine to address the muscarinic effects, which should be titrated until clearing of the secretions. Pralidoxime is given to address the nicotinic effects. Midazolam can be used to treat seizures.

17. **The answer is D**. (Chapter 9) Persons exposed to suspected anthrax (but not currently symptomatic) should be started on oral ciprofloxacin (and prophylaxis should continue for 60 days). If active systemic or pulmonary disease is suspected, the patient should be admitted to the hospital and antibiotic coverage should be broadened to include IV antibiotics. For patients who are critically ill, anthrax immunoglobulin should be considered as adjunctive therapy. Anthrax vaccination has not been well studied in terms of efficacy but may be recommended to high-risk first responder or military personnel in certain settings.

18. **The answer is A**. (Chapter 9) During an outbreak, critical information that a public health system should provide includes a case definition for the particular agent in the question. A case definition imparts definitive clinical and diagnostic criteria for an individual patient. Within the case definition, criteria should be supplied that define "presumptive" or "suspect" cases for patients awaiting confirmatory testing.

19. **The answer is B**. (Chapter 10) Following an exposure to ionizing radiation, a lymphocyte count is among the most useful prognostic and diagnostic indicators, as its level at different times following the procedure can provide an estimate of relative dose received as well as an accurate prognostic indicator of mortality.

20. **The answer is C**. (Chapter 10) Because radioactive contamination is never immediately life threatening, treatment of life-threatening injuries (such as significant trauma or respiratory distress) should not be delayed while awaiting or performing decontamination. So, as long as treating providers are wearing sufficient protective gear, decontamination may be delayed until after treatment is rendered.

Resuscitation

2

QUESTIONS

1. A 45-year-old Japanese man presents to the emergency department after he had a witnessed syncopal event. The patient denies any prodromal symptoms prior to the event nor injuries secondary to the event. He denies recent illness, chest pain before or after the event, bloody or back bowel movements, shortness of breath, recent surgeries, or lower extremity swelling. He has no significant past medical history or social history and he takes no medications. He is adopted and does not know his family history. Physical examination including vital signs are unremarkable. Laboratory evaluation shows no abnormalities. Chest x-ray shows no acute abnormalities. ECG was performed and is shown in Figure 2.1. What is the appropriate NEXT step in care for this patient?
   (A) Consult cardiology for automatic implantable cardioverter-defibrillator (AICD) placement
   (B) Consult cardiology for emergent cardiac catheterization
   (C) Discharge patient home with outpatient follow-up with his primary care physician
   (D) Order a CT angiogram to rule out pulmonary embolism

2. A 46-year-old woman presents to the emergency department with severe pneumonia and septic shock. She is given antibiotics, is intubated, and a central line is placed. Despite appropriate fluid resuscitation, the patient remains with mean arterial pressures below 65. The decision is made to initiate vasopressor therapy. Which vasopressor agent is considered first line for septic shock?
   (A) Dopamine
   (B) Epinephrine
   (C) Norepinephrine
   (D) Vasopressin

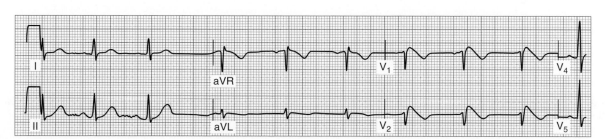

FIGURE 2.1 Reproduced with permission from J.E. Tintinalli, J.S. Stapczynski, O.J. Ma, D. Yealy, G.D. Meckler, D.M. Cline: Tintinalli's Emergency Medicine: A Comprehensive Study Guide, 9th Edition. McGraw-Hill Education; 2020.

3. A 24-year-old man presents to the emergency department after a high-speed motorcycle crash. He is intubated in the field and brought into the emergency. He arrives to the department with the following vital signs: T 35°C, HR 120, BP 60/40, and RR 20. He has equal breath sounds bilaterally, with a normal chest x-ray, but has a notably distended abdomen. A FAST (focused assessment with sonography for trauma) examination is performed which is positive. Unfortunately, there is a delay in going to the operating room and the patient requires extended resuscitation. Massive transfusion protocol is initiated after he received a 1-L bolus of isotonic crystalloid fluid with transient response, and he is given four units of packed red blood cells, four units of fresh frozen plasma, and one pack of platelets. His vital signs are now the following: T 35°C, HR 90, BP 90/60, and RR 20. His labs show no abnormalities in his coagulation panel, platelets, hematocrit, or hemoglobin. His lactate is 2.0 and his arterial blood gas is the following: pH 7.36, bicarbonate 26, pCO₂ 39, and pO₂ 200. What places him at risk for trauma-induced coagulopathy?
   (A) Hypothermia
   (B) Inappropriate blood pressure post massive transfusion protocol
   (C) Inappropriate ratio of blood products
   (D) Isotonic crystalloid use

4. What is the MOST common symptom in patients with anaphylaxis?
   (A) Diarrhea
   (B) Dyspnea
   (C) Hypotension
   (D) Urticaria

5. A 24-year-old woman presents to the emergency department with a chief complaint of tongue and lip swelling. She reports that she had a minor fall off a step stool yesterday evening but without any serious injury. She additionally reports that she feels as if she is having some swelling in her throat and feels slightly dyspneic. Her vital signs are the following: T 97.9°F, HR 80, BP 110/80, and RR of 19. On examination, she has moderate swelling of her upper and lower lip as well as her tongue. Despite this, she is able to speak full sentences easily. Her lungs are clear to auscultation bilaterally. She has no skin rashes on examination. She takes no medications. There have been no new environmental exposures. She does report however that these exact symptoms have happened once in the past and that she was recently diagnosed with hereditary angioedema. Which of the following treatments will shorten the duration of her attack?
   (A) Corticosteroids
   (B) Epinephrine
   (C) Plasmapheresis
   (D) Transfusion of fresh frozen plasma

6. What does the section marked with the letter X on the end-tidal capnogram represent (Figure 2.2)?
   (A) End-tidal concentration
   (B) Expiratory plateau
   (C) Expiratory upstroke
   (D) Inspiratory baseline

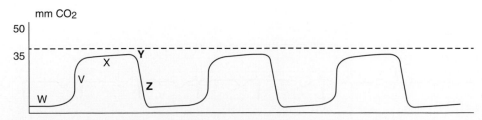

FIGURE 2.2 Reproduced with permission from J.E. Tintinalli, J.S. Stapczynski, O.J. Ma, D. Yealy, G.D. Meckler, D.M. Cline: Tintinalli's Emergency Medicine: A Comprehensive Study Guide, 9th Edition. McGraw-Hill Education; 2020.

7. A 70-year-old woman with dementia presents with signs and symptoms consistent with acute gastroenteritis for the past 4 days. Her caregivers report that she has been unable to eat or drink due to her severe vomiting and has also had profuse diarrhea. On examination, she is notably dehydrated, tachycardic, and lethargic. Her labs reveal a sodium level of 165 mEq/L. Her prior sodium level 3 months prior was 150 mEq/L. Her caregivers state that her by mouth intake is poor at baseline due to her dementia and she usually has chronic mild hypernatremia. She is admitted for IV fluid resuscitation and correction of her sodium level. She is started on high-volume D5 water IV fluids. Twelve hours later, she becomes acutely unresponsive and has to be intubated. Repeat labs reveal a sodium level of 135. Based on this information, what is your diagnosis as the cause of her change in mental status?
   (A) Acute intracerebral hemorrhage
   (B) Central pontine myelinolysis
   (C) Cerebral edema
   (D) Osmotic demyelination syndrome

8. A 65-year-old man presents to the emergency department complaining of coughing, increased sputum production, and dyspnea with exertion. He has a past medical history of coronary artery disease, hypertension, hyperlipidemia, and chronic obstructive pulmonary disease. On examination, he is mildly tachypneic, speaks short sentences, and has wheezing in bilateral lung fields. He has a new oxygen requirement and is placed on 2L nasal cannula. He is tachycardiac, afebrile, with normal blood pressure. A rhythm strip is obtained which reveals the following (Figure 2.3). What is the APPROPRIATE management of this patient?
   (A) Amiodarone 150 mg bolus
   (B) Bronchodilators, steroids, antibiotics, and hospital admission
   (C) IV diltiazem 15 to 20 mg bolus
   (D) IV metoprolol 5 mg

9. For which of the following conditions is digoxin contraindicated?
   (A) Atrial fibrillation
   (B) Atrial flutter
   (C) Congestive heart failure
   (D) Ventricular tachycardia

10. Which of the following vasopressors is NOT recommended for cardiogenic shock due to its potential to cause reflex bradycardia and subsequent decreased cardiac output?
   (A) Dobutamine
   (B) Epinephrine
   (C) Norepinephrine
   (D) Phenylephrine

11. What is the MOST common adverse reaction in patients treated with hyperbaric therapy?
   (A) Middle ear barotrauma
   (B) Nuclear cataract development
   (C) Oxygen toxicity
   (D) Progressive myopia

12. A 22-year-old woman who is 38 weeks pregnant is visiting her grandfather who is a current patient in the emergency room. While talking to her grandfather and eating her lunch, she suddenly begins to choke on a chicken nugget. She grabs her neck with both hands and staff quickly recognizes the universal sign for an airway obstruction. Initially, she is able to cough and speak, and the staff encourages her to continue her spontaneous efforts to clear the obstruction. However, she soon develops an ineffective cough, is no longer able to speak, becomes dyspneic and cyanotic, but she is still awake and alert. The physician is then called to bedside. What is the NEXT appropriate course of action?
   (A) Continue to encourage the patient's spontaneous efforts to clear the obstruction
   (B) Perform a blind finger sweep
   (C) Start performing the Heimlich maneuver, using chest thrusts
   (D) Start performing the Heimlich maneuver, using subdiaphragmatic abdominal thrusts

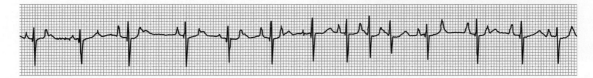

FIGURE 2.3 Reproduced with permission from J.E. Tintinalli, J.S. Stapczynski, O.J. Ma, D. Yealy, G.D. Meckler, D.M. Cline: Tintinalli's Emergency Medicine: A Comprehensive Study Guide, 9th Edition. McGraw-Hill Education; 2020.

13. Both during cardiac arrest and afterward with return of spontaneous circulation, hyperventilation is not recommended. The pathophysiology that occurs from hyperventilation (and thus why it is not recommended) is which of the following?
    (A) Hyperventilation causes decreased intrathoracic pressure and decreased venous return with resulting decreased cardiac output.
    (B) Hyperventilation causes decreased intrathoracic pressure and increased venous return and with resulting decreased cardiac output.
    (C) Hyperventilation causes increased intrathoracic pressure and decreased venous return and with resulting decreased cardiac output.
    (D) Hyperventilation causes increased intrathoracic pressure and increased venous return and with resulting decreased cardiac output.

14. Which of the following represents the physiologic changes that occur during pregnancy?
    (A) Decreased cardiac output
    (B) Decreased plasma volume
    (C) Increased minute ventilation
    (D) Increased peripheral vascular resistance

15. Which of the following statements is TRUE regarding post arrest targeted temperature management (TTM)?
    (A) Aim for a core temperature of less than 32°C when cooling a patient.
    (B) Bradycardia is common when starting TTM.
    (C) Clinical neurologic reflexes post arrest are predictive of cardiac arrest outcome.
    (D) Pregnant women should be excluded from TTM.

16. How should one measure when deciding on the appropriate size of this airway adjunct (Figure 2.4)?

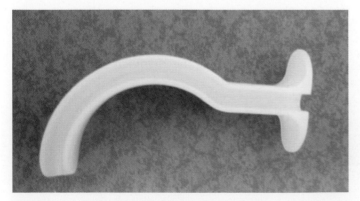

FIGURE 2.4 An oral airway. Reproduced with permission from J.E. Tintinalli, J.S. Stapczynski, O.J. Ma, D. Yealy, G.D. Meckler, D.M. Cline: Tintinalli's Emergency Medicine: A Comprehensive Study Guide, 9th Edition. McGraw-Hill Education; 2020.

(A) Corner of the mouth to the angle of the mandible
(B) Corner of the mouth to the ear pinna
(C) Middle of the mouth to the angle of the mandible
(D) Middle of the mouth to the ear pinna

17. A 48-year-old woman presents to the department in respiratory distress. She has a history of myasthenia gravis and is having a myasthenia crisis. Decision is made to intubate the patient using rapid sequence intubation (RSI) with etomidate and succinylcholine. After administration of these medications, the patient subsequently goes into cardiac arrest. She is intubated quickly and easily but despite resuscitative efforts, the patient expires. Which of the following adverse medication reactions listed below from the RSI medications MOST LIKELY resulted in her cardiac arrest?
    (A) Adrenal insufficiency
    (B) Hyperkalemia
    (C) Hypotension
    (D) Vomiting with resulting massive aspiration

18. A 7-year-old female patient of normal body mass index (BMI) presents to the emergency department after she was hit by a car while riding her bike. She has significant facial fractures and noted blood and swelling of her airway. Attempts at oral intubation fail and she additionally cannot be oxygenated or ventilated using bag valve mask ventilation. A 16-gauge catheter is inserted percutaneously through her cricothyroid membrane and jet ventilation is initiated. Which of the following represents the CORRECT psi of oxygen to deliver?
    (A) Until adequate chest rise and fall is noted, which in children is typically is usually <30 mm Hg.
    (B) Until adequate chest rise and fall is noted, which in children is typically is usually <50 mm Hg.
    (C) Until adequate chest rise and fall is noted, which in children is typically is usually <75 mm Hg.
    (D) Until adequate chest rise and fall is noted, which in children is typically is usually <100 mm Hg.

19. All of the following when present can signal a potential airway management difficulty EXCEPT:
    (A) Beard
    (B) Large chin
    (C) Male sex
    (D) Mallampati score of 4

20. A 70-year-old male patient presents with an acute change in mental status and hypertension with a blood pressure of 200/110. A CT head is obtained and a spontaneous intracranial hemorrhage in the basal ganglia is identified. The decision is made to lower his blood pressure to a systolic goal of less than 140. An arterial line is placed in the right radial artery. A square wave flush test is performed, and the number of oscillations is measured at two. What does this indicate about the blood pressure values obtained?
  (A) The waveform is optimally dampened, and the blood pressure values obtained are accurate.
  (B) The waveform is overdampened, and the systolic blood pressure is underestimated.
  (C) The waveform is under dampened, and the systolic blood pressure is overestimated.
  (D) The waveform is under dampened, and the systolic blood pressure is underestimated.

21. A 50-year-old woman who has end-stage renal disease and is dialysis-dependent presents with a chief complaint of weakness, mild dyspnea, mild chest pain, and dizziness. Her vital signs are as follows: HR 130, BP 80/60, RR 20, SpO$_2$ 99%, and a T 37.6°C. On examination, she is pale and diaphoretic. A chest x-ray is performed and is shown in Figure 2.5. Which of the following should be performed to treat this patient?

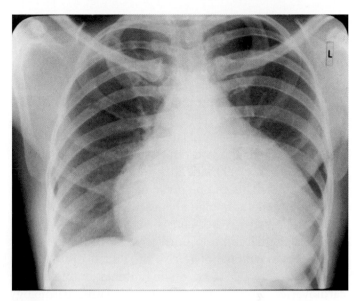

FIGURE 2.5 Reproduced with permission from Sorajja P: Pericardial disease, in Hall JB, Schmidt GA, Kress JP (eds): Principles of Critical Care, 4th ed. New York: McGraw-Hill, Inc.; 2015.

  (A) Amiodarone to control tachycardia with a goal heart rate of less than 100
  (B) Esmolol bolus to control tachycardia with a goal heart rate between 60 and 80
  (C) Intravenous fluid bolus to improve right ventricular function and consider preparations for a pericardiocentesis
  (B) Intravenous furosemide bolus and initiation of noninvasive positive pressure ventilation

ANSWERS

1. **The answer is A.** (Chapter 11) The ECG shown is consistent with Brugada's syndrome. In leads V_1 and V_2, it displays the typical downsloping ST-segment elevation and additionally the QRS morphology mimics a right bundle branch block pattern. This syndrome commonly affects men of Southeast Asia and Japanese descent, is autosomal dominant genetically, and results in sodium channel dysfunction. It is crucial to identify due to the risk of sudden cardiac death. This can be prevented by placement of an internal automatic implantable cardioverter-defibrillator. The ECG pattern is not consistent with an ST-elevated myocardial infarction so emergent cardiac catheterization is not warranted. The risk of sudden death that is preventable by insertion of an automatic implantable cardioverter-defibrillator (AICD) mandating cardiology involvement and not simply follow-up with a primary care physician. Nothing in the history of present illness, physical examination, laboratory evaluation, or ECG suggests a pulmonary embolus as the cause of the patient's syncope.

2. **The answer is C.** (Chapter 12) Norepinephrine primarily acts on alpha-1 receptors (and some beta-1 activation as well), which induces smooth muscle and vessel constriction. This medication is thus exceptionally useful in shock where venous tone predominates, such as septic shock. Norepinephrine is considered a first-line agent for most types of shock, including sepsis of which it has a demonstrated mortality benefit. Dopamine is considered to be second-line therapy for septic shock due to its association with adverse events, such as its potential to induce tachydysrhythmias. Epinephrine is also not first line for sepsis due to its potential side effects of increased lactic acidosis, hyperglycemia, and tachydysrhythmias. Finally, vasopressin is not considered a first-line agent for septic shock as it does not have a mortality benefit as has been proven for norepinephrine. This medication is usually not titrated due to its potent splanchnic vasoconstriction.

3. **The answer is A.** (Chapter 13) Often referred to as the lethal triad, the development of hemodilution (coagulopathy), acidosis, and hypothermia results in trauma-induced coagulopathy. Acidosis in this setting occurs when pH decreases below 7.0. This triad can be caused by ongoing blood loss in the setting of iatrogenic effects of resuscitation. To prevent coagulopathy, massive transfusion protocols often provide platelets, packed red blood cells, and fresh frozen plasma in a 1:1:1 fashion. One pack of platelets equates to 4 to 6 units of platelets. The patient in the question stem received 1:1:1 blood transfusion. Current trauma recommendations include providing crystalloid solution, either 1 to 2 L depending on the guideline followed, prior to initiating blood product transfusion. This patient appropriately received crystalloid fluids and then was switched to blood products, especially in the setting of known ongoing bleeding with delay in operating room availability. Finally, in terms of target hemodynamics for resuscitation, systolic blood pressure goals for trauma patients are 80 to 90. This lower systolic target is to prevent higher blood pressure, which could raise hydrostatic pressure and disrupt the clot in a noncompressible hemorrhage location.

4. **The answer is D.** (Chapter 14) Urticaria and/or angioedema have the most common incidence in anaphylaxis patients. The next most common symptom is pharyngeal or laryngeal edema, with an approximate incidence of 50% to 60%. Hypotension has an incidence of 30% to 50%, dyspnea 45% to 50%, and diarrhea 25% to 30%.

5. **The answer is D.** (Chapter 14) Hereditary angioedema (HAE) is a rare autosomal dominant disorder in which patients either have a deficiency in C1 esterase inhibitor or have a dysfunctional C1 esterase enzyme. Minor trauma is known to precipitate episodes and symptoms include acute edema involving the upper respiratory system, gastrointestinal tract, or extremity soft tissues. The traditional treatment for anaphylaxis of epinephrine, corticosteroids, and antihistamines is ineffective. Treatment for HAE attacks includes a C1 esterase inhibitor, a bradykinin-2 receptor antagonist, or a kallikrein inhibitor. However, if a C1 esterase is not available, fresh frozen plasma can be used. Plasmapheresis has not been studied for use in this disorder and thus is not the correct answer.

6. **The answer is B.** (Chapter 16) W portion represents inspiratory baseline. The V portion represents expiratory upstroke. The X portion represents expiratory plateau. The Y portion represents end-tidal concentration. The Z portion of the capnogram represents inspiratory downstroke.

7. **The answer is C.** (Chapter 17) In patients who have acute hypernatremia, and the adaptation of brain cells is thus incomplete, correction of sodium levels can be performed at the rate of 1 mEq/L/h. However, in patients of whom hypernatremia is chronic, onset >48 hours, the rate of correction should be lower, no more than 0.5 mEq/L/h with a total maximum correction in 24 hours no more than 10 to 12 mEq. The patient in this question stem had her sodium dropped 30 points within 12 hours, which is

much too fast. As a result, this patient has developed diffuse cerebral edema with resulting neurologic changes. Osmotic demyelination syndrome occurs after the rapid correction of low sodium levels. Central pontine myelinolysis is the old former term used for what is now called osmotic demyelination syndrome, which again occurs in the setting of rapid correction of hyponatremia. Acute intracerebral hemorrhage is not the correct diagnosis as this is not the known complication from rapid correction of sodium levels.

8. **The answer is B.** (Chapter 18) This is a patient whose rhythm strip displays multifocal atrial tachycardia (MAT). MAT has three or more distinct p-wave morphologies. This irregular rhythm is most often found in elderly patients with decompensated chronic lung disease, but it may also be present in patients with heart failure and/or sepsis. Treatment for MAT is directed toward the underlying disorder, which is why answer B that focuses on treatment for the patient's chronic obstructive pulmonary disease (COPD) exacerbation is the correct answer. Antidysrhythmic treatment is not indicated for MAT, which is why the other answers are all incorrect.

9. **The answer is D.** (Chapter 19) Digoxin use is contraindicated for ventricular arrhythmias. Ventricular tachycardia is an adverse side effect of digoxin use and thus using it as treatment for this condition would likely worsen the ventricular tachycardia. Digoxin is indicated for rate control for atrial fibrillation or atrial tachycardia, but it is not considered first-line therapy. Digoxin is also used for symptom control in congestive heart failure when symptoms are unrelieved by diuretics and angiotensin-converting enzyme inhibitors.

10. **The answer is D.** (Chapter 20) Phenylephrine is a selective alpha-1 adrenergic agonist and lacks any beta-adrenergic activity. Thus, phenylephrine causes systemic arterial vasoconstriction without any direct effects in heart rate. This increase in afterload without the beta-adrenergic activity to the failing heart can result in reflex bradycardia and subsequent reduction in cardiac output. Dobutamine is a potent inotropic agent with resulting increased contractility and heart rate, and it is thus indicted for short-term management of patients with acute cardiac decompensation. Norepinephrine stimulates both alpha-adrenergic and beta-adrenergic receptors resulting in peripheral vasoconstriction and inotropic stimulation of the heart. Epinephrine similarly stimulates both alpha- and beta-adrenergic receptors and thus also increases systemic vascular resistance, heart rate, and cardiac output.

11. **The answer is A.** (Chapter 21) Middle ear barotrauma is the most common adverse effect of hyperbaric oxygen treatment (HBO). As the ambient pressure within the hyperbaric chamber increases, the patient must equalize the pressure within the middle ear. If the patient is unable to achieve this, tympanostomy tubes must then be placed in order for HBO therapy to continue. Nuclear cataract can occur when treatment hours exceeds 150 to 200 hours. Progressive myopia may occur in patients who undergo prolonged daily HBO therapy, but typically it reverses within 6 weeks after termination of treatments. Finally, acute oxygen toxicity is also a known complication of HBO, occurring in one to four times per 10,000 patient treatments and usually manifests as grand mal seizures.

12. **The answer is C.** (Chapter 22) In the patient who is choking, if they are able to speak, cough, and exchange air, then he or she should be encouraged to continue their spontaneous efforts to clear the obstruction. However, once air exchange becomes inadequate, such as when the individual is cyanotic or unable to speak, then immediate intervention is required. In the awake patient, a blind finger sweep should never be attempted. While for the majority of patients, the Heimlich maneuver consists of subdiaphragmatic abdominal thrusts; for some patients, it is impossible for the rescuer to reach around to the patient's abdomen. Pregnancy and morbid obesity are two common examples. In these circumstances, a chest thrust maneuver should be used instead. Because the patient in this scenario is 38 weeks pregnant, chest thrusts should be used instead of subdiaphragmatic abdominal thrusts.

13. **The answer is C.** (Chapter 24) Hyperventilation is not routinely recommended because it can increase intrathoracic pressure and decrease venous return with resulting decreased cardiac output. Additionally, the hypocarbia resulting from hyperventilation results in decreased blood flow to the brain, thus worsening anoxic brain injury. In the postarrest patient, physicians should target normocapnia (pCO_2 35–45), which is usually achieved with 10 to 12 ventilations per minute. In the patient who is in cardiac arrest and has an advanced airway, the provided breaths should be no more than 10 per minute. If the patient does not have an advance airway, the compression to breath ratio is 30:2.

14. **The answer is C.** (Chapter 25) Pregnant patients have larger tidal volume ventilation, which results in increased minute ventilation. This is necessary due to increased carbon dioxide increase, especially by the third trimester and during labor, and also due to progesterone directly

stimulating the central respiratory center. It is thus not uncommon to see in a healthy pregnant patient, an arterial blood gas with mild respiratory alkalosis. Both cardiac output and plasma volume increase by 30% to 50%. Peripheral vascular resistance decreases by 20%.

15. **The answer is B.** (Chapter 26) Bradycardia is common with targeted temperature management (TTM) and can be pronounced with induction but is usually of little clinical consequence and requires no treatment. It is important to note that the clinical neurologic reflexes arc not predictive of cardiac arrest outcomes. There is still considerable debate about the exact targeted core temperature for postarrest cooling. Recommendations range from 32 to 36°C but not lower than 32°C. TTM for pregnant patient varies among institutions. Several case reports have demonstrated good outcomes for postarrest pregnant patients.

16. **The answer is A.** (Chapter 28) Oropharyngeal airways are rigid, curve devices that help prevent the base of the tongue from blocking the airway via occlusion of the hypopharynx. It should only be used in the comatose or obtunded patient who does not have a gag reflex. Properly sized oral airways should reach from the corner of the mouth to the angle of the mandible.

17. **The answer is B.** (Chapter 29) Succinylcholine is a depolarizing paralytic agent that has rapid onset after IV administration. While in most patients the serum potassium only rising 0.5 mEq/L without clinical impact, in some patient populations this response is clinically significant or exaggerated. Succinylcholine is contraindicated in patients with myasthenia gravis, myopathies, or preexisting hyperkalemia/renal failure. It is also contraindicated in patients who 5 days prior or longer suffered a burn, denervation, or crush injury. Hypotension can theoretically occur after any induction agent, but it is much less common with etomidate and is less likely to have caused this patient's demise. While etomidate has been demonstrated to result in transient cortisol inhibition, there is no current evidence that this worsens patient outcomes. Vomiting with aspiration is a risk with any emergent rapid-sequence intubation (RSI), but there was no indication that this occurred.

18. **The answer is A.** (Chapter 30) In children younger than 12 years, especially younger than 8 years, in whom the physician cannot oxygenate or ventilate and cannot achieve oral intubation and a surgical airway is needed, a cricothyrotomy is not recommended. Young children are more likely to have late complications, especially stenosis, as their larynx is more easily damaged with this procedure. A tracheotomy is preferred but this is out of

TABLE 2.1	Factors Associated With Airway Management Difficulty
• Obesity
• Facial hair
• Edentulous anatomy
• History of snoring/sleep apnea
• Short neck
• Limited neck mobility
• Small or large chin
• Prominent incisors
• High arched palate
• Facial or airway trauma
• Head and neck tumors
• Angioedema
• Ludwig's angina
• Inflammation of the airway (e.g., airway burns)

Reproduced with permission from J.E. Tintinalli, J.S. Stapczynski, O.J. Ma, D. Yealy, G.D. Meckler, D.M. Cline: Tintinalli's Emergency Medicine: A Comprehensive Study Guide, 9th Edition. McGraw-Hill Education; 2020.

the scope of an emergency physician's practice. Thus, jet ventilation is used to help bridge the gap until a definitive surgical airway can be achieved. Jet ventilation when used in a child, the recommended psi to start with is 0.5 psi/kg and increased until chest rise and fall is achieved. In teenagers and adults, the psi to achieve this is typically 35 to 50. In children, because of their smaller body habitus, they typically require a psi of <30. In very young children and infants, their psi is usually <20.

19. **The answer is C.** (Chapter 29A) Sex of a patient alone does not identify patients that may be challenging airway management cases. Facial hair can make it difficult to bag a patient because of difficulty getting a seal on the mask. The same holds true for a small or large chins. There are multiple factors associated with airway management difficulties as noted in Table 2.1. Mallampati scores help to identify patients that may be challenging to intubate. The lower the score, the better view of the posterior pharynx (Figure 2.6).

20. **The answer is A.** (Chapter 32) During a flush bolus of the catheter tubing of an arterial line, a square wave is observed and the number of oscillations at the end of the

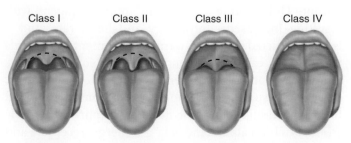

Class I   Class II   Class III   Class IV

FIGURE 2.6 Reproduced with permission from J.E. Tintinalli, J.S. Stapczynski, O.J. Ma, D. Yealy, G.D. Meckler, D.M. Cline: Tintinalli's Emergency Medicine: A Comprehensive Study Guide, 9th Edition. McGraw-Hill Education; 2020.

bolus prior to returning to the blood pressure tracing may result in overestimated or underestimated blood pressure. The optimally damped arterial line has 1.5 to 2 oscillations before returning to tracing, indicating that the values are accurate. The underdamped arterial waveform has more than 2 oscillations, which result in overestimated systolic pressure. Additionally, diastolic pressure may be underestimated. The arterial waveform that is overdamped has less than 1.5 oscillations, which results in underestimation of systolic blood pressure. In the overdamped waveform, diastolic pressure may not be affected (Figure 2.7).

21. **The answer is C.** (Chapter 34) This is a patient who is exhibiting signs and symptoms consistent with pericardial tamponade. Renal failure is a known condition that predisposes patients to this condition. There are a number of symptoms that are associated with pericardial effusion and tamponade, including, but not limited to, dyspnea, chest pain, lethargy, fever, weakness, and palpitations. Physical examination findings include pulsus paradoxus >10 mm Hg in 82% of patients, jugular venous distension in 76% of patients, tachycardia in 77% of patients, muffled heart sounds in 26% of patients, and hypotension in 26%. The chest x-ray shown displays enlarged cardiac silhouette, rounded in its lower portion and tapers at the base of the heart, which is consistent with a pericardial effusion. While answer B would be correct if the patient had an isolated aortic dissection, lowering heart rate in this patient would drop the cardiac output and result in worsening shock and thus this answer is incorrect. The use of

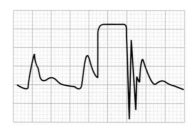

Optimally damped:
1.5–2 oscillations before returning to tracing. Values obtained are accurate.

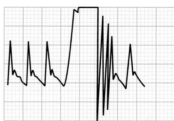

Underdamped:
>2 oscillations. Overestimated systolic pressure, diastolic pressure may be underestimated.

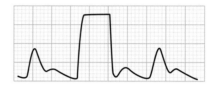

Overdamped:
<1.5 oscillations. Underestimation of systolic pressure, diastolic may not be affected.

FIGURE 2.7 Reproduced with permission from J.E. Tintinalli, J.S. Stapczynski, O.J. Ma, D. Yealy, G.D. Meckler, D.M. Cline: Tintinalli's Emergency Medicine: A Comprehensive Study Guide, 9th Edition. McGraw-Hill Education; 2020.

amiodarone is incorrect for similar reasons in that dropping the tachycardia would worsen the patient's shock. The patient has clear lung fields on the chest x-ray without signs of pulmonary edema or congestive heart failure. There is thus no indication for furosemide or noninvasive positive pressure ventilation.

Analgesia, Anesthesia, and Procedural Sedation

3

QUESTIONS

1. A 46-year-old man presents complaining of low back pain and has received pain medication. When you walk into the room, he is lying on the bed with his eyes closed. He has normal vital signs. Which of the following is the MOST effective method to assess his current pain?
   - (A) Ask the patient to quantify the pain based on a numeric or visual pain scale
   - (B) Ask the patient to quantify the pain using simple descriptors such as "a little" or "an awful lot"
   - (C) Ask the patient whether he or she requires more analgesic
   - (D) Assess the patient's pain based on vital signs, grimacing and agitation

2. A 20-year-old healthy woman presents with 10 out of 10 acute abdominal, back, and leg pain after a motor vehicle collision. The patient is hemodynamically stable. She reports only minimal pain relief after receiving 50 mcg fentanyl intravenously. She has a history of developing a rash after taking hydrocodone. What is the NEXT BEST step in pain management for this patient?
   - (A) Administer a dose of hydromorphone
   - (B) Administer a dose of morphine
   - (C) Administer another dose of fentanyl
   - (D) Apply a transdermal fentanyl patch

3. Which of the following is TRUE regarding nonsteroidal anti-inflammatory drugs (NSAIDs)?
   - (A) Ibuprofen has a greater risk of gastrointestinal bleeding than ketorolac.
   - (B) Ketorolac is limited to 7 days intravenously (IV) or 14 days orally.
   - (C) NSAIDs decrease the risk of cardiac death in people with ischemic heart disease.
   - (D) NSAIDs exert their analgesic effect by decreasing the excitability of dorsal horn neurons via inhibition of cyclooxygenase-2 enzyme in the spinal cord.

4. Which of the following is TRUE of ketamine?
   - (A) Ketamine is contraindicated in trauma patients because it will increase intracranial pressure.
   - (B) Ketamine typically preserves a patient's respiratory effort and has minimal effect on blood pressure.
   - (C) A typical ketamine dose for analgesia is a loading dose of 1 mg/kg IV over 10 minutes followed by an infusion if desired.
   - (D) Laryngospasm is more common in adults than children.

5. An 85-year-old man with a history of stage 5 chronic kidney disease, metastatic prostate cancer, and history of exploratory laparotomy for a gunshot wound presents with acute sharp left lower quadrant abdominal pain. He does not take any medications. Vital signs are BP 130/70, HR 80, RR 14, SpO$_2$ 95% on RA, T 37.9°C. Examination is notable for tenderness to palpation to the left lower quadrant. Laboratory studies show a glomerular filtration rate (GFR) of <15 mL/min/1.73 m^2. Which of the following is the MOST APPROPRIATE initial pharmacotherapy for this patient?
   (A) Fentanyl 100 mcg nasal spray in each nostril
   (B) Hydromorphone 0.0075 mg/kg IV
   (C) Ibuprofen 800 mg orally
   (D) Morphine patient-controlled analgesia

6. A 45-year-old man presents with a 20-cm superficial laceration to the thigh after a work-related injury. Two percent lidocaine without epinephrine is injected locally into the wound in preparation for wound repair. Subsequently, the patient reports tongue numbness, blurred vision, and tinnitus. He is noted to become somnolent and develops muscle twitching. His heart rate is 147 with significant ectopy and QRS widening noted on the monitor. Which medication class would be MOST APPROPRIATE for immediately treating this patient?
   (A) β-Blocker
   (B) Calcium channel blocker
   (C) GABA receptor modulator
   (D) Lipid emulsion

7. Which of the following actions may have helped prevent this patient's response to the administration of lidocaine?
   (A) Add sodium bicarbonate to the local anesthetic
   (B) Premedicate the patient with diphenhydramine
   (C) Premedicate the patient with lipid emulsion
   (D) Use lidocaine with epinephrine

8. Which of the following steps can reduce the pain of needle puncture and local anesthetic injection?
   (A) Applying a topical anesthetic prior to injection
   (B) Avoiding insertion of the needle at large pores or hair follicles
   (C) Cooling the local anesthetic agent
   (D) Inserting the needle with bevel down position

9. Which of the following is TRUE regarding regional anesthesia?
   (A) Bupivacaine requires 15 to 30 minutes to achieve optimal anesthesia.
   (B) Lidocaine is significantly less cardiotoxic than levobupivacaine and ropivacaine.
   (C) Lidocaine offers a longer duration of action than levobupivacaine and ropivacaine.
   (D) Loss of touch and deep pressure sensation are affected first, followed by pain and temperature sensation.

10. A 10-year-old girl presents with a 3-cm laceration to the thenar eminence of the right hand. Which of the following describes the appropriate location for a regional nerve block?
    (A) Insert the needle between the palmaris longus and flexor carpi radialis tendons at the level of the proximal wrist crease.
    (B) Insert the needle horizontally beneath the carpi ulnaris tendon.
    (C) Insert the needle on the dorsal surface of the proximal first phalanx and advance toward the volar surface staying tangential to the phalanx and repeat on the other side.
    (D) Insert the needle over the lateral aspect of the radial styloid just proximal to the anatomic snuffbox.

11. Which of the following is TRUE regarding hematoma blocks?
    (A) Hematoma blocks are performed by injecting 5 to 20 mL of local anesthetic solution into the fracture site.
    (B) Hematoma blocks increase the risk of infection.
    (C) Hematoma blocks may be performed through an open fracture.
    (D) Local anesthetic should not be injected if blood is aspirated.

12. Which of the following is TRUE regarding procedural sedation monitoring?
    (A) Capnography is recommended for prolonged deep sedation.
    (B) End-tidal carbon dioxide >50 mm Hg indicates hyperventilation.
    (C) Monitoring is no longer necessary upon completion of the procedure.
    (D) Ventilation can be monitored via pulse oximetry.

13. A patient presents after an automobile versus pedestrian accident and is found to have an open ankle fracture dislocation with diminished distal pulses. The patient is prepped for an emergent reduction under procedural sedation. He is placed on a cardiac monitor with capnography and pulse oximetry. His vital signs are within normal limits, and his oxygen saturation is 100%. Airway equipment is available at the bedside. Which of the following describes the NEXT step?
    (A) Administer fentanyl IV
    (B) Administer hydromorphone IV
    (C) Sedate with etomidate IV
    (D) Remove supplemental oxygen as it can delay the recognition of respiratory suppression

14. A 3-year-old boy weighing 16 kg presents with a crush injury to the left upper extremity and is given a rapid bolus of 50 mcg IV fentanyl for acute traumatic pain. Moments later he is noted to be apneic and cannot be effectively ventilated. Which of the following is the definitive step in management of this patient?
    (A) Administer IV flumazenil
    (B) Administer IV naloxone
    (C) Insert oral airway and continue bag valve mask ventilation
    (D) Perform rapid sequence intubation (RSI)

15. Which of the following should be corrected prior to the administration of propofol?
    (A) Acidosis
    (B) Hyperkalemia
    (C) Hypovolemia
    (D) Tachycardia

16. An 85-year-old man presents with a hip dislocation after a fall at home. Which of the following is TRUE regarding procedural sedation in this patient?
    (A) Etomidate has analgesic properties; therefore, co-administration of opioids is not necessary.
    (B) Etomidate should be avoided in the elderly due to its increased cardiovascular side effects.
    (C) Propofol may be administered at typical IV bolus doses in the elderly.
    (D) The risk of respiratory depression from all agents is increased in this elderly patient.

17. Which of the following is TRUE regarding chronic pain syndromes?
    (A) Allodynia is an exaggerated response to a normally painful stimulus.
    (B) Fibromyalgia is characterized by muscular pain involving multiple body areas without alterations in sleep or cognition.
    (C) Hyperalgesia is pain from a normally nonpainful stimulus.
    (D) Transformed migraine is a syndrome in which classic migraine headaches change over time and develop into a chronic pain syndrome, most commonly from medication overuse.

18. A 45-year-old woman presents for acute on chronic right-sided neck pain that is constant, dull and occasionally shooting. She has not had any trauma. She has point tenderness that produces reproducible pain in the right trapezius muscle, no muscle atrophy and poor range of motion in the right shoulder due to pain. History and examination are otherwise unremarkable. You review the patient electronic medical record and see that she has recently had X-rays and magnetic resonance imaging (MRIs) of the cervical spine and right shoulder that were normal. You perform a trigger point injection, which provides some pain relief to the patient. The patient requests a pain medication prescription for discharge and states that scheduled oral nonsteroidal anti-inflammatory drugs (NSAIDs) have not been controlling her pain. Which of the following is the MOST APPROPRIATE medication for this patient?
    (A) Amitriptyline
    (B) Oxycodone
    (C) Topical diclofenac patch
    (D) Topical fentanyl patch

19. A 50-year-old woman with poorly controlled type 2 diabetes mellitus presents with bilateral chronic foot pain described as constant burning and aching pain. On examination, gentle touch to the feet produces severe reproducible pain. The patient has decreased two-point discrimination. Which of the following is the primary pharmacologic treatment for this patient?
    (A) Carbamazepine
    (B) Duloxetine
    (C) Gabapentin
    (D) Pregabalin

20. Which of the following is TRUE regarding aberrant drug-related behavior?
    (A) A personal history of illicit drug and alcohol abuse is the only consistent predictor of aberrant drug-related behavior in chronic pain patients.
    (B) Dental pain is a common complaint of patients who attempt to obtain opioids from the emergency department .
    (C) "Drug-seeking behavior" is an appropriate way to document concerns about opioid misuse in a patient's chart.
    (D) Teens trying illicit drugs for the first time are equally likely to try prescription opioids as to try marijuana.

21. A 30-year-old man presents with acute dental pain. He reports that his oxycodone prescription from another hospital was stolen and requests a refill. Examination is unremarkable. Which of the following describes a recommended practice for appropriate opioid prescribing in the emergency department when you suspect aberrant drug-related behavior?
    (A) Prescribe opioids to patients whose medications were stolen, as this was not their fault.
    (B) Provide an opioid prescription for a patient presenting with dental pain whose examination demonstrates dental caries only.
    (C) Refill a prescription for a patient who has lost their opioid prescription.
    (D) Search for the patient's name in a prescription drug monitoring database prior to prescribing opioids.

ANSWERS

1. **The answer is C.** (Chapter 35) The patient's subjective reporting of pain, not the physician's impression, is the basis for pain assessment and treatment. There is weak correlation between nonverbal signs such as tachycardia, tachypnea, and changes in patient expression and movements and the patient's report of pain. The patient's subjective reporting should be the basis for assessment and management. Several self-report instruments are valid in patients with acute pain and include numeric, visual analog and adjective rating scales. However, once it is determined that the patient needs pain medication, asking if the patient requires more analgesic may be simpler and more efficient than using any standardized pain evaluation tool.

2. **The answer is C.** (Chapter 35) As much as possible, avoid using multiple agents, and titrate a single drug to effect. When used in equianalgesic doses, there is no compelling evidence to recommend one opioid over another. Thus, a larger dose of fentanyl is preferable to administering morphine or hydromorphone. Furthermore, hydromorphone and hydrocodone are both semisynthetic alkaloids. Although there is minimal evidence of cross-sensitivity within opioid classes, it is prudent to choose a drug from a different class if a patient develops a hypersensitivity reaction or has a history of hypersensitivity. Last, transdermal formulations are not useful for acute pain treatment because of delayed onset and prolonged duration of action.

3. **The answer is D.** (Chapter 35) Nonsteroidal anti-inflammatory drugs (NSAIDs) are well known for their anti-inflammatory effect due to decreased production of prostanoids and arachidonic acid-mediated inflammatory peptides generated at the site of tissue injury. They also exert a centrally mediated analgesic effect by decreasing the excitability of dorsal horn neurons that produce hyperalgesia and allodynia. Ketorolac has a greater risk of gastrointestinal bleeding than ibuprofen and is limited to 3 days IV or 5 days orally. All NSAIDs increase the risk of cardiac death in patients with ischemic heart disease, although cyclooxygenase-2–specific agents such as celecoxib appear to carry higher risk than the nonselective agents.

4. **The answer is B.** (Chapters 35 and 37) Ketamine is a phencyclidine derivative that produces analgesia and anxiolysis at low doses, and can also produce sedation, amnesia, and dissociative anesthesia at larger doses, with the advantage of causing minimal to no respiratory depression or hemodynamic instability with usual doses. Ketamine is safe for use in trauma patients and will often result in a lower opioid requirement for pain control. There is no clear evidence that ketamine is harmful in patients with potential head injury; however, it should be avoided in patients with eye injuries or glaucoma due to its effect on increasing intraocular pressure. Ketamine dosing for analgesia is 0.15 to 0.4 mg/kg IV over 10 minutes, which can be followed by an infusion at 0.1 to 0.2 mg/kg/h. Sedative doses of ketamine are 1 mg/kg IV. Laryngospasm is more common in children than adults. Children with significant upper respiratory infectious symptoms should not receive ketamine due to a possible increased risk of laryngospasm.

5. **The answer is B.** (Chapter 35) In patients with renal failure, hydromorphone and fentanyl are the preferred opioids. In addition, opioid-naïve elderly patients are more sensitive to the analgesic effect of opioid drugs because they experience a higher peak and longer duration of pain relief. Thus, initial IV opioid doses in the elderly are typically half (0.0075 mg/kg IV hydromorphone) those used in younger adults (0.015 mg/kg IV hydromorphone). Thus, the best initial pharmacotherapy in this elderly, opioid-naïve patient with renal failure is a low dose of hydromorphone IV. Intranasal or buccal fentanyl is useful for breakthrough pain in opioid-tolerant cancer patients. Since this patient is elderly and opioid-naïve, a lower dose of 50 mcg IN in one nostril may have also been a suitable therapy. Patient-controlled IV analgesic systems are particularly effective for emergency department patients with acute abdominal pain; thus, a low-dose hydromorphone or fentanyl patient-controlled analgesia in this patient with renal failure may be another alternative. Oral medications should be avoided in a patient with abdominal pain with a concern for bowel obstruction. Ibuprofen, an NSAID, should not be given to a patient with kidney disease. Of note, early administration of IV opioids is safe for the treatment of acute abdominal pain in the emergency department and does not affect the accuracy of diagnosis or management.

6. **The answer is D.** (Chapter 36) This patient developed classic effects of systemic local anesthetic toxicity including tongue numbness, lightheadedness, visual and auditory disturbances, twitching, loss of consciousness, and tachyarrhythmias. These can progress to seizures, coma, and respiratory and cardiac arrest. Systemic local anesthetic toxicity is treated with IV 20% lipid emulsion. Local anesthetics are highly lipid soluble. Typical agents used to treat cardiac arrest (e.g., vasopressin) and tachyarrhythmias (e.g., β-blockers and calcium channel blockers)

should be avoided in the setting of local anesthetic systemic toxicity. Seizures due to neurologic toxicity should be treated with benzodiazepines.

7. **The answer is D.** (Chapter 36) The addition of epinephrine to the injected local anesthetic solution increases the duration of anesthesia, helps to control wound bleeding, and slows the systemic absorption. Using a lower concentration of lidocaine (e.g., 1% vs. 2%) will decrease the total dose given. In order to avoid systemic local anesthetic toxicity, calculate the maximum safe dose of local anesthetic that may be used, especially when treating smaller patients or tending to large wounds. Consider the use of procedural sedation, regional anesthesia, systemic analgesics, or anxiolytics when the use of a large quantity of local anesthetic is unavoidable. The addition of sodium bicarbonate to local anesthetics shortens the onset of action by raising tissue pH and reduces the pain of injection. Sodium bicarbonate does not reduce systemic toxicity. Premedicating with diphenhydramine or lipid emulsion are not effective methods of preventing systemic toxicity from local anesthetics.

8. **The answer is A.** (Chapter 36) A variety of techniques are used to reduce the pain of needle puncture and local anesthetic injection: application of a topical anesthetic prior to injection, warming the local anesthetic agent, stretching the skin at the puncture site, vibrating the skin adjacent to the area, talking during the process to distract the patient, inserting the needle through enlarged pores or hair follicles, inserting the needle with bevel up position, or numbing the skin with an aerosol refrigerant.

9. **The answer is A.** (Chapter 36) Peripheral nerve blocks require time to achieve optimal analgesia, approximately 10 to 20 minutes for lidocaine and 15 to 30 minutes for bupivacaine. Although lidocaine continues to be the most popular agent, bupivacaine, levobupivacaine, and ropivacaine offer a longer duration of action, with levobupivacaine and ropivacaine being significantly less cardiotoxic. Pain and temperature sensation are affected first, followed by loss of touch, deep pressure, and then motor function.

10. **The answer is A.** (Chapter 36) Innervation to the thenar eminence is provided by the median nerve. The median nerve is blocked by inserting the needle between the palmaris longus and flexor carpi radialis tendons. The radial nerve block begins with an injection over the lateral aspect of the radial styloid. See Figure 3.1. An ulnar nerve block is performed by inserting the needle under the flexor carpi ulnaris tendon to an additional 5 to 10 mm past the edge of the tendon. To perform a digital nerve

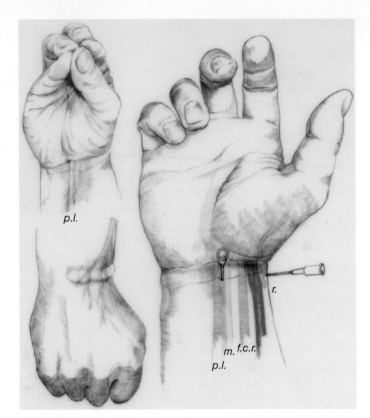

FIGURE 3.1

block, insert the needle on the dorsal surface of the proximal phalanx, advance toward the volar surface staying tangential to the phalanx and repeat on the other side. A digital nerve block would not be useful in this scenario because the wound is located proximal to the digit.

11. **The answer is A.** (Chapter 36) Hematoma blocks are commonly performed for fracture reduction, utilizing the hematoma formation around the fracture to deliver anesthetic to the fracture site, most commonly for distal radius fractures. When performing a hematoma block, the needle is inserted directly into the hematoma, aspiration of blood aids in confirmation of needle position, although care should be taken to avoid regional vessels. Five to 20 mL of local anesthetic solution is then injected into the fracture site. It is a misconception that hematoma blocks dramatically increase the risk of infection. However, this procedure should not be performed through a contaminated wound or an open fracture.

12. **The answer is A.** (Chapter 37) Ventilation can be electronically monitored using capnography, the measurement of the partial pressure of carbon dioxide in exhaled breath. Capnography should be considered for moderate sedation and is recommended for prolonged deep sedation given the increased risk for respiratory depression. End-tidal carbon dioxide >50 mm Hg or an

increase in end-tidal carbon dioxide >10 mm Hg indicates hypoventilation. Patients are at the highest risk of hypoxia and hypoventilation during the period immediately after IV medication administration and during the immediate postprocedure period (when external stimuli are discontinued and the stimulating pain of the procedure has subsided). Pulse oximetry is not a substitute for monitoring ventilation, as hypoventilation or apnea develop before oxygen saturation decreases.

13. **The answer is A.** (Chapter 37) It is appropriate to administer a short-acting analgesic agent prior to the procedure when time permits. Shorter-acting agents (such as fentanyl and morphine) are preferred to drugs with a longer duration of action (such as hydromorphone) to minimize postprocedure respiratory depression. Begin procedural sedation after the last dose of analgesic has reached its peak effect (3–5 minutes for IV morphine and 2–3 minutes for IV fentanyl). Despite its potential to delay the recognition of respiratory suppression, supplemental oxygen reduces the incidence of hypoxemia and has no adverse clinical effects and should therefore be utilized in procedural sedation.

14. **The answer is D.** (Chapter 37) This child developed rigid chest syndrome, a rare complication characterized by spasm of the respiratory muscles leading to respiratory depression or apnea. This is seen when high doses (3–5 mcg/kg) of fentanyl are given by rapid IV bolus. In small children, this syndrome may be precipitated by rapidly flushing the IV line. Administration of fentanyl (1–3 mcg/kg over 5 minutes) followed by slow and careful flushing of the IV line can prevent rigid chest syndrome. Rigid chest syndrome may not be reversible with opioid receptor antagonists such as naloxone, and bag valve mask ventilation may not provide adequate ventilation. Intubation with rapid-sequence induction and pharmacologic paralysis is usually required to ventilate a patient in this situation. Flumazenil is a benzodiazepine receptor antagonist and would not be indicated in this situation.

15. **The answer is C.** (Chapter 37) Propofol can produce hypotension as a result of both negative inotropy and vasodilatation. Hypotension is more common in hypovolemic patients and those with severe systemic disease or multiple comorbidities. Hypovolemia should be corrected before propofol administration.

16. **The answer is D.** (Chapter 37) The risk of respiratory depression from all agents is increased in the elderly population due to reduced ventilatory drive, decreased ability to maintain a patent airway, underlying comorbidities, and hepatic or renal insufficiency. Etomidate is

a good sedative agent in the elderly and in hypotensive patients who require sedation for an emergency procedure because of its minimal cardiovascular effects. For painful procedures, opioids may be necessary, as etomidate has no analgesic effect. Propofol produces greater peak plasma concentrations after an IV bolus dose in the elderly, therefore producing a greater risk of respiratory depression and apnea. To counteract this, the initial and subsequent doses should be 50% of those recommended for younger adults, and more cautious titration is needed.

17. **The answer is D.** (Chapter 38) Transformed migraine is a syndrome in which common migraine headaches transform into a chronic pain syndrome, most commonly from medication overuse, including barbiturates, opioids, and NSAIDs. Pain may be more similar to tension headache with tenderness and tension of scalp musculature. Fibromyalgia is widespread muscular pain involving greater than six body areas out of 19 total regions and a symptom severity score of 5 or more for fatigue, sleep disturbance, and cognitive dysfunction (e.g., forgetfulness, inability to concentrate or recall simple words or numbers, confusion, and associated nonmuscle pain symptoms). Hyperalgesia is an exaggerated response to a normally painful stimulus. Allodynia is pain from a normally nonpainful stimulus.

18. **The answer is C.** (Chapter 38) This patient has a myofascial pain syndrome. Pain symptoms include constant, dull, occasionally shooting pain, which does not typically follow nerve distribution. Signs include trigger points in area of pain, absence of muscle atrophy and poor range of motion in the involved muscle. Primary treatment for myofascial pain syndromes includes oral NSAIDs and topical diclofenac patch for single site of pain. Secondary treatment is amitriptyline. Long-acting controlled-release opioids for noncancer pain such as OxyContin, fentanyl patches, or methadone should not be prescribed from the emergency department. Outpatient opioids for patients with acute exacerbation of chronic noncancer pain should be avoided in the emergency department.

19. **The answer is B.** (Chapter 38) This patient has painful diabetic neuropathy. The symptoms of painful diabetic neuropathy are symmetric numbness associated with burning, electrical, or stabbing pain in lower extremities. Patients may have hyperesthesia, dysesthesias, and/or deep aching pain. Pain may be provoked with a gentle touch to the skin in the areas of abnormal sensation. Duloxetine is the primary treatment for diabetic neuropathy. Pregabalin and gabapentin are secondary treatments of painful diabetic neuropathy. Carbamazepine is the primary treatment for trigeminal neuralgia.

20. **The answer is A.** (Chapter 38) A systematic review of the literature found that the only consistent predictor of aberrant drug-related behaviors in chronic pain patients is a personal history of illicit drug and alcohol abuse. The most common complaints of patients who attempt to obtain opioids from the emergency department are (in order of highest to lowest frequency) back pain, headache, extremity pain, and dental pain. When aberrant drug-related behavior is confirmed or suspected in the emergency department, it should be documented in the chart, stating only the facts. Concerns about opioid overuse can be documented without diagnosing the patient with "drug-seeking behavior," which may not be appropriate without evidence of illegal behavior. In 2012, 17% of the teens trying illicit drugs for the first time used prescription opioids, second only to marijuana.

21. **The answer is D.** (Chapter 38) It can be challenging to identify patients with aberrant drug-related behavior. The patients with this disorder may present with a wide range of complaints including back pain, headache, tooth pain, extremity pain, and panic attack to name a few. Practitioners are encouraged to review the prescription drug monitoring program database before prescribing a discharge medication in order to help identify patients who are abusing or overusing prescription drugs. Other strategies for managing aberrant drug-related behavior in the emergency department include the following. Inform patients that report their prescription or pill bottle was stolen that this is a police issue and recommend that the patient call the police to rectify the matter. Perform a local nerve block and refer to a dentist any patient presenting with dental pain whose examination demonstrates dental caries only. Establish a policy that no lost opioid prescriptions will be filled and notify patients of this policy as they receive prescriptions.

Wound Management

4

QUESTIONS

1. Which of the following is TRUE with respect to sutures?
   (A) Absorbable verses nonabsorbable suture material for percutaneous repairs in the ED for most cases is clinically irrelevant.
   (B) Larger-diameter suture material is preferred.
   (C) Nonabsorbable sutures retain their tensile strength for 30 days.
   (D) Tensile strength increases with the gauge size of the suture material.

2. Which of the following is TRUE with respect to wound location and infection risk?
   (A) Highly vascular areas have low risk of infection even when grossly contaminated with human or animal feces.
   (B) There is conclusive evidence to support the use of antibiotics for intraoral lacerations.
   (C) Highest baseline skin bacterial counts are found on the upper arms, legs, and torso.
   (D) Facial and scalp wounds with heavy contamination have a low rate of infection regardless of degree of intensity of cleaning.

3. Which of the following is the MOST IMPORTANT part of hand examination prior to administration of anesthesia?
   (A) Capillary refill
   (B) Motor and tendon function
   (C) Two-point sensation of hands and fingers
   (D) Quality of pulses distal to injury

4. A 40-year-old right-hand dominant man presents with curvilinear puncture wounds over his fourth and fifth metacarpal phalangeal joints on his right hand. Which of the following organisms are you concerned about and want to make sure antibiotics you prescribe will cover?
   (A) *Eikenella*
   (B) *Pasteurella*
   (C) *Pseudomonas*
   (D) *Staph aureus*

5. Which suturing technique is MOST APPROPRIATE for closing long simple linear lacerations with minimal time and even distribution of tensile force on the skin?
   (A) Continuous percutaneous suture
   (B) Continuous subcuticular suture
   (C) Half-buried horizontal mattress
   (D) Horizontal mattress suture

6. What is the primary disadvantage of using staples for wound closure?
   (A) High cost.
   (B) Higher infection rate.
   (C) Least precise wound closure.
   (D) Removal of hair is required.

7. In which of the following situations would cyanoac-rylate be LEAST EFFECTIVE for closing a wound?
   (A) Short simple pediatric facial laceration
   (B) Superficial wound oriented parallel to line of tension
   (C) Used in conjunction with tape
   (D) Wound with varying dynamic tension

8. A 25-year-old man is hit in the right eye by a fist with ring on it. There is mild swelling, no orbital step-offs, and a superficial eyelid laceration 6 mm away from the medial canthus. Globe is intact, vision is normal, and no extraocular muscle entrapment is noted. What should appropriate emergency department management be?
   (A) Primary closure in the emergency department with 7-0 nonabsorbable suture
   (B) Primary closure in the emergency department with tissue skin adhesive
   (C) Referral to ophthalmologist or oculoplastic specialist
   (D) Wound healing by secondary intent

9. What is the BEST WAY to repair laceration shown in Figure 4.1?

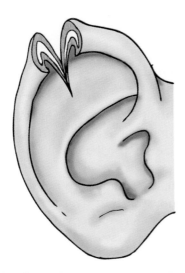

FIGURE 4.1 Reproduced with permission from J.E. Tintinalli, J.S. Stapczynski, O.J. Ma, D. Yealy, G.D. Meckler, D.M. Cline: Tintinalli's Emergency Medicine: A Comprehensive Study Guide, 9th Edition. McGraw-Hill Education; 2020.

   (A) Close skin layer only with 6-0 nonabsorbable sutures
   (B) Debride the skin edges
   (C) Remove loose pieces of cartilage
   (D) Two-layer closure

10. A 28-year-old man has sustained a laceration from a knife to his left cheek 3 cm anterior to the earlobe attachment and just inferior to the zygoma. Which of the following should raise suspicion of parotid duct injury?
    (A) Arterial bleeding
    (B) Paralysis of lower eyelid
    (C) Ptosis
    (D) Sensory loss in the V^2 branch of the trigeminal nerve

11. You are staffing a small critical access hospital. A distal fingertip amputation less than 1 cm^2 in an 11-year-old child is noted on examination. There is no involvement of the nail bed and no exposed bone. Which of the following is the recommended treatment?
    (A) Immediate transfer to tertiary care center 3 hours away for reimplantation by a hand surgeon
    (B) Healing by secondary intent with nonadherent dressing changes
    (C) Replacement of the amputated tip as a full-thickness skin graft after defatting and cleaning
    (D) V-Y advancement flap closure

12. A partial flexor tendon injury is identified on a volar hand laceration affecting the palm of the hand. The patient is able to flex all digits at the metacarpophalangeal, proximal interphalangeal, and distal interphalangeal joints. Which of the following is the MOST APPROPRIATE management?
    (A) Hand surgeon consultation for follow-up in 2 to 3 days with splinting
    (B) Immediate operative repair
    (C) Primary wound closure after tendon repair by emergency physician
    (D) Superficial laceration repair with 4 weeks of position of function splinting

13. Which of the following could aid in the detection of a joint capsule laceration of the knee?
    (A) Fluorescein saline injection into the wound to visualize leaking joint fluid
    (B) Methylene blue injection into joint capsule
    (C) Probe exploration of capsule
    (D) Saline load test of joint capsule

14. Which of the following will LIKELY yield a false negative for detection of an Achilles tendon laceration?
    (A) Active plantar flexion
    (B) Direct examination
    (C) Thompson test
    (D) Ultrasound

15. Which of the following foreign bodies should be removed promptly?
    (A) Glass in the arm after motor vehicle accident
    (B) Metal needle in the arm of IV drug user
    (C) Plastic wire in the hand from industrial injury
    (D) Wood splinter in the foot of a diabetic patient

16. Which of the following might ultrasound have difficulty localizing?
    (A) Broken needle in the arm
    (B) Glass in the forehead
    (C) Plastic earing backing
    (D) Palmar thorn

17. Prophylactic use of which of the following classes of antibiotics may be used in immunosuppressed patients who are bitten by a dog?
    (A) Clindamycin
    (B) Fluoroquinolone
    (C) Lincomycin
    (D) Penicillin

18. A 45-year-old painter presents with the wound shown below on his index finger. He was using a trigger activated paint sprayer and injured it 2 hours prior to arrival. Initially, the patient had minimal pain and bleeding. Pain is now becoming severe (Figure 4.2). What is the INITIAL STEP in management?

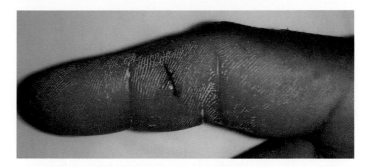

FIGURE 4.2 Photo contributed by J. S. Stapczynski, MD.

    (A) Broad-spectrum antibiotics
    (B) Digital nerve block for pain control
    (C) Pain management with IV opioids
    (D) Splinting and referral to hand surgeon for recheck the following day

19. A 32-year-old female farmer sustained a laceration on a rusty nail protruding from a barn stall door while cleaning animal stalls. Last tetanus immunization was 7 years ago. The patient reports a severe local reaction at that time with significant swelling and pain at the sight of injection. What is the APPROPRIATE management with respect to the concern for exposure to tetanus?
    (A) Administer tetanus toxoid
    (B) Administer tetanus toxoid and tetanus immune globulin
    (C) No prophylaxis is needed
    (D) Watch for signs of tetanus and treat if they develop

20. Which of the following has the biggest impact on wound infection rates?
    (A) Bio-occlusive dressing use for 72 post wound repair
    (B) Compulsive wound cleaning with tap water and soap
    (C) Prophylactic oral antibiotics
    (D) Routine application of topical antibiotic ointment

ANSWERS

1. **The answer is A.** (Chapter 41) The use of absorbable verses nonabsorbable suture material for percutaneous repairs in the emergency department for most cases is clinically irrelevant. The use of absorbable suture material can be especially helpful in children who might be traumatized by manipulating the wound again to remove the sutures. Nonabsorbable sutures retain their tensile strength for 60 days, whereas absorbable sutures lose most of their tensile strength in less than 60 days. Thinner suture material is generally preferred over larger-diameter suture material as it produces less damage to tissues and leaves a smaller hole in the skin. The higher the gauge size, the lower the tensile strength of the suture material.

2. **The answer is D.** (Chapters 39 and 42) Due to their vascularity, scalp and facial wounds have a very low infection rate, degree of cleaning has not been shown to have an impact on this rate. In fact, in resource poor situations, facial and scalp wounds have been repaired with adhesive strips without prior cleaning and irrigation. Fecal contamination is always associated with a high risk of infection. Lowest baseline skin bacterial counts are on the upper arms, legs, and torso; highest are in moist areas such as axilla, perineum, intertriginous areas, and toe web spaces. Oral antibiotics while traditionally recommended for intraoral lacerations have inconclusive evidence to support their use.

3. **The answer is C.** (Chapters 40 and 43) All represent important parts of the examination that should be completed prior to anesthesia. Complete evaluation of sensation including two-point discrimination should always be accomplished prior to initiation of anesthesia. Normal two-point discrimination is less than 6 mm. Motor function may be impaired by pain from the injury and better assessed afterwards. Distal pulses and capillary refill should not be affected by anesthetic application proximal to the wound. Be sure to assess tendons after anesthetizing the wound. The patient may have tendon function but have a tendon injury that you would not be able to detect without visualizing the tendon through the wound opening throughout the range of motion.

4. **The answer is A.** (Chapter 43) The scenario describes the classic "fight bite" or puncture wounds/lacerations caused by striking another person's teeth with a clenched fist, *Eikenella* is the organism of concern and amoxicillin/clavulanate would be antibiotic of choice. *Pasturella* would be primary concern for animal bites and again amoxicillin/clavulanate would be agent of choice. *Pseudomonas* would be of concern for puncture through a shoe or fresh water contamination and ciprofloxacin or other

antpseudomonal coverage would be needed. *Staph aureus* remains the concern for skin source infection, and first-generation cephalosporin or other beta-lactam is first-line agent despite methicillin resistance increasing prevalence.

5. **The answer is A.** (Chapter 41) Continuous (running) percutaneous sutures are the most time efficient sutures for long simple lacerations not requiring detailed approximation. Continuous subcuticular are the most complex suture to place but can yield very good approximation and cosmetic results often with out superficial closure being required. Horizontal mattresses are good for wounds that require very low tension to prevent suture from causing wound edge necrosis and tearing trough fragile skin. Half-buried horizontal mattress is a technique of closing complex stellate laceration and tip of flap laceration where the needle and suture pass through only the dermal layer of tissue when traversing the tip of the flap or a stellate prong.

6. **The answer is C.** (Chapter 41) Staples have the advantage of being quick and cost-effective, easier to find in hair-covered areas for removal, and generally do not require hair removal to place as the hair can be held out of the way by hand or antibiotic ointment. Infection rates and cosmetic appearance are comparable to sutures. It is, however, the least precise method of closure, not suitable for the face, and prone to downward displacement of wound edges if too much pressure is used in placing staples.

7. **The answer is D.** (Chapter 41) Cyanoacrylate is similar to 4-0 absorbable subcuticular sutures in strength but not as strong as staples. It is well suited for superficial lacerations under low tension. Works well for children's facial lacerations that are easily approximated, as it does not require removal, generally sloughing off in 5 to 10 days. It forms its own bio-occlusive dressing. It can be used in conjunction with paper tape closures for added strength to thin layer skin closures. It is not well served for closing areas of high skin tension, widely gaping wounds, or areas of varying tension such as over joints.

8. **The answer is C.** (Chapter 42) Eyelid lacerations within 6 to 8 mm of the medial canthus are at risk of injury to the canalicular system. This risk increase when there is an associated medial wall orbital blow out fracture, this combination of injuries should prompt a referral to an ophthalmologist or oculoplastic specialist. Other high-risk injuries prompting a referral include injuries to the tarsal plate, lid margin, inner surface of the lid, lacrimal duct, or injuries with associated ptosis. A careful provider may repair superficial lacerations limited to outer

lid surface not involving the aforementioned structures, using magnification (loops) and 6-0 or 7-0 nonabsorbable suture material. Lacerations less than 1 mm in length will close well by secondary intent.

9. **The answer is A.** (Chapter 42) Auricular lacerations involving the cartilage often can be closed in the emergency department by simply closing the overlying skin with interrupted 6-0 nonabsorbable sutures. Care should be taken to include the thin layer of perichondrium when placing skin sutures, as well as ensuring any loose cartilage fragments are kept in place for possible later reconstruction if needed. This will provide adequate support for cartilage healing. Skin should not be cut nor should loose pieces of cartilage removed. An auricular pressure dressing should be applied for 24 hours and rechecked to ensure there is no hematoma development that may cause ear deformation from cartilage damage in the healing process. If hematoma develops, sutures are removed hematoma drained, resutured, and pressure reapplied with another recheck in 24 hours. Very complex lacerations, those extending into the canal, significant tissue loss, or involvement of the tympanic membrane are best referred to a specialist (Figure 4.3).

10. **The answer is A.** (Chapter 42) A branch of the facial artery along with the buccal branch of the facial nerve travel with the parotid duct. The presence of arterial bleeding or paralysis of the cheek should raise significant concern with any injury occurring in a zone posterior to a line drawn vertically through the lateral canthus and inferiorly to a line drawn from frenulum to tragus. See Figure 4.4. Ptosis of the upper lid would be from injury to oculomotor nerve, and the lower lid is innervated from zygomatic branch of the facial nerve. Mandibular branch (V^2) of the trigeminal nerve travels above the zygoma.

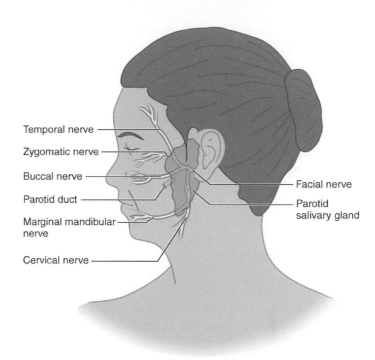

FIGURE 4.4 Reproduced with permission from J.E. Tintinalli, J.S. Stapczynski, O.J. Ma, D. Yealy, G.D. Meckler, D.M. Cline: Tintinalli's Emergency Medicine: A Comprehensive Study Guide, 9th Edition. McGraw-Hill Education; 2020.

11. **The answer is B.** (Chapter 43) Healing by secondary intent is the preferred method of treatment with better cosmetic appearance, sensation, and functional outcomes. Daily cleaning, soaks, and dressing change is all that is needed when no bone is exposed and nail bed is intact especially for wounds 1 cm^2 or less in size. The use of defatted amputated tissue as a full-thickness graft may be helpful for larger tissue defects. The flap may develop necrosis and fall of as the underling tissues heal. V-Y flap, generally done by the hand surgeon, may be used in closing an amputation through the nail bed with exposed tuft. This will require shorting of the bone with the use of a rongeur to adequately cover the defect.

12. **The answer is A.** (Chapter 43) Most hand surgeons prefer to repair full-thickness flexor tendon injuries within 24 hours. If delayed, they should be seen within 2 to 3 days for repair within 7 days, beyond 10 to 14 days post injury scaring and tendon retraction complicate repair. Splinting should be done with flexion at the wrist and metacarpophalangeal joint and extension at distal and proximal interphalangeal joints. Partial flexor tendon injuries should be seen by a hand surgeon for timely follow-up and may require repair, especially flexor digitorum superficialis that may cause trigger finger if unrepaired. And experienced emergency physician may undertake repair of partial or complete extensor tendon lacerations on the dorsum of the hand located between the distal wrist and metacarpophalangeal joint.

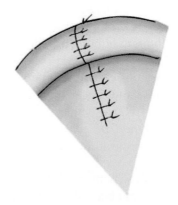

FIGURE 4.3 Reproduced with permission from J.E. Tintinalli, J.S. Stapczynski, O.J. Ma, D. Yealy, G.D. Meckler, D.M. Cline: Tintinalli's Emergency Medicine: A Comprehensive Study Guide, 9th Edition. McGraw-Hill Education; 2020.

13. **The answer is D.** (Chapter 44) Articular capsule lacerations are extremely difficult to detect on examination. Gas in a joint space on a plain radiograph is diagnostic. When gas is not present, saline load test is the best method of determining joint integrity. Injection of enough saline into the joint space to demonstrate leakage into the wound is a positive test, and false negative may occur if too little saline is injected. Installation of 60 to 100 mL of saline into the knee joint may be required to avoid a false-negative test. Fluorescein may be added to saline injected to aid in detection, and methylene blue should not be added as it does not add accuracy and will cause staining of joint structures complicating intraoperative repair of intra-articular injuries.

14. **The answer is A.** (Chapter 44) Direct examination and exploration as the foot is put through range of motion is good method for detecting lacerations, a "catch" may be felt for partial tendon injury. Ultrasound allows direct examination of the entire tendon. Thompson test, squeezing the calf as the patient lies prone with the knee bent and lower leg up should produce plantar flexion, comparing to the opposite side may help detect subtle injuries. Active plantar flexion may yield a false negative as the tibialis posterior muscle also plantar flexes the foot at the ankle.

15. **The answer is D.** (Chapter 45) Foreign body removal need not be done emergently, particularly for inert substances such as metal, plastics, and glass. If it is readily identified and localized, removal can be done in the emergency department. However, it may be easier to find under operative exploration with good regional anesthesia, exposure, and lighting in a bloodless field. Hand foreign bodies are best explored by a hand surgeon owing to complex anatomies and easily injured surrounding structures. Organic foreign bodies such as splinters, thorns, spines, or teeth should be removed as promptly as possible. Patients with immunodeficiency are at highest risk of secondary infection.

16. **The answer is D.** (Chapter 45) High-resolution ultrasound can detect the widest array of foreign bodies with greater than 90% sensitivity for object greater than 4 to 5 mm. It is useful for directing removal of objects identified by other modalities in place of fluoroscopy. Frequency affects both depths of penetration and resolution; high-frequency probes have better resolution and can detect multiple small objects close together but are unable to penetrate deep tissues. Low frequency lacks resolution but can image deeper levels. Optimal evaluation for an object would be to scan with both high- and low-frequency probes. Other limitations include areas dense in echogenic structures such as the hands and feet with close bones and tendons, which may interfere with interpretation. Ultrasound is also dependent on skill and experience of the operator.

17. **The answer is D.** (Chapter 46) *Capnocytophaga* infection is rare but rapidly progressive systemic illness in immunocompromised patients with dog bites. Patients with prior splenectomy, diabetes, immunosuppression, and alcoholics are at highest risk of this disease. Systemic illness may occur in the absence of local wound infection. Penicillin class antibiotics should be routinely considered for this group of patients. While lincomycin class (clindamycin) does cover *Capnocytophaga*, it does not provide adequate coverage of *Pasturella* and should not be used alone for dog and cat bites.

18. **The answer is C.** (Chapter 46) High-pressure injections should prompt immediate referral to the hand specialist for exploration and debridement. Initial injury may appear relatively innocuous, often starting with minimal pain but will likely have significant underlying injury including fractures, tendon and ligament disruption, and foreign material travel throughout fascial plains. Digital nerve block should be avoided due to potential for worsening of compartment pressure and ischemia; pain control should be accomplished with parenteral opioids. Antibiotics should cover skin flora, and tetanus prophylaxis should be given. Debridement within 6 hours significantly lowers risk of subsequent amputation.

19. **The answer is A.** (Chapter 47) Tetanus toxoid prophylaxis should be given if the patient has had primary (more than three doses) immunization more than 10 years previous for a clean wound or more than 5 years for a contaminated or high-risk wound. Tetanus immunoglobulin should be given for patient with high risk wound and incomplete (less than three doses) or no previous immunization with tetanus toxoid. Tetanus toxoid is only contraindicated for history of previous neurologic reaction or systemic reaction. Local reaction is common and not a contraindication to vaccination. Patients with history of severe local reaction often have a history of frequent previous vaccinations and have a high serum tetanus antitoxin level; they should not be vaccinated more frequently than every 10 years. Tetanus immunoglobulin should be given to patients with high-risk injuries that are contraindicated for tetanus toxoid.

20. **The answer is B.** (Chapter 47) Routine use of prophylactic antibiotics has not been shown to reduce the rates of wound infection over that of simple wound care with frequent cleaning with soap and tap water. High-risk injuries

such as bite and heavily contaminated wounds should have antibiotic choice tailored base on presumed pathogen. Bio-occlusive dressings may aid in wound healing by providing a moist environment to promote reepithelialization; however, benefit is limited beyond 24 to 48 hours.

Antibiotic ointment is an alternative for a wound dressing especially for wounds that it is difficult to place a dressing on. Antibiotic ointment aid in maintaining wound moisture and decrease scab formation when applied for 3 to 4 days post injury.

Cardiovascular Disorders

5

QUESTIONS

1. What is the BEST predictor of syncope recurrence?
   (A) Age >65
   (B) Chest pain prior to syncopal event
   (C) Syncopal episodes lasting >1 minute
   (D) Syncope in the preceding year

2. An 82-year-old woman with a history of coronary artery disease, hypertension, and chronic kidney disease presents with several months of progressive exertional dyspnea. Her symptoms have become so severe she can no longer walk across the room without getting light-headed. On review of systems, she admits to orthopnea but denies chest pain. She is well appearing on examination and in no acute distress. She has a thin body habitus with no peripheral edema. Her lungs are clear to auscultation and equal bilaterally. She has a faint mid-diastolic murmur on cardiac auscultation. She has equal pulses in all extremities. Vital signs are HR 88, BP 170/98, RR 20, and T 36.8°C. ECG is shown in Figure 5.1. Laboratory analysis reveals sodium 138 mEq/L, potassium 3.9 mEq/L, bicarbonate 24 mEq/L, creatinine 1.6 mg/dL, glucose 144 mg/dL, white blood cell count 9.1, hemoglobin 12.4 g/dL, platelet count 223 k/μL, troponin T <0.01 ng/mL, and B-type natriuretic peptide (BNP) 46 pg/mL. Chest x-ray shows straightening of the left heart border. Which of the following is the BEST NEXT step in her management?
   (A) Admit for an echocardiogram
   (B) Consult cardiology for cardiac catheterization
   (C) Discharge her home with outpatient cardiology follow-up
   (D) Obtain a CT pulmonary angiogram

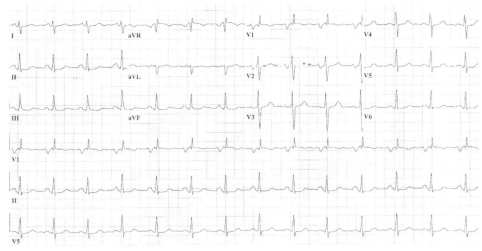

FIGURE 5.1 Reproduced with permission from J.E. Tintinalli, J.S. Stapczynski, O.J. Ma, D. Yealy, G.D. Meckler, D.M. Cline: Tintinalli's Emergency Medicine: A Comprehensive Study Guide, 9th Edition. McGraw-Hill Education; 2020.

3. Which of the following is NOT included within the thrombolysis in acute myocardial infarction (TIMI) score?
   (A) Age
   (B) History
   (C) Risk factors
   (D) Troponin

4. A 54-year-old woman is brought to the emergency department by Emergency Medical Services for respiratory distress. The patient's vital signs are HR 107, BP 170/95, RR 32, SpO$_2$ 86%, and T 37.2°C. Her examination is remarkable for tachypnea, rales bilaterally on auscultation, and jugular venous distension. She is sitting up on the stretcher, pulling off her cardiac monitor leads, and not answering questions or following commands. IV access has been obtained. What is the BEST NEXT step?
   (A) Obtain a stat ECG and chest x-ray
   (B) Place the patient on a non-rebreather, administer IV furosemide, and start a nitroglycerin infusion
   (C) Place the patient on bilevel positive airway pressure (BiPAP)
   (D) Prepare for emergent intubation

5. A 67-year-old woman presents to the emergency department with an acute myocardial infarction. She had a full physical and cardiac workup 6 months prior with normal echocardiogram, chest x-ray, and normal laboratory studies including renal function. On examination, the patient has rales in the bilateral lower lung fields. She is short of breath with oxygen saturation of 90% on room air. Which medication will reduce this patient's chance of developing long-term congestive heart failure associated with the acute myocardial infarction?
   (A) Angiotensin-converting enzyme (ACE) inhibitors
   (B) β-Blockers
   (C) Calcium channel antagonists
   (D) Oxygen

6. Which of the following is TRUE with respect to intra-aortic balloon pump counterpulsation?
   (A) Augments diastolic perfusion pressure and unloads the left ventricle
   (B) Can be used long term to support cardiac perfusion
   (C) Decreases coronary artery blood flow due to the positioning of the balloon in the aorta
   (D) Increases afterload and diastolic blood pressure

7. A 41-year-old man with no past medical history presents to the emergency department with significant chest pain and diaphoresis. The patient takes no medications and has no allergies. He is tachycardic, diaphoretic, and hypertensive. The patient's ECG demonstrates no significant ST or T-wave abnormalities and is notable only for his heart rate. The patient admits to using cocaine prior to presenting to the emergency department. Which is the NEXT APPROPRIATE step in management?
   (A) Administer 324 mg of chewable aspirin, 0.4 mg sublingual nitroglycerin, and 1 mg of IV lorazepam, and admit to observation for serial cardiac enzymes.
   (B) Complete a thrombolysis in acute myocardial infarction (TIMI) score in order to guide treatment and management.
   (C) Consult cardiology and administer 1 mg/kg of subcutaneous enoxaparin.
   (D) Obtain an echocardiogram, administer 5 mg metoprolol IV, and admit to observation for serial ECGs and cardiac enzymes.

8. Which statement concerning mitral valve prolapse is TRUE?
   (A) Antithrombotic therapy is routinely recommended.
   (B) Most patients are symptomatic with exertion.
   (C) Patients with mitral valve prolapse and concomitant mitral regurgitation require endocarditis prophylaxis.
   (D) The classic auscultatory finding is a pansystolic murmur.

9. Which of the following patients has the highest likelihood of a major adverse cardiac event in the next 30 days?
   (A) A 32-year-old man with a history of diabetes, hypertension, tobacco use, and family history of early myocardial infarction who presents to the emergency department with an acute onset of sharp chest pain for the past 15 minutes. The patient has a normal ECG and normal troponin.
   (B) A 50-year-old woman with no past medical history and no family history presents to the emergency department with pressure-like chest pain for the past 2 hours that radiates to both arms. She has no other symptoms or physical examination findings. Her ECG has nonspecific repolarization abnormalities. A troponin is normal.

(C) A 67-year-old man with a history of diabetes, hypertension, hypercholesterolemia, and family history of early myocardial infarction who presents to the emergency department with pressure-like chest pain but no other symptoms or physical examination findings. His ECG shows ST depression. A troponin is normal.

(D) An 88-year-old woman with hypertension, hypercholesterolemia, and no significant family history presents to the emergency department with 30 hours of constant, sharp, nonexertional, nonpleuritic, and nonpositional pain. She has hypertension and mild edema on examination. Her ECG shows nonspecific repolarization abnormalities. Her troponin in normal.

10. Which of the following correctly lists the mortality risk associated with syncope etiology from highest to lowest?
(A) Cardiac, neurologic, unknown, vasovagal
(B) Cardiac, neurologic, vasovagal, unknown
(C) Neurologic, cardiac, unknown, vasovagal
(D) Unknown, cardiac, neurologic, vasovagal

11. A 72-year-old man presents to the emergency department in severe respiratory distress. Emergency Medical Services reports his wife called due to gradually increased work of breathing throughout the day. They report the patient has a history of hypertension, chronic obstructive pulmonary disease (COPD), congestive heart failure, and osteoarthritis. On examination you see a morbidly obese man in moderate respiratory distress. His lung sounds are coarse diffusely. You decide to utilize bedside ultrasound to help differentiate whether his symptoms are due to a heart failure exacerbation or a COPD exacerbation. Which of the following is considered pathologic for alveolar and interstitial edema?

(A) Detection of A-lines with the absence of B-lines
(B) Loss of "seashore" sign in M-mode
(C) More than one B-line seen in three or more sonographic windows on the anterior or anterolateral chest
(D) More than three B-lines seen in one or more sonographic windows on the anterior or anterolateral chest

12. Which statement regarding physical examination findings in patients with acute myocardial infarction is correct?
(A) Distant low-pitched rattling breath sounds are often heard with patient's presenting with ischemia-induced congestive heart failure.
(B) Patient who present with acute coronary syndrome are almost always tachycardic and hypertensive.
(C) Physical examination findings most strongly associated with acute coronary syndrome are hypotension and diaphoresis.
(D) Reproducible chest pain, tenderness to the chest wall with palpation, has been reported with the diagnosis of acute myocardial infarction in 40% of patients.

13. Heart failure has a poor prognosis with approximately 50% of patients diagnosed dying within what period of time?
(A) 2 years
(B) 5 years
(C) 10 years
(D) 20 years

14. A 47-year-old man presents to the emergency department with severe chest pain that is worse when lying supine. Three days ago he had a pacemaker placed for symptomatic bradycardia. The patient is in moderate distress, slightly altered, and slow to respond. His vital signs are BP 76/60, HR 110, RR 22, SpO$_2$ 96% on RA, and T 37.3°C. His ECG shows sinus tachycardia, not paced, with normal intervals and no significant ST or T-wave abnormalities. Bedside point-of-care echocardiogram is performed. The parasternal long- and short-axis views are shown in Figure 5.2. The patient's inferior vena cava collapses 10% with forced inspiration. What is the NEXT BEST step in management?

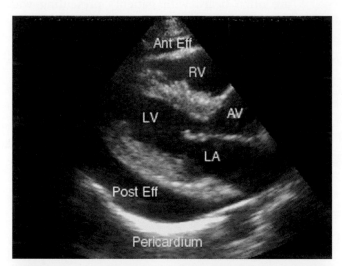

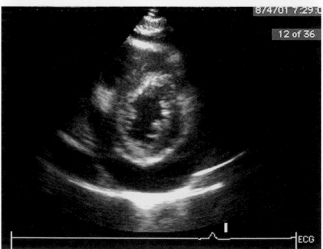

FIGURE 5.2 Reprinted with permission from Reardon RF, Joing SA: Cardiac, in Ma OJ, Mateer JR, Blaivas M (eds): Emergency Ultrasound, 2nd ed. Copyright © 2008, The McGraw-Hill Companies, Inc., all rights reserved.

(A) Dobutamine 5 mcg/kg/min IV
(B) Emergent pericardiocentesis
(C) Emergent thoracostomy
(D) Heparin 500 units IV bolus

15. Which of the following statements regarding CT coronary angiography is TRUE?
(A) Approximately 20% of patients will have a non-diagnostic CT coronary angiography and thus require additional testing.
(B) CT coronary angiography provides adequate assessment of cardiac function and offers superior information compared to traditional testing for patients with known coronary artery disease.
(C) Patients undergoing cardiac evaluation with CT coronary angiography had a similar length of stay in the emergency department compared to patients undergoing a traditional stress test.
(D) The cost of cardiac evaluation with CT coronary angiography far exceeds the cost of a cardiac evaluation with traditional stress test.

16. A 54-year-old woman presents with crushing chest pain, shortness of breath, and diaphoresis for the past 2 hours. The patient has no past medical history, home medications, or allergies. An ECG shows an anterior ST-elevation myocardial infarction. The patient's vital signs are BP 135/72, HR 86, and SpO$_2$ 97% on RA. You obtain IV access and administer 324 mg of chewable aspirin. Percutaneous coronary intervention (PCI) is not available at your hospital, and it will take over 2 hours to transfer the patient to a center with PCI capability. Which of the following is the BEST course of treatment for this patient?
(A) Administer a 1-L normal saline bolus, 0.4 mg sublingual nitroglycerin, 4 L/min oxygen by nasal canula, 75 mg oral clopidogrel, and transfer the patient for PCI as soon as possible.
(B) Administer 75 mg oral clopidogrel, 180 mcg/kg bolus of eptifibatide, and IV heparin 60 units/kg bolus followed by an infusion. Admit the patient to the hospitalist at your facility.
(C) Administer 75 mg oral clopidogrel, 1 mg/kg subcutaneous enoxaparin, 50 mg IV tissue plasminogen activator, and transfer the patient for PCI as soon as possible.
(D) Administer 50 mg IV tissue plasminogen activator, 4 L/min nasal canula oxygen, 0.4 mg sublingual nitroglycerin, and admit the patient to the hospitalist at your facility.

17. While evaluating a 57-year-old man in the emergency department, you auscultate a new cardiac murmur. The murmur is quiet but heard immediately with your stethoscope placed on the chest wall. What is the grade of this murmur?

(A) I
(B) II
(C) III
(D) VI

18. Which of the following patients would be MOST APPROPRIATE for an ECG exercise stress using a treadmill?

    (A) A 42-year-old man with a history of a previous myocardial infarction and stent placement presenting with 3 days of chest pain and two sets of normal cardiac enzymes. Laboratory studies demonstrate significant hypokalemia. The patient has normal vital signs and a normal examination.

    (B) A 50-year-old man with a history of hypertension and tobacco use who presents to the emergency department with 6 hours of chest pain that has now resolved. The patient takes a daily aspirin. He has normal vital signs and a normal physical examination. ECG shows no abnormalities. The patient has one normal troponin and is now pain free.

    (C) A 63-year-old woman with a history of symptomatic aortic stenosis but no previous cardiac disease. Her thrombolysis in acute myocardial infarction (TIMI) score is zero. The patient has normal serial cardiac markers spaced 6 hours apart and is now pain-free.

    (D) A 75-year-old man with no past medical history who takes no medications. The patient has normal vital signs and physical examination. The patient's ECG demonstrates a right bundle branch block. Serial cardiac markers are negative and he is pain-free.

19. The symptom with the highest sensitivity for heart failure is which of the following?

    (A) Dyspnea on exertion
    (B) Edema
    (C) Orthopnea
    (D) Paroxysmal nocturnal dyspnea

20. A 80-old-man with a history of diabetes, hypertension, and tobacco use presents to the emergency department with chest pain, nausea, vomiting, and shortness of breath. He takes a daily aspirin and insulin. His blood pressure is 84/65 with a heart rate of 74. He appears diaphoretic and distressed. You obtain this ECG (Figure 5.3). Which artery is occluded?

    (A) Left circumflex artery
    (B) Obtuse marginal artery
    (C) Proximal left anterior descending artery
    (D) Right coronary artery

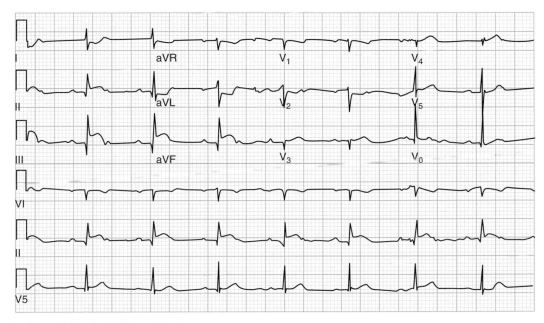

FIGURE 5.3 Courtesy of David M. Cline, MD, Wake Forest University.

21. Which of the following is considered first-line treatment for nitroglycerin-associated headache?
    (A) Acetaminophen
    (B) Caffeine
    (C) Morphine
    (D) Prochlorperazine

22. Which of the following is the MOST helpful in the diagnosis of syncope?
    (A) ECG
    (B) History
    (C) Labs
    (D) Orthostatic vital signs

23. A 56-year-old woman presents to the emergency department with fatigue, mild shortness of breath, diaphoresis, and overall feeling unwell. She has no prior past medical history. The patient has no chest pain or abdominal pain. The ECG shows ST elevation in the anterior leads concerning for acute myocardial infarction. What percentage of women who present with acute cardiac ischemia have no chest pain?
    (A) Approximately 5%
    (B) Approximately 15%
    (C) Approximately 25%
    (D) Approximately 35%

24. Which of the following is TRUE regarding syncope in the elderly?
    (A) Due to calcification of vessels, orthostatic syncope is less common in the elderly.
    (B) Postprandial syncope is less common.
    (C) Risk is not increased until age 65.
    (D) Vasovagal syncope decreases with increasing age.

25. You are examining a 74-year-old man in the emergency department who tells you he has a cardiac valve that was replaced several years ago. On chest auscultation you hear a loud, clicking metallic sound associated with S_1. Which of the following is TRUE regarding mechanical valves when compared to bioprosthetic valves?
    (A) Mechanical valves are more frequently rejected by the host immune system.
    (B) Mechanical valves carry an increased risk of stroke.

(C) Mechanical valves fail more frequently.
(D) Mechanical valves require surgical replacement more frequently.

26. Which of the following conduction disturbances has the worst prognosis for a patient with an acute myocardial infarction?
    (A) Accelerated idioventricular rhythm
    (B) Premature ventricular contractions
    (C) Sinus bradycardia with normal blood pressure
    (D) Sinus tachycardia with normal blood pressure

27. A 55-year-old man presents to the emergency department in cardiogenic shock after suffering an acute myocardial infarction. The patient has no significant past medical history and takes no medications. Vital signs are BP 68/44, HR 82, RR 14, T 37.1°C, and SpO_2 98% on RA. The patient receives a 1-L normal saline bolus with no significant change in blood pressure. He has a Glasgow coma scale (GCS) of 15, mildly coarse breath sounds at the lung bases, no murmurs, and equal femoral pulses. What is the NEXT BEST step?
    (A) Dobutamine 2 mcg/kg/min titrated up to 20 mcg/kg/min
    (B) Dobutamine 2 mcg/kg/min titrated up to 20 mcg/kg/min and norepinephrine 2 mcg/min
    (C) Dopamine 3 mcg/kg/min titrated up to 50 mcg/kg/min
    (D) Milrinone 0.5 mcg/kg/min

28. Which of the following murmurs is paired INCORRECTLY with the valve deficiency?
    (A) Harsh systolic murmur best heard in the left second intercostal space—pulmonic stenosis
    (B) High-pitched blowing diastolic murmur immediately after S_2—aortic regurgitation
    (C) Mid-diastolic rumble, crescendos into S_2—mitral valve prolapse
    (D) Soft, blowing, holosystolic—tricuspid valve regurgitation

29. A 68-year-old woman with a past medical history of coronary artery disease, paroxysmal atrial fibrillation, a cerebral vascular accident, and rheumatoid arthritis presents following a syncopal episode while sitting at dinner with family. She has no complaints on arrival. Vital signs are HR 82, BP 150/85, RR 16, SpO$_2$ 100%, and T 36.9°C. Her ECG shows a left bundle branch block, which is unchanged from a prior ECG. Laboratory analysis is significant for sodium 136 mEq/L, potassium 4.1 mEq/L, chloride 100 mEq/L, bicarbonate 23 mEq/L, creatinine 0.8 mg/dL, glucose 128 mg/dL, white blood cell count 8.4, hemoglobin 10.2 g/dL, hematocrit 29%, and platelet count 188 k/μL. Which of the following makes this patient a high risk for serious outcome according to the San Francisco syncope rule?
    (A) Age of 68
    (B) Hematocrit of 29%
    (C) History of paroxysmal atrial fibrillation
    (D) Left bundle branch block on ECG

30. What percentage of patients who present with undifferentiated chest pain will have either an ECG consistent with acute ischemia/infarction or initially positive cardiac biomarkers?
    (A) 10%
    (B) 25%
    (C) 50%
    (D) 75%

31. Emergency medical services (EMS) responds to a call for a 75-year-old man with no known past medical history who is prescribed no medications. He complains of chest pain and mild shortness of breath. The patient's vital signs are BP 75/45, HR 102, RR 22, SpO$_2$ 97% on RA, and T 37°C. The patient has clear lung sounds and faint equal radial and femoral pulses. EMS established an IV and obtained an ECG that demonstrates ST elevation in the inferior leads with ST depression in leads 1 and aVL. You are contacted to provide medical command. Which of the following is the BEST prehospital advice for this patient?
    (A) Administer 324 mg chewable aspirin, a 500-mL IV normal saline bolus, and transfer to the closest emergency department 5 minutes away that does not have percutaneous coronary intervention (PCI)
    (B) Administer 324 mg chewable aspirin, a 500-mL IV normal saline bolus, and transfer to an emergency department 15 minutes away that does have PCI and cardiac revascularization capability
    (C) Administer 324 mg of chewable aspirin, 500-mL IV normal saline bolus, 5 mg IV metoprolol, and transfer to the closest emergency department 5 minutes away that does not have PCI
    (D) Administer 324 mg chewable aspirin, 500-mL IV normal saline bolus, 5 mg IV metoprolol, and transfer to an emergency department 15 minutes away that does have PCI and cardiac revascularization capability

32. A 65-year-old woman with a history of diabetes presents to the emergency department with an anterior ST-elevation myocardial infarction. She is taken for percutaneous coronary intervention (PCI) with successful stenting. However, 6 hours after this procedure she develops hypotension and shortness of breath. The patient's echocardiogram demonstrates impaired ejection fraction of 20%, and her chest x-ray shows signs of congestive heart failure. Which of the following MOST CLOSELY estimates her risk of mortality?
    (A) 20% total risk of mortality and 20% of deaths occur within 48 hours.
    (B) 20% total risk of mortality and 50% of deaths occur within 48 hours.
    (C) 50% total risk of mortality and 20% of deaths occur within 48 hours.
    (D) 50% total risk of mortality and 50% of deaths occur within 48 hours.

33. Which of the following elements of a patient's history would be MOST typical for the diagnosis of classic cardiac chest pain?
    (A) Constant pain lasting 10 minutes
    (B) Constant pain lasting 24 hours
    (C) Pain lasting 30 seconds
    (D) Sharp, shooting pain that is well localized

34. Which of the following cardiomyopathies is the leading cause of sudden death in competitive athletes?
    (A) Arrhythmogenic right ventricular cardiomyopathy
    (B) Brugada syndrome
    (C) Dilated cardiomyopathy
    (D) Hypertrophic cardiomyopathy

35. Which of the following ECG findings is indicative of hypertrophic cardiomyopathy?
    (A) Electrical alternans
    (B) Inferior T-wave inversions
    (C) Large septal Q waves
    (D) Poor R-wave progression

36. A middle-aged man presents with chest pain. He has a history of coronary artery disease and has a left ventricular assist device. As you are examining him, he suddenly collapses, is not breathing, and does not have a blood pressure. Which of the following is relatively contraindicated?
    (A) Amiodarone
    (B) Cardioversion
    (C) Chest compressions
    (D) Defibrillation

37. A 16-year-old patient presents with light headedness. You notice a systolic murmur on examination and an irregular cardiac shadow on his chest x-ray. You suspect he may have hypertrophic cardiomyopathy. Which of the following would increase the intensity of the murmur?
    (A) A fluid bolus of normal saline
    (B) Hand grip maneuver
    (C) Passive leg raise
    (D) Standing

38. A 35-year-old woman without any significant past medical history presents with dyspnea on exertion that has progressed over the last week. She denies any family history of cardiac disease, and her review of systems is negative for any infectious symptoms. She does admit to daily cigarette use and is using birth control. On examination her lungs are clear and a murmur is not appreciated. An ECG is obtained (Figure 5.4). Which of the following is the MOST LIKELY diagnosis?
    (A) Acute coronary syndrome
    (B) Bronchitis
    (C) Pericarditis
    (D) Pulmonary embolism

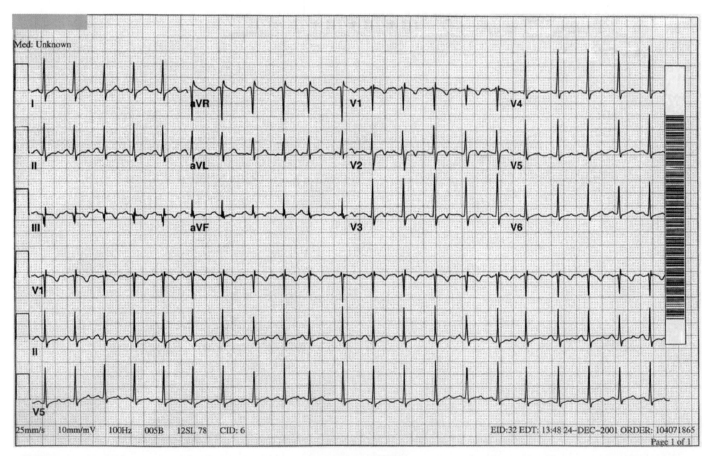

FIGURE 5.4 Image contributed by Department of Emergency Medicine, Wake Forest Baptist Hospital.

39. A patient presents with a history mildly concerning for pulmonary embolism. He has a resting heart rate of 105 and recently had a cast removed from his leg. His leg is not tender or swollen. Which is the BEST initial diagnostic test of choice?
    (A) D-dimer assay
    (B) Pulmonary angiography
    (C) Pulmonary embolism rule out criteria
    (D) Ventilation-perfusion lung scanning

40. You are considering ordering a D-dimer on a patient. However, you remember there are conditions that can falsely elevate or lower the test. Which of the following factors could cause a false negative test?
    (A) Age >70
    (B) Pregnancy
    (C) Lipemia
    (D) Liver disease

41. A 70-year-old man presents with chest pain and shortness of breath. A D-dimer is ordered and results at 750 ng/mL. Which of the following formulas can be used to age adjust the D-dimer to determine if further diagnostic testing is necessary?
    (A) Age × 10 ng/mL
    (B) (Age/2) × 10 ng/mL
    (C) D-dimer result × 10/age
    (D) Age × D-dimer result/100

42. A patient presents with chest pain and shortness of breath. A D-dimer is obtained and is elevated. CT angiogram demonstrates a segmental pulmonary embolism. Which of the following patients would be MOST APPROPRIATE for outpatient treatment?
    (A) A 35-year-old homeless man that is otherwise well and does not want to be admitted
    (B) A 37-year-old man with normal oxygen saturations and respiratory rate but with a heart rate of 112
    (C) A 65-year-old woman with a resting heart rate of 85 and oxygen saturation of 94% on room air
    (D) An 82-year-old woman with normal labs and vital signs who lives with her two children

43. A 29-year-old man presents with pleuritic chest pain. He has no significant medical history and denies recent surgery, trauma, long plane trips, or immobilization. There is no family history of a coagulopathy.

The rest of his review of systems is negative aside from a nonproductive cough 1 week ago that is now improved. On examination, his heart rate is 75, saturations are 97% on room air without tachypnea, and his blood pressure is 135/70. His legs are not swollen or tender and are symmetric. Which is the MOST APPROPRIATE INITIAL diagnostic test to rule out pulmonary embolism in this gentleman?
    (A) CT angiography
    (B) D-dimer
    (C) Pulmonary embolism rule-out criteria
    (D) Ventilation-perfusion lung scanning

44. A 53-year-old man presents to the emergency department with chest pain. His blood pressure is 250/170. Due to his severe hypertension and concerning description of the pain, he is immediately started on an antihypertensive medication. Five hours later the admitting team mentions that they are concerned about cyanide toxicity if the patient stays on the medication too long. Which medication was started?
    (A) Amlodipine
    (B) Esmolol
    (C) Nesiritide
    (D) Nitroprusside

45. A patient presents to the emergency department with a blood pressure of 235/140. He states that his blood pressure has never been this high before. Upon further questioning, he admits to running out of his antihypertensive medication 2 days ago. Which medication was he MOST LIKELY taking?
    (A) Amlodipine
    (B) Clevidipine
    (C) Clonidine
    (D) Enalapril

46. A 39-year-old woman without a significant medical history is referred from a health fair for hypertension. She denies chest pain, shortness of breath, headaches, light headedness, or vision changes. Ninety minutes later, her blood pressure remains elevated at 210/100. Which of the following is the BEST treatment recommendation?
    (A) Amlodipine
    (B) Initiation of medication is not indicated
    (C) Labetalol
    (D) Nitroglycerin

47. A 25-year-old man presents with acute agitation, diaphoresis, and mydriasis. His blood pressure is 190/100. Which medication should be avoided?
    (A) Clonidine
    (B) Lorazepam
    (C) Metoprolol
    (D) Nitroglycerin

48. Which of the following is the BEST initial diagnostic test to assess pulmonary hypertension in the emergency department?
    (A) B-type natriuretic peptide (BNP)
    (B) Chest x-ray
    (C) Transthoracic echocardiography
    (D) Troponin

49. A 75-year-old woman with chronic obstructive pulmonary disease on home oxygen presents with weakness and shortness of breath. Physical examination demonstrates jugular venous distension and hypotension so a bedside echocardiogram is obtained. The echocardiogram demonstrates adequate left ventricular function but shows a dilated, hypertrophied right ventricle with decreased contractility. Which is the BEST strategy to treat her hypotension?
    (A) Bolus 2 L of normal saline
    (B) Initiate a low-dose dobutamine infusion
    (C) Initiate a low-dose dopamine infusion
    (D) Initiate a low-dose phenylephrine infusion

50. Emergency Medical Services transports a 65-year-old woman with severe pulmonary hypertension to the emergency department. The patient was lethargic, and they placed her on oxygen. On arrival to the emergency department, she remains hypoxic with shallow respirations, so a decision is made to intubate her. What should you tell your respiratory therapist regarding her ventilator settings?
    (A) Start with low tidal volume such as 6 mL/kg ideal body weight
    (B) Titrate oxygen to keep her saturations over 95%
    (C) Use high amounts of positive end-expiratory pressure to maintain saturations
    (D) Use low respiratory rates and tolerate significant permissive hypercapnia

51. A 45-year-old man with coronary artery disease, hypertension, diabetes, and pulmonary hypertension presents with severe chest pain. You notice that his blood pressure is elevated. He took a baby aspirin, tadalafil, and enalapril this morning. As he describes his pain, you are worried about unstable angina. Which medication should be avoided in this patient?
    (A) Clopidogrel
    (B) Full-dose aspirin
    (C) Labetalol
    (D) Nitroglycerin

52. A 65-year-old patient with severe pulmonary hypertension presents after a fall. While in the emergency department, he begins to complain of shortness of breath. You notice that his continuous infusion pump is beeping and are concerned that it may be malfunctioning, possibly due to the fall. He tells you that he receives a continuous infusion of epoprostenol through the pump and gives you his pulmonologist's card. What should you do first?
    (A) Call the pulmonologist on call for further advice
    (B) Place a central line to administer the epoprostenol
    (C) Start a norepinephrine infusion to prevent hypotension
    (D) Switch the epoprostenol to a peripheral intravenous catheter until you can determine why the pump is malfunctioning

53. A 50-year-old man with chronic hypertension presents with chest pain described as sudden in onset and radiating to his back. You are worried about aortic dissection. Which of the following tests can BEST rule out an aortic dissection?
    (A) Chest CT
    (B) Chest radiograph (x-ray)
    (C) D-dimer
    (D) ECG

54. Which of the following classification systems is NOT paired correctly?
    (A) DeBakey type 1: Dissection involving the ascending aorta, the arch, and the descending aorta
    (B) DeBakey type 2: Dissection involving only the descending aorta
    (C) Stanford A: Aortic dissection involving the ascending aorta
    (D) Stanford B: Aortic dissection only involving the descending aorta

55. A 55-year-old man presents with chest pain described as sudden in onset and radiating to his back and then to his abdomen. His examination is notable for hypertension and abnormal pulses. You have high suspicion for aortic dissection and want to initiate therapy immediately while you confirm the diagnosis. Which medication should be initiated first?
    (A) Diltiazem
    (B) Esmolol
    (C) Nicardipine
    (D) Nitroglycerin

56. While rare, aortic dissection can occur during pregnancy. Which of the following statements about aortic dissection in pregnancy is CORRECT?
    (A) A bicuspid aortic valve is not a risk factor for aortic dissection.
    (B) A CT scan should not be used to make the diagnosis.
    (C) It usually occurs in the third trimester or postpartum period.
    (D) Nitroglycerin should not be administered in pregnancy.

57. A 45-year-old woman presents to the emergency department with chest pain. She says that it started suddenly, is tearing in quality, and radiates to her back. You are worried she may have an aortic dissection. Aside from hypertension, what physical examination finding would you expect to find on examination?
    (A) Aortic insufficiency murmur
    (B) Most patients have a relatively normal examination
    (C) Neurologic deficits
    (D) Pulse deficit

58. Which of the following is a risk factor for an abdominal aortic aneurysm?
    (A) Age over 50
    (B) Female gender
    (C) Sedentary life style
    (D) Smoking

59. What is Cullen's sign?
    (A) Biphasic femoral artery pulsations
    (B) Flank ecchymosis
    (C) Pain upon extension of the hip
    (D) Periumbilical ecchymosis

60. A 45-year-old man with a past history of abdominal aortic aneurysm with an aortic graft presents with abdominal pain. He denies a history of peptic ulcer disease, liver disease, hepatitis B or C, intravenous drug use, or alcoholism. He denies burning pain or pain that is worse with eating. While evaluating him, he develops a sudden and large upper gastrointestinal bleed. What is the MOST LIKELY diagnosis?
    (A) Aortoenteric fistula
    (B) Arteriovenous fistula
    (C) Esophageal varices
    (D) Gastric ulcer

61. A patient presents with abdominal pain. An abdominal ultrasound is obtained (Figure 5.5). What landmark shown on the ultrasound can help to distinguish between the aorta and inferior vena cava?

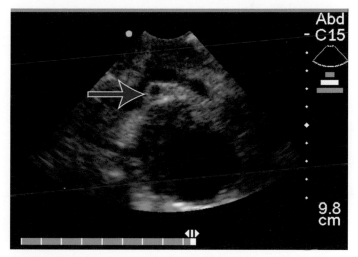

FIGURE 5.5 Reproduced with permission from J.E. Tintinalli, J.S. Stapczynski, O.J. Ma, D. Yealy, G.D. Meckler, D.M. Cline: Tintinalli's Emergency Medicine: A Comprehensive Study Guide, 9th Edition. Copyright © McGraw-Hill Education. All rights reserved.

    (A) Liver
    (B) Proper hepatic artery
    (C) Superior mesenteric artery
    (D) Uterus

62. A 65-year-old man presents with sudden onset of abdominal pain that is ripping in nature. His vital signs are normal with a heart rate of 75 and a blood pressure of 130/75. There is no rebound or guarding on examination, but the patient is diffusely tender to palpation. A CT scan demonstrates a 5.3-cm abdominal aortic aneurysm that is not ruptured. Which is the NEXT step in management?
    (A) β-Blocker administration
    (B) Blood transfusion
    (C) Serial examinations
    (D) Surgical evaluation

63. A patient presents with progressive pain in his legs while walking that improves with rest. His examination is notable for delayed capillary refill. An ankle-brachial index is ordered due to concerns for peripheral arterial disease. What is the normal value for an ankle-brachial index?
    (A) 0.4
    (B) 0.8
    (C) 1.2
    (D) 1.4

64. A 56-year-old man with diabetes presents with pain and swelling in his legs. His symptoms improve with hanging his foot over his bed. On examination he is noted to have an irregular heart rhythm with pallor and diminished pulses to his leg. He is diagnosed with acute embolic limb ischemia from atrial fibrillation. Atrial fibrillation is the most common cause of acute embolic limb ischemia, but what is the second most common cause?
    (A) Atrial myxomas
    (B) Mural thrombus
    (C) Prosthetic heart valve
    (D) Vegetations from valve leaflets

65. A 43-year-old woman with paroxysmal atrial fibrillation on warfarin presents with pain to her feet in the middle of summer. Physical examination reveals a regular cardiac rhythm with warm feet and palpable pulses. A few toes are noticed to be dusky, cool, and tender with delayed cap refill. She has a normal ankle-brachial index and an unremarkable cardiac echocardiogram. What is the cause of her abnormal examination finding?

    (A) Atheroembolic disease
    (B) Embolic cardiac disease
    (C) Hemolytic disease
    (D) Vasospasm

66. A 56-year-old man presents with leg pain. The pain is brought on by exercise and relieved by rest and reoccurs at a consistent walking distance. Which of the following may help differentiate the pain of spinal stenosis from the pain caused by vascular claudication?
    (A) Bilateral leg pain
    (B) Pain improves with rest
    (C) Relieved with lumbar spine flexion
    (D) Worsening pain with walking

67. Which set of findings is classically associated with acute limb ischemia?
    (A) Pain, pallor, palpitations
    (B) Pain, pallor, petechiae
    (C) Paralysis, paresthesias, polar
    (D) Pulselessness, edema, sensory loss

68. A patient presents with symptoms concerning for peripheral artery disease. Which one of the following factors is MORE consistent with a thrombotic as opposed to an embolic cause of disease?
    (A) Gradual onset of pain
    (B) History of atrial fibrillation
    (C) No history of claudication
    (D) Normal contralateral leg

ANSWERS

1. **The answer is D.** (Chapter 52) A history of any previous syncope in the preceding year was associated with a 1-year probability of 46% for syncope recurrence, compared to 7% syncope recurrence for patients without a previous history.

2. **The answer is A.** (Chapter 54) The patient has symptomatic mitral stenosis, which will be diagnosed by echocardiography. While the most common cause worldwide remains rheumatic heart disease, risk factors for nonrheumatic mitral stenosis are female gender, age, hypertension, and chronic renal failure. Examination is remarkable for a mid-diastolic rumbling murmur with crescendo toward S_2. Though nondiagnostic, left atrial enlargement and right axis deviation, as seen in this patient's ECG, is consistent with mitral stenosis. Due to left atrial enlargement, the cardiac silhouette will show straightening of the left heart border. While coronary artery disease remains on the differential, she does not need emergent percutaneous coronary intervention with a nonischemic ECG, normal troponin, and no active chest pain. Pulmonary embolism is less likely given the chronic progressive presentation of her symptoms and associated diastolic murmur and left atrial enlargement. This patient should not be discharged home because her disease has progressed to the point that she cannot walk around her house without significant dyspnea, placing her at high risk of falling.

3. **The answer is B.** (Chapter 51) The components that make up the thrombolysis in acute myocardial infarction (TIMI) score are as follows: Age greater or equal to 65, more than three risk factors for coronary artery disease, known coronary artery disease with stenosis greater than 50%, aspirin use in the past 7 days, severe angina with two or more episodes in the past 24 hours, ST changes on ECG greater than or equal to 0.5 mm, and positive cardiac markers. The HEART Score, in contrast, does use history as part of its scoring system.

4. **The answer is D.** (Chapter 53) The patient is in severe respiratory distress secondary to a heart failure exacerbation. The patient is not following commands, agitated, hypoxic, and uncooperative with altered mental status. The correct course of action is emergent intubation. BiPAP is contraindicated in patients who are unable to protect their airway due to poor mental status. Placing a non-rebreather is also not going to protect the patient's airway, and given her respiratory status, she will benefit from positive pressure ventilation to correct her hypoxia and work of breathing. Administration of furosemide

and nitroglycerin may be helpful in her management but are not the first priority in a patient with an unprotected airway.

5. **The answer is A.** (Chapter 49) In the setting of acute myocardial infarction (MI), angiotensin-converting enzyme (ACE) inhibitors have been shown to reduce the development of congestive heart failure. An ACE inhibitor should be given to the patient within 24 hours of presentation but do not necessarily need to be given emergently in the emergency department. β-Blockers help reduce the risk of reinfarction but are not immediately indicated in the setting of acute congestive heart failure after MI. Calcium channel antagonists do not reduce the risk of developing chronic heart failure after MI. Oxygen would be indicated in this setting given the patient saturation is 90% on room air but does not lead directly to a reduction in congestive heart failure in the same way as ACE inhibitor treatment.

6. **The answer is A.** (Chapter 50) An intra-aortic balloon pump provides short-term hemodynamic support by decreasing afterload and increasing diastolic blood pressure. This change in physiology lowers oxygen demand and increases coronary perfusion. The balloon of the device is inflated during diastole and increases blood flow back through the coronary arteries. The device does augment diastolic perfusion pressure and unloads the left ventricular pressure to improve survival in the short term until definitive therapy can be initiated. There have been no long-term benefits demonstrated at this time for this device.

7. **The answer is A.** (Chapter 49) Acute myocardial infarction (MI) occurs in approximately 6% of patients, who present to the emergency department with chest pain after using cocaine. An ECG is only 36% sensitive for identifying cocaine induce MI. Cardiac troponin is the most sensitive biomarker for this type of ischemia. The initial evaluation is the same as with any other patient presenting with chest pain. The thrombolysis in acute myocardial infarction (TIMI) score is not useful for patients that use cocaine and does not help risk stratify this patient population. The initial mainstay of treatment for cocaine-induced chest pain is aspirin, nitroglycerin, and benzodiazepines. β-Blockers such as metoprolol are contraindicated in this patient population. The 1-year rate of MI after a negative chest pain observation evaluation for patients with cocaine-induced chest pain is less than 1%, so cardiology consultation and enoxaparin administration

are not indicated unless the patient has abnormal cardiac troponin results.

8. **The answer is C.** (Chapter 54) Patients who undergo dental procedures that involve manipulation of gingival tissue, the periapical region of the teeth or perforation of oral mucosa should have prophylaxis for endocarditis if they have BOTH mitral valve prolapse AND concomitant mitral regurgitation. Antithrombotic therapy is not recommended unless the patient has other indications such as transient ischemic attacks, stroke, or atrial fibrillation. Most patients are asymptomatic, and morbidity increases if symptoms are present with exercise. The classic finding on auscultation is a midsystolic click; pansystolic murmurs are typically associated with aortic stenosis.

9. **The answer is C.** (Chapter 51) The question is based on the HEART score for cardiac risk stratification of patients presenting with chest pain. A has a HEART score of 2 with slightly suspicious history (0), normal ECG (0), age <45 (0), three or more risk factors (2), and normal troponin (0). B has a HEART score of 4 with highly suspicious history (2), nonspecific ECG (1), age between 45 and 65 (1), no risk factors (0), and normal troponin (0). Choice C has a HEART score of 7 with moderately suspicious history (1), significant ST depression (2), age >65 (2), three or more risk factors (2), normal troponin (0). D has a HEART score of 5 with moderately suspicious history (1), nonspecific ECG (1), age >65 (2), 2 risk factors (1), normal troponin (0).

10. **The answer is A.** (Chapter 52) The Framingham study showed that cardiac syncope doubled the risk of death, neurologic syncope increased the risk of death by 50%, and unknown cause of syncope increased the risk of death by 30%. Vasovagal syncope carried no increase in risk of death when compared to the general population.

11. **The answer is D.** (Chapter 53) When evaluating for pulmonary edema using ultrasound, the presence of three or more B-lines in any one sonographic window along the anterior and anterolateral chest is considered pathologic and specific for alveolar and interstitial edema. Occasional B-lines are considered normal. A-lines are not associated with pulmonary edema. A loss of the "seashore" sign is associated with pneumothorax on thoracic ultrasound.

12. **The answer is C.** (Chapter 49) The most common physical examination findings associated with acute myocardial infarction (MI) are hypotension, S_3 gallop, and diaphoresis. Distant low-pitched rattling breath sounds are often heard with patient's presenting with chronic obstructive pulmonary disease (COPD). Reproducible chest pain, tenderness to the chest wall, has been reported with the diagnosis of acute MI in 15% of patients.

13. **The answer is B.** (Chapter 53) According to the American Heart Association 2014 Heart Disease statistics, survival after heart failure diagnosis has improved over time. However, the death rate remains high; approximately 50% of people diagnosed with heart failure will die within 5 years.

14. **The answer is B.** (Chapter 50) The patient presents to the emergency department with cardiac tamponade, as evidenced by positional chest pain, hypotension, and narrow pulse pressure. The ultrasound also helps demonstrate tamponade with a pericardial effusion and hypotension in the setting of minimally collapsible IVC. Given that that patient is hemodynamically unstable, an emergent pericardiocentesis is indicated.

15. **The answer is A.** (Chapter 51) CT coronary angiography allows for rapid evaluation of the coronary arteries with the use of peripheral IV contrast. Images are improved with a heart rate <65 and more advanced CT scanner equipment. Studies have shown that no significant disease was missed on CT coronary testing, but approximately 20% of patients have a nondiagnostic result and thus are required to complete traditional stress testing. The test provides very limited assessment of cardiac function and is not as valuable for patients with known coronary artery disease. Studies have shown that CT coronary angiography can decrease length of stay for emergency department patients but does result in significant radiation exposure for the patient. Overall cost of CT coronary angiography is similar to traditional coronary artery testing.

16. **The answer is C.** (Chapter 49) In the setting of acute ST-elevation myocardial infarction, the American Heart Association goal for treatment is 90 minutes for patients who arrive at a hospital with percutaneous coronary intervention (PCI) and 120 minutes for patients who arrive at a hospital that requires transfer. The benefit of fibrinolytic therapy is for patients who arrive with less than 12 hours of symptoms. If given within 3 hours >30 lives were saved per 1000 patients. The loss of benefit is 1.6 lives/1000 patients per hour delay. There is improved outcome with initial tissue plasminogen activator (TPA) therapy with delayed PCI when transport time is greater than 120 minutes. Optimal antithrombin therapy and dual antiplatelet therapy lead to improved outcomes. Patients treated with TPA may still require rescue PCI and should still be transferred to a facility with PCI capability even if they demonstrate improvement with initial thrombolytic therapy.

TABLE 5.1	A Grading System for Murmurs
Grade	Description
1	Faint, may not be heard in all positions
2	Quiet, but heard immediately with stethoscope placement onto the chest wall
3	Moderately loud
4	Loud
5	Heard with stethoscope partly off the chest wall
6	Heard when stethoscope is entirely off the chest wall

Reproduced with permission from J.E. Tintinalli, J.S. Stapczynski, O.J. Ma, D. Yealy, G.D. Meckler, D.M. Cline: Tintinalli's Emergency Medicine: A Comprehensive Study Guide, 9th Edition. McGraw-Hill Education; 2020.

17. **The answer is B.** (Chapter 54) Murmurs are graded on a scale from 1 to 6 (Table 5.1).

18. **The answer is B.** (Chapter 51) The absolute contraindications to ECG stress test are acute myocardial infarction within the past 2 days, high-risk unstable angina, uncontrolled dysrhythmias, symptomatic aortic stenosis, pulmonary embolus/infarction, acute myocarditis/pericarditis, or aortic dissection. The relative contraindications are left main coronary disease, stenotic valvular heart disease, severe hypertension (>200 systolic, >110 diastolic), tachy/brady dysrhythmias, hypertrophic cardiomyopathy, electrolyte abnormalities, physical impairment to exercise, or high-degree atrioventricular block. Treadmill ECG stress tests are less useful in patients with a baseline abnormal ECG, such as a bundle branch block, that may make the results difficult to interpret.

19. **The answer is A.** (Chapter 53) While paroxysmal nocturnal dyspnea, orthopnea, and edema are the most specific symptoms, the symptom with the highest sensitivity is dyspnea on exertion (84%).

20. **The answer is D.** (Chapter 49) The ECG demonstrates ST elevation in the inferior leads. The elevation is greater in lead III than in lead II with ST depression in the high lateral leads of I and aVL. A left circumflex myocardial infarction (MI) will cause ST elevation in leads I, aVL, V5, and ST depression in leads V_1, V_2, and V_3. An obtuse marginal artery MI will cause similar findings to a circumflex MI given that it is a branch originating from the circumflex artery. A left anterior descending artery MI will cause ST elevation in V_1, V_2, V_3, and ST depression in leads II, III, and aVF.

21. **The answer is A.** (Chapter 53) Headache is a common side effect following administration of nitroglycerin due to vasodilation in cerebral circulation. The first-line treatment is acetaminophen that has been shown to usually be adequate as monotherapy. Caffeine is often used for post lumbar puncture headaches or tension headaches, but in the setting of heart failure or ischemic chest pain will increase oxygen demand and thus not be an appropriate choice. Opiates are not considered first-line treatment for headaches. Prochlorperazine is used to treat nausea, vomiting, and off-label treatment of migraines.

22. **The answer is B.** (Chapter 52) Most diagnostic tests have a low diagnostic yield in the workup for syncope. History should be obtained from the patient and witnesses. One should record premonitory symptoms such as headache, diplopia, vertigo, or focal weakness, length of unconsciousness, and symptoms occurring after gaining consciousness. Concerning symptoms include chest pain (acute myocardial infarction), aortic dissection, pulmonary embolism, aortic stenosis), palpitations (dysrhythmia), shortness of breath (pulmonary embolism, congestive heart failure), headache (subarachnoid hemorrhage), and abdominal or back pain (leaking abdominal aortic aneurysm, ruptured ectopic pregnancy). Further testing should be directed by the history.

23. **The answer is D.** (Chapter 49) As many as 37.5% of women and 27.4% of men with a confirmed diagnosis of myocardial infarction (MI) present without chest pain to the emergency department. Also, as many as 30% of patients have silent, clinically unrecognized MI and do not seek medical care at the time of the event.

24. **The answer is D.** (Chapter 52) Vasovagal syncope actually decreases with age, in part as a consequence of the decreased responsiveness of the autonomic nervous system. There is a continuum of increasing risk with increasing age; however, cardiovascular risk factors appear to be a better predictor than age itself. Postprandial syncope is more common in the elderly, especially nursing home patients, and is thought to be due to a rapid rate of nutrient delivery from the stomach into the small intestine. Due to calcification of vessels, a less sensitive thirst mechanism, and decreased endocrine responsive to volume depletion, orthostatic syncope is more common in the elderly.

25. **The answer is B.** (Chapter 54) Mechanical valves are more durable with lower failure rates, but they do carry a higher risk for thromboembolic complications. Antiplatelet therapy is recommended for all patients with prosthetic valves; however, for patients with mechanical valves lifelong anticoagulation is recommended. The risk of valve thrombosis or thromboembolism is about 8% and falls to 1% to 2% per year with anticoagulation.

26. The answer is D. (Chapter 49) There are many conduction disturbances that worsen the prognosis for patients suffering from an acute myocardial infarction. However, accelerated idioventricular rhythms, sinus bradycardia, and ventricular premature contractions are not associated with worse outcomes. Sinus tachycardia is associated with increased morbidity and mortality and should be treated in the acute setting. The cause of tachycardia may be pain, anxiety, left ventricular failure, atrial infarction, or medications. The cause should be determined and effort made to resolve it. Heart block, ventricular tachycardia, and new bundle branch blocks also have increased morbidity and mortality.

27. The answer is B. (Chapter 50) The patient presents in cardiogenic shock with no response to IV fluid bolus and mild pulmonary congestion on examination. Therefore, inotrope therapy is appropriate. Dobutamine is the mainstay of pharmacologic treatment. It increases cardiac contractility and should be considered as individual agent when a patient's blood pressure is greater than 90 systolic. Dobutamine has vasodilatory properties and therefore should not be used alone in the setting of hypotension. Dopamine may increase cardiac work by increasing heart rate and also increase LV end-diastolic pressure by its β-agonist effect. This agent would be better used in combination with dobutamine than alone as a single agent. Milrinone is a selective phosphodiesterase inhibitor and is considered a second-line agent for this clinical picture or could be used if dobutamine combinations are ineffective. Combining dobutamine with norepinephrine or dopamine has more effect on peripheral vasoconstriction than either agent by itself. When a patient's blood pressure is less than 70 systolic, norepinephrine is the better choice to combine with dobutamine given its pressor effect.

28. The answer is C. (Chapter 54) A mid-diastolic rumble, crescendoing into S_2 is associated with mitral stenosis, whereas mitral valve prolapse is associated with a click that may be followed by a late systolic murmur that crescendos into S_2.

29. The answer is B. (Chapter 52) Any of the following make a patient high risk according to the San Francisco Syncope rules: history of congestive heart failure, hematocrit less than 30%, ECG abnormalities (including changes from baseline or any nonsinus rhythm), shortness of breath, or systolic blood pressure less than 90 in the emergency department.

30. The answer is A. (Chapter 51) Of emergency department patients with undifferentiated chest pain, 7% will have ECG findings consistent with acute ischemia or infarction, and 6% to 10% of those in whom cardiac markers are ordered will have initially positive results. The other approximately 90% of patients will be classified as low probability or possible acute coronary syndrome.

31. The answer is B. (Chapter 50) The patient presents with cardiogenic shock due to ischemia. The most important intervention for ischemic-related cardiogenic shock is emergent revascularization. Stabilization in the emergency department is temporizing, and the ultimate goal is definitive therapy as fast as possible. In the prehospital setting, Emergency Medical Services should direct any suspected cardiogenic shock to a facility that has 24-hour emergency cardiac revascularization capability. Therefore, answers A and C are incorrect because the 10 minutes saved in transport do not make up for the patient benefit of presenting to the facility that can manage his specific disease. Answer D is incorrect because metoprolol is contraindicated in a patient presenting with cardiogenic shock.

32. The answer is D. (Chapter 50) During the past decade, percutaneous coronary intervention (PCI) and coronary bypass surgery have decreased the incidence and mortality of post myocardial infarction (MI) cardiogenic shock. However, despite these advances, the mortality remains high at 50%, with half of these deaths occurring within 48 hours of presentation. The risk factors for cardiogenic shock are elderly age, female, impaired ejection fraction, extensive infarct, proximal left anterior descending occlusion, multivessel disease, previous MI, previous congestive heart failure, and diabetes.

33. The answer is A. (Chapter 48) Classic chest pain is retrosternal left anterior chest crushing, squeezing, tightness, or pressure. Traditional teaching is that angina chest pain lasts 2 to 10 minutes, unstable angina pain lasts 10 to 30 minutes, and pain from acute MI often lasts longer than 30 minutes. It is important to remember that many patients with confirmed acute coronary syndrome never report "classic" symptoms.

34. The answer is D. (Chapter 55) Hypertrophic cardiomyopathy is the second most common cause of sudden cardiac death in the adolescent population and the leading cause of sudden death in competitive athletes. Common clinical features include chest pain, dyspnea on exertion, syncope, and a systolic ejection murmur. Overall, dilated cardiomyopathy is the most common cardiomyopathy. It can present with systolic and diastolic dysfunction and regurgitant murmurs. Brugada syndrome and arrhythmogenic right ventricular cardiomyopathy can predispose to arrhythmias and have specific findings on the ECG.

35. **The answer is C.** (Chapter 55) As emergency access to echocardiogram may not be readily available in many emergency departments, it is important to recognize signs of hypertrophic cardiomyopathy on an ECG. Both left ventricular hypertrophy and large septal Q waves may be present, both of which would be very abnormal in an otherwise young and healthy patient. Septal Q waves are >0.3 mV and similar Q waves can be located in the anterior, lateral, or inferior leads. T waves in those leads are normally upright. The other answer choices are ECG findings but do not carry a relationship to hypertrophic cardiomyopathy.

36. **The answer is C.** (Chapter 55) Left ventricular assist devices augment left ventricular output due to severe cardiomyopathy. There are also right ventricular and biventricular devices. Most contemporary devices use continuous flow so these patients may not have a pulse. Additionally, patients with left ventricular assist devices still rely on right ventricular function, which can be impeded if they are in an arrhythmia. Amiodarone, cardioversion, and defibrillation can all be administered if the patient is in a life-threatening arrhythmia or has arrested. It is recommended not to place defibrillator pads over the driveline. Performing chest compressions on a patient with a left ventricular assist device can dislodge the device from the heart and aorta. There are some newer models where this may not be the case, but you should be sure about this prior to initiating compressions due to the otherwise high risk of dislodgement.

37. **The answer is D.** (Chapter 55) Interventions that decrease left ventricular filling and the distending pressure in the left ventricular outflow tract or that increase the force of myocardial contraction accentuate the murmur of hypertrophic cardiomyopathy. These interventions include standing and the strain phase of the Valsalva maneuver. Maneuvers that increase left ventricular filling such as squatting, passive leg raise elevation, hand grip decrease the murmur. A fluid bolus would also be expected to increase the ventricular filling.

38. **The answer is D.** (Chapter 56) All four answers could potentially cause dyspnea on exertion. All estrogen-containing contraceptives increase the risk of venous thromboembolism. Smoking does not increase the probability of venous thromboembolism in the emergency department, but it is a population risk factor. Her ECG demonstrates sinus tachycardia and signs of right heart strain including an incomplete right bundle-branch block, an S1-Q3-T3 pattern, and anterior t-wave inversions, all features of a severe pulmonary embolism. Her lungs are clear, and she denies infectious symptoms making

bronchitis less likely. She does not have ECG findings such as PR depression or ST changes that might be expected in pericarditis. Given the lack of risk factors, lack of family history, and ECG findings, pulmonary embolism is a more likely diagnosis than acute coronary syndrome.

39. **The answer is A.** (Chapter 56) Pulmonary embolism cannot be excluded by the pulmonary embolism rule out criteria as the patient is tachycardic. By Well's criteria the patient has a score of 3 (tachycardia and immobilization in the last 4 weeks) which places him at moderate risk for a pulmonary embolism. In patients in whom clinical suspicion is low or moderate based on gestalt estimation, a Well's score ≤4, or has a "safe" designation by the Charlotte rule, an age-adjusted quantitative D-dimer can effectively rule out a pulmonary embolism. While pulmonary angiography can be ordered it is invasive, associated with radiation exposure and complications, and not always available. Ventilation-perfusion is also an option but is not always diagnostic. Given that a negative D-dimer would result in a posttest probability of <2% for this patient, it is the preferred test.

40. **The answer is C.** (Chapter 56) Multiple factors can cause a false-negative as well as a false-positive D-dimer. Age >70, pregnancy, active malignancy, surgical procedure in the last week, liver disease, infections, and trauma can all cause a false positive. Warfarin, symptoms lasting over 5 days, small clots, a small isolated pulmonary infarction, and lipemia can cause false negatives.

41. **The answer is A.** (Chapter 56) D-dimer increases with age. The most common formula studied is age × 10 ng/mL. When used with a Well's score of ≤4 or a simplified Geneva score <5, this resulted in a false-negative rate of 0.3% in one large study. This assumes the D-dimer is adjusted from a conventional cutoff of 500 ng/mL. In this patient's case, the age adjusted D-dimer cutoff would have been 700 ng/mL (70 × 10 ng/mL).

42. **The answer is C.** (Chapter 56) Like patients with deep vein thrombosis, low-risk patients with a pulmonary embolism, and adequate home support and follow-up can be discharged on anticoagulation. In the properly selected population, short-term mortality and bleeding risk are low; additionally, the cost of care is also decreased with this strategy. Patients can be stratified using either the Hestia criteria or the Simplified Pulmonary Embolism Severity Index. Additional, high-risk features include an elevated troponin, B-type natriuretic peptide (BNP) >100 pg/mL, pulmonary arterial hypertension on the ECG, and elevated bleeding risks. Patients A and D are high risk by the Simplified Pulmonary Embolism Criteria due to a pulse

>110 and age >80. Even though the patient in scenario B is otherwise well and wants to be discharged, his social situation and lack of follow-up make him inappropriate for this strategy. The rest of the Simplified Pulmonary Embolism Severity Index include history of cancer, history of heart failure or chronic lung disease, systolic blood pressure <100, and oxygen saturation <90%.

43. **The answer is C.** (Chapter 56) This patient presented with pleuritic chest pain. While a pulmonary embolism is possible, it is unlikely and he has a pretest probability of <15%. In this situation, it is recommended to initially use the pulmonary embolism rule-out criteria. In this case, he is negative for all the pulmonary embolism rule-out criteria meaning that his probability for a pulmonary embolism is <2%. Multiple publications demonstrate that when combined with low gestalt pretest probability, the pulmonary embolism rule-out criteria is 100% sensitive. The other three options could be used but would not significantly change your posttest probability and carry risk. CT scans carry risk of radiation and contrast exposure, D-dimers can have false positives leading to imaging studies, and the ventilation-perfusion scanning causes radiation exposure. As the pulmonary embolism rule-out criteria can successfully rule out pulmonary embolism in this patient, it should be the initial diagnostic test.

44. **The answer is D.** (Chapter 57) Patients on nitroprusside can develop cyanide toxicity. Patients with renal dysfunction or on high doses are at a higher risk of developing this complication. It occurs when the nitroprusside molecule releases cyanide ions. None of the other three answers are associated with the development of cyanide toxicity. Amlodipine is an oral calcium channel antagonist. As this patient requires emergent blood pressure control, they should receive intravenous medication. Esmolol is a β-blocker. It can cause bronchospasm in patients with chronic obstructive pulmonary disease or asthma. Additionally, β-blockers can cause worsening hypertension in patients with an acute sympathetic crisis due to unopposed α-agonism. Nesiritide is a recombinant form of B-type natriuretic peptide (BNP). It can be administered to patient with acute hypertensive pulmonary edema. However, at least some data associate it with increased morbidity and mortality.

45. **The answer is C.** (Chapter 57) Clonidine is an α_2-agonist. Abrupt cessation can cause significant rebound hypertension. Abrupt cessation of amlodipine or enalapril can cause a recurrence of the patient's hypertension but would not be expected to cause rebound hypertension. Amlodipine and clevidipine are both calcium channel antagonists. Clevidipine is ultra-short acting and only

administered intravenously. Enalapril is an angiotensin-converting enzyme inhibitor and should be avoided in pregnancy.

46. **The answer is A.** (Chapter 57) Patients with asymptomatic hypertension due not necessarily require extensive evaluation in the emergency department. For patients with persistently elevated blood pressure or a blood pressure >180/110, initiating therapy in the emergency department should be considered. This can be done via an oral route and not by intravenous administration. Initial recommendations for nonblack individuals include a thiazide diuretic, angiotensin-converting enzyme inhibitor, or calcium channel antagonist. In African Americans, a thiazide diuretic or calcium channel antagonist is recommended.

47. **The answer is C.** (Chapter 57) This patient is presenting with an acute sympathetic crisis. It may be due to a drug such as cocaine or amphetamine. Though controversial, there is concern that administration of a β-blocker such as metoprolol can result in unopposed α-agonism, potentiating vasoconstriction, and hypertension. While labetalol has both β- and α-antagonism, it should be administered with a vasodilator due to the limited α-antagonism. Lorazepam and nitroglycerin would both be indicated. There is no contraindication to clonidine, although it would be difficult to administer an oral medication to this patient.

48. **The answer is C.** (Chapter 58) Transthoracic echocardiography allows estimation of the pulmonary artery systolic pressure and detection of decreased right ventricular function, right atrial and ventricular hypertrophy, and leftward deviation of the intraventricular septum that are indicative of more severe disease. The other diagnostics can all be abnormal with pulmonary hypertension but do not necessarily assess the degree of severity of the disease, although troponin elevations are associated with increased morbidity and mortality.

49. **The answer is B.** (Chapter 58) This patient has severe pulmonary hypertension causing right ventricular dysfunction, likely due to the chronic pulmonary obstructive disease. While intravenous fluids can be administered, this should be done as serial small boluses with frequent reexamination as too much fluid can cause worsening right ventricular dysfunction by displacing the intraventricular septum and further compromise the patient's cardiac output. Dopamine and phenylephrine should be avoided because they can precipitate tachydysrhythmias, elevate pulmonary artery pressure and pulmonary vascular resistance, and worsen right coronary artery perfusion. Dobutamine is the preferred agent as it can improve

ventricular function and increase cardiac output. The infusion should be titrated to a dose less than 10 mcg/kg/min to avoid worsening hypotension. Milrinone is also a viable alternative.

50. **The answer is A.** (Chapter 58) In patients with severe pulmonary hypertension, intubation, and ventilation can increase intrathoracic pressure from positive-pressure ventilation leading to rapid cardiovascular collapse. The ventilator settings should maintain low airway pressures. This can be done using lung protective settings such as low tidal volumes (6 mL/kg of ideal body weight), setting the lowest positive end expiratory pressure (PEEP), and titrating her oxygen to maintain saturations greater than 90%. Using large amounts of oxygen to obtain saturations between 95% and 100% can lead to damage from hyperoxia. While her respiratory rate should be monitored to avoid stacking and increasing intrathoracic pressures, given the low tidal volumes the patient will most likely need a higher respiratory rate to avoid hypercapnia that can lead to increased pulmonary vascular resistance, higher pulmonary pressures, and right ventricular strain.

51. **The answer is D.** (Chapter 58) The patient is on a phosphodiesterase 5 inhibitor (tadalafil). When taken in combination with nitrates, it can precipitate severe hypotension. If you are worried about acute coronary syndrome, it would be recommended to give the patient a full dose of aspirin even if they took a baby aspirin this morning. While β-blockers are not routinely recommended in the emergency department evaluation of acute coronary syndrome, they are recommended for patients with hypertension and acute coronary syndrome. Neither labetalol nor clopidogrel would be contraindicated.

52. **The answer is D.** (Chapter 58) Prostanoids (epoprostenol, treprostinil, and iloprost) are potent vasodilators indicated for pulmonary arterial hypertension and right ventricular failure. While unlikely to be started in the emergency department, patients may present who are receiving these medications at home, much like patients on home dobutamine infusions. The first step when these patients present is to immediately confirm that the catheter and pump are functioning correctly. If there is concern for a malfunction, both epoprostenol and treprostinil can be administered via a peripheral intravenous catheter. This is particularly important as epoprostenol only has a half-life of 2 to 5 minutes. You do not need a central line to administer epoprostenol. Although the primary provider should be contacted for long-term management in the event of a pump malfunction, given the short half-life of the drug, it is important not to delay resuming the infusion prior to consultation. If the patient became

hypotensive, norepinephrine may improve blood pressure and right coronary artery perfusion. However, it should not be administered prophylactically.

53. **The answer is A.** (Chapter 59) Chest CT is the diagnostic test of choice and can accurately rule out aortic dissection. In addition to diagnosing dissection, it can diagnose other pathology such as intramural hematoma or penetrating atherosclerotic ulcer. The other diagnostics listed can be abnormal in patients with aortic dissection but cannot be used to exclude the diagnosis. Between 12% and 37% of chest x-rays will not have abnormalities. Recently, D-dimer has been investigated to rule out this disease in order to decrease costs and radiation and contrast exposures. However, guidelines recommend against this practice. D-dimer may have a false-negative rate as high as 18%. Young patients with a short dissection length and thrombosed false lumen may be particularly at risk for this. Patients may have abnormal ECGs, but the findings are nonspecific and can be normal in 19% to 31% of patients.

54. **The answer is B.** (Chapter 59) There are two common classification schemes used to characterize aortic dissection, Stanford and DeBakey. Stanford divides dissections into types A and B. Type A includes dissections that involve the ascending aorta while type B only involves the descending aorta. DeBakey is divided into three types. Type 1 involves the ascending aorta, descending aorta, and the arch; type 2 only involves the ascending aorta; and type 3 only involves the descending aorta.

55. **The answer is B.** (Chapter 59) A negative inotropic agent should be initiated first in order to lower blood pressure without increasing the shear force on the intimal flap of the aorta. Ideally, this should be initially accomplished with a short-acting β-blocker such as esmolol. If there is a contraindication to a β-blocker, centrally acting calcium channel antagonists can be administered, but experience with them in this setting is limited. Vasodilators such as nitroglycerin, nitroprusside, or nicardipine should be started after administration of the negative inotropic agent. Nicardipine is a peripherally acting calcium channel antagonist that acts as a vasodilator and does not cause sufficient negative inotropy.

56. **The answer is C.** (Chapter 59) Aortic dissection normally occurs in the third trimester or postpartum period. A bicuspid aortic valve, connective tissue disorders, hypertension, and family history are all risk factors for aortic dissection. Nitroglycerin can be safely administered in pregnant patients. While radiation exposure to the fetus should be minimized, aortic dissection is a life-threatening disease and a CT scan may be appropriate to

exclude the diagnosis, especially if the patient is not stable to go to MRI.

57. **The answer is B.** (Chapter 59) For most patients, their examination will be relatively normal. Symptoms of an aortic dissection depend on the site of the initial disruption. Dissection near a carotid artery can present with stroke-like symptoms while proximal dissection can cause cardiac tamponade. An aortic insufficiency murmur occurs in 32% of patients while a pulse deficit occurs in only 15% of patients. Only 20% of patients with a type A dissection have neurologic abnormalities.

58. **The answer is D.** (Chapter 60) Smoking is a risk factor for abdominal aortic aneurysms. The risk decreases with the number of years since quitting smoking. Other risk factors include being male and age over 60. Eighteen percent of patients with an abdominal aortic aneurysm have a first-degree relative with an aortic aneurysm compared to <3% without an aneurysm.

59. **The answer is D.** (Chapter 60) Periumbilical ecchymosis from retroperitoneal or intra-abdominal bleeding is known as Cullen's sign. It is not specific for a ruptured abdominal aortic aneurysm. It can also occur in pancreatitis or ruptured ectopic pregnancy. Grey Turner's sign is flank ecchymosis. An iliopsoas sign is pain upon extension of the hip, which can occur due to retroperitoneal blood irritating the psoas muscle. While blood can compress the femoral nerve causing a neuropathy, abdominal aortic aneurysms do not typically alter femoral arterial pulsations. It is important to note that external signs of an acute rupture of an abdominal aortic aneurysm are not reliably found and their absence does not exclude the disease.

60. **The answer is A.** (Chapter 60) This patient has a history of an aortic graft placement with sudden, massive upper gastrointestinal bleeding that should worry the provider for the development of an aortoenteric fistula. These fistulas frequently involve the duodenum. Mild bleeding may be the first sign but massive, life-threatening bleeding is common. Aortic aneurysms can erode into vasculature forming an arteriovenous fistula. These patients present with high-output cardiac failure and decreased arterial blood flow distal to the fistula. This patient does not have liver disease or a history of peptic ulcer disease. While both are still possible, given this patient's history and the high mortality associated with it, aortoenteric fistula needs to be ruled out first.

61. **The answer is C.** (Chapter 60) The patient has an abdominal aortic aneurysm as defined as an aneurysm

≥3.0 cm in diameter when measured from the outside margin of one wall to the outside margin of the opposite wall. A technically adequate ultrasound has >90% sensitivity for demonstrating an aneurysm. This ultrasound also demonstrates the superior mesenteric artery, which can distinguish the aorta from the vena cava. The other three answer choices would not be useful to distinguish between the two and are not demonstrated in the picture.

62. **The answer is D.** (Chapter 60) Abdominal aortic aneurysms ≥5 cm in diameter are at risk of rupture and require surgical evaluation. All symptomatic aneurysms require emergency surgical consultation while asymptomatic aneurysms should follow up in the next few days. As it is not ruptured and the patient is not hypotensive, the patient does not require a transfusion. Perioperative β-blocker administration in nonruptured aneurysms reduces dysrhythmias and myocardial ischemia but does not affect mortality or length of hospitalization. Given the normal blood pressure, this can likely wait until after discussing management with the surgeon. As the history and examination are concerning with imaging demonstrating an aneurysm >5 cm, the patient should receive surgical consultation and serial examinations will not change that.

63. **The answer is C.** (Chapter 61) The ankle-brachial index is the ratio of the systolic blood pressure with the cuff just above the malleolus to the highest brachial pressure in either arm. Patients with peripheral arterial disease have an ankle-brachial ratio <0.9. Values <0.25 are concerning for limb-threatening vascular disease. Normal values are between 0.91 and 1.3. An index >1.3 is likely from a noncompressible vessel, which may be seen in patients with severe vascular calcifications. Segmental blood pressures can also be obtained to determine if the patient has peripheral arterial disease. A difference of 30 mm Hg or more between two adjacent areas on the leg (e.g., below the knee and above the knee) suggest obstructing disease.

64. **The answer is B.** (Chapter 61) Acute limb ischemia due to embolism is less common than occlusion from thrombosis. This is in part due to the decline in rheumatic heart disease and the improvement in the management of patients with atrial fibrillation. Even with this improvement, atrial fibrillation is still the leading cause of embolic ischemic disease. The second most common source is from a mural thrombus that forms in the ventricle after a recent myocardial infarction (MI). This accounts for approximately 20% of all limb emboli. Heart valves, myxomas, and vegetations are rare causes of embolic disease.

65. **The answer is A.** (Chapter 61) The patient has blue toe syndrome, which is also known as trash foot or purple

toe syndrome. It is most commonly caused by atheroemboli formed by plaque fragmentation causing obstruction of the microcirculation. The atheroemboli consist of cholesterol-laden debris and platelet aggregates. In addition to thrombi, blue toe syndrome is associated with warfarin. Embolic cardiac disease generally causes limb ischemia, although if the embolus fragments, it is possible to cause obstruction in the microcirculation. With a normal cardiac examination and normal echocardiogram, this would be less likely. Vasospasm such as occurs in Raynaud's disease would be expected to cause the skin to turn white or pale prior to turning blue or purple. It normally occurs in response to cold temperatures and stress. Treatment generally includes warming the extremity.

66. **The answer is C.** (Chapter 61) Pain from spinal stenosis can mimic the pain from peripheral arterial disease. Some refer to the pain as neurogenic claudication or pseudoclaudication as they can be so similar. Classically, the pain from spinal stenosis is relieved by lumbar spine flexion and worsened by standing or spine extension. Pain from vascular claudication is improved by standing. Pain from either vascular or neurologic claudication is worse with movement and improves with rest. Vascular claudication can cause bilateral pain if the occlusion occurs in a more proximal vessel.

67. **The answer is C.** (Chapter 61) Acute limb ischemia is classically associated with the "six P's": pain, pallor, paralysis, pulselessness, paresthesias, and polar (for cold; may also be called poikilothermia). While these are the classic findings, the absence of any or all of the "six P's" does not exclude limb ischemia. Pulselessness is generally a late finding in acute disease and not always a useful finding in chronic disease. Pallor is one of the first skin changes followed by mottled skin, cyanosis, and petechiae and blisters. Muscle weakness and ischemic neuropathy presenting as either hypoesthesia or hyperesthesia are early findings. Preservation of light touch on skin testing is a good guide to tissue viability. Some of these findings are included in the Rutherford criteria, which provides prognostic information in patients with peripheral artery disease.

68. **The answer is A.** (Chapter 61) Limb ischemia can be caused by thrombotic and embolic disease. Patients without a history of claudication, with a normal contralateral leg, with sudden onset of pain, and with minimal peripheral disease and no collateral circulation on imaging are more likely to have embolic disease. Atrial fibrillation is the most common cause of ischemia from embolic disease. Patients with claudication are more likely to have thrombotic disease from atherosclerotic plaques that either rupture or propagate. Claudication is a cramp-like pain, ache, or tiredness worsened by exercise and improved by rest. It is reproducible and generally resolves in minutes. Patients with thrombotic disease are likely to have findings of peripheral arterial disease to both extremities, have gradual onset of pain, and have widespread disease with collaterals on imaging. Nonembolic ischemia from chronic occlusion may also be clinically silent if a significant collateral network has formed.

Thoracic-Respiratory Disorders

QUESTIONS

1. A 62-year-old man with a past medical history of obesity, hypertension, dyslipidemia, myocardial infarction, heart failure with preserved ejection fraction, smoking (30 pack-years), chronic obstructive pulmonary disease (COPD), and obstructive sleep apnea on continuous positive airway pressure (CPAP) at night presents with several months of dyspnea lasting for 4 to 6 hours per day. Symptoms worsen with exertion, are accompanied by a nonproductive cough and fatigue, do not improve with albuterol, and are not associated with fevers, hemoptysis, or weight loss. Vital signs are T 36°C, HR 96, BP 158/90, RR 20, and SpO_2 92% on RA. Physical examination reveals an overweight patient sitting upright, with crackles, plus occasional end-expiratory wheezes on auscultation. Medications include albuterol as needed, lisinopril, hydrochlorothiazide, atorvastatin, carvedilol, aspirin, nitroglycerin, and amiodarone. Which of this patient's medications is the MOST LIKELY contributor to his dyspnea?
   (A) Amiodarone
   (B) Atorvastatin
   (C) Carvedilol
   (D) Lisinopril

2. A 45-year-old woman with past medical history of dilated cardiomyopathy and an ejection fraction of 35% presents complaining of 6 hours of dyspnea and cough productive of white frothy sputum that began after she exercised on a treadmill. The patient has a history of malignant hypertension for which she is on a four-drug regimen, but she reports limited adherence to all four medications. Vitals are T 37°C, HR 110, BP 210/130, RR 28, and SpO_2 92% on RA. Physical examination is notable for crackles in all lung fields but no peripheral edema or jugular venous distention (JVD). Which of the following is the MOST definitive method to assess this patient's volume status related to her pulmonary examination?
   (A) Chest x-ray
   (B) NT-pro-BNP
   (C) Physical examination
   (D) Thoracic ultrasound

3. A 40-year-old patient is found down, without identification or medical alert bracelet. No history is available. Vital signs are T 39°C, HR 110, BP 140/76, RR 28, and SpO_2 79% on RA. Physical examination is notable for rhonchi on the right. An Emergency Medical Technician applies 100% O_2 by nonrebreather and the patient's SpO_2 rises to 85%. Which of the following is the MOST LIKELY cause of this patient's presentation?
   (A) Asphyxia
   (B) Chronic obstructive pulmonary disease
   (C) Pneumonia
   (D) Pulmonary embolus

4. A 20-month-old infant with family history of asthma and atopic disease presents to the emergency department with 3 days of worsening upper respiratory congestion, cough, wheezing, and fevers. The parents say there have been many sick contacts at daycare this winter. Vital signs reveal T 38°C, HR 140, BP 96/50, RR 40, and SpO_2 94% on RA. Physical examination is notable for scattered end-expiratory wheezing in all fields, crackles in the bilateral central lung fields, occasional cough, and supraclavicular retractions. There is no stridor. The patient is treated with albuterol with limited response. Which of the following is the MOST LIKELY diagnosis?
   (A) Asthma
   (B) Bronchiolitis
   (C) Croup
   (D) Epiglottitis

5. A 37-year-old man with no significant past medical history presents to the emergency department for evaluation of a chronic nonproductive cough, which has persisted for the past 8 weeks. He denies any fevers, chest pain, hemoptysis, weight loss, dyspnea, or lower extremity edema. He does not smoke or take any chronic medications and has never traveled outside the Northeastern United States. He works from home as an accountant. His vital signs are within normal limits and his cardiopulmonary examination is unremarkable except for occasional coughing. He saw his primary care physician 1 week ago for these symptoms and had a two-view chest x-ray is normal. What is the NEXT BEST step in his management?
   (A) Chest CT
   (B) Prescribe an oral antihistamine/decongestant
   (C) Prescribe baclofen
   (D) Referral for outpatient polysomnography

6. In adults, which of the following is the MOST common cause of pleural effusions with a pH of 7.3, pleural lactate dehydrogenase <200, and pleural protein <50% of serum protein level?
   (A) Cirrhosis
   (B) Heart failure
   (C) Nephrotic syndrome
   (D) Pneumonia

7. A 34-year-old-woman with no significant past medical history presents to the emergency department with new onset bloody cough. She describes 3 days of nasal congestion and blood-tinged sputum for 1 day. She is a smoker, does not use illicit drugs, has had no international travel, and denies night sweats, weight loss, or hematuria. Vital signs include T 98.6°F, RR 14, and SpO_2 of 96% on RA. On examination, she has hyperemic nasal turbinates, a clear oropharynx, no cardiac murmurs, and scattered wheezing to auscultation. Which of the following is the MOST APPROPRIATE initial diagnostic test?
   (A) Bedside ultrasound
   (B) Chest x-ray
   (C) Computed tomography angiography (CTA)
   (D) Multidetector computed tomography (CT)

8. A 69-year-old man with hypertension, chronic obstructive pulmonary disease, and lung cancer presents with bloody sputum. His vital signs are RR 22, HR 106, BP 92/50, and SpO_2 89% on RA. An emesis basin contains about 200 mL of blood clots that his nurse says he coughed up. What is the NEXT BEST procedure indicated for this patient?
   (A) Fiberoptic bronchoscopy
   (B) Interventional embolization
   (C) Operative exploration
   (D) Rigid bronchoscopy

9. What is the BEST postintubation position for a patient with massive hemoptysis?
   (A) Bleeding lung dependent
   (B) Head elevated at 30 degrees
   (C) Prone
   (D) Trendelenburg

10. A 32-year-old male smoker presents with 7 days of cough productive of yellow sputum, worse in the morning, and clearing over the day, accompanied by 4/10 substernal chest pain, which is worse with coughing. He states that his symptoms originally began with a runny nose and sore throat 10 days prior. He denies fevers and reports no prior medical history or medication use. Vital signs are within normal limits. A physical examination is notable for diffuse rhonchi that clear with coughing. Which of the following is the MOST LIKELY diagnosis?
   (A) Acute bronchitis
   (B) Chronic bronchitis
   (C) Chronic obstructive pulmonary disease exacerbation
   (D) Pneumonia

11. A 10-year-old boy is brought to the emergency department with 3 weeks of cough productive of yellow sputum. Parents state his symptoms began with an upper respiratory infection. He was febrile with a runny nose, sore throat, and cough for 1 week; his symptoms have since transitioned to episodes of coughing. He was seen in an outpatient clinic and diagnosed with bronchitis. He has had no sick contacts. He was born in India and missed his early vaccinations; he has not yet caught up on vaccines. Which historical feature in this case MOST warrants further testing or evaluation?
    (A) Birth in India
    (B) Duration of symptoms
    (C) History of fever
    (D) Missed vaccinations

12. A 21-year-old man presents to the emergency department with a 3-day history of cough productive of yellow sputum, sore throat, fevers, and myalgia. He describes sharp, substernal chest pain when coughing and with breathing. Vital signs are T 38°C, HR 110, BP 118/70, RR 22, and SpO_2 100% on RA. Physical examination is notable for diffuse rhonchi. Which of the following is the BEST NEXT step in management?
    (A) Admit and prescribe ceftriaxone and azithromycin
    (B) Discharge and prescribe acetaminophen and benzonatate
    (C) Order a chest x-ray
    (D) Order a complete blood count and blood cultures

13. A 36-year-old woman presents with cough productive of yellow sputum, subjective fevers, and pleuritic chest pain 2 days after having symptoms of an upper respiratory infection. Her vital signs are notable for temperature of 37.5°C and are otherwise within normal limits. Her physical examination is nonfocal. She is diagnosed with acute bronchitis. Which of the following is the BEST choice of treatment for this patient?
    (A) Albuterol
    (B) Azithromycin
    (C) Diphenhydramine
    (D) Supportive care

14. Which of the following patients would MOST benefit from treatment if diagnosed with influenza?
    (A) An adult older than 65 years on chronic low-dose steroid therapy with a history of epilepsy
    (B) An adult older than 65 years with human immunodeficiency virus (HIV), a recent CD4 count of 216, and a history of emphysema
    (C) An otherwise healthy child, age 5
    (D) An otherwise healthy woman who is 5 weeks postpartum

15. A 35-year-old man presents with 2 weeks of cough, which is worse at nighttime and described as "fits of coughing that last for a few minutes at a time." His symptoms began with low-grade fevers, rhinorrhea, sore throat, and a nonproductive cough. He has not seen a doctor in 20 years but believes he had all of his childhood vaccines. He works as a social worker in a home for disadvantaged children, many of whom have been sick lately. His primary care physician suspects that his immunity to pertussis has waned and sends a swab for culture. What would MOST LIKELY be seen on this patient's chest x-ray?
    (A) Airspace disease
    (B) Cavitary lesion with calcification, upper lobes
    (C) Ground glass infiltrates and hilar prominence
    (D) No acute cardiopulmonary process

16. A 65-year-old obese man with no recent illnesses was admitted to the hospital 2 days ago after an elective total knee replacement. He was extubated postprocedure and spent one night in the hospital. He did not use his continuous positive airway pressure (CPAP) machine at night, and he had restless sleep during his 24-hour hospitalization due to his sleep apnea. One day after discharge he developed fatigue, productive cough, fever, shortness of breath, and pleuritic chest pain. What is the MOST LIKELY mechanism responsible for his medical condition?
    (A) Aspiration
    (B) Endothelial damage from surgery
    (C) Hematogenous spread
    (D) Inhalation

17. A 55-year-old African-American man presents to the emergency department with 1 day of fever to 102.5°F, chills, productive cough, sputum streaked with dark brown blood, and pleuritic chest pain. He has had no recent hospitalizations or sick contacts. Laboratory testing reveals a leukocytosis. His chest x-ray is shown in Figure 6.1. What is the MOST LIKELY etiology of this patient's pneumonia?

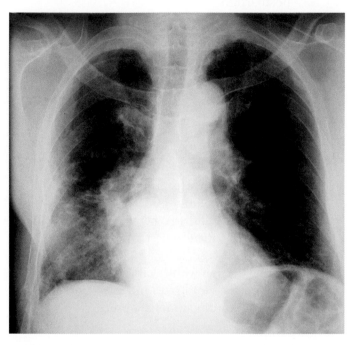

(A) *Haemophilus influenzae*
(B) *Mycoplasma pneumoniae*
(C) *Pseudomonas aeruginosa*
(D) *Streptococcus pneumoniae*

18. A 56-year-old woman presents to the emergency department with 4 days of multiple complaints. She visited a local spa with friends last week and had a massage, steam shower, and soaked in a hot tub. The patient has fever, chills, headache, muscle aches, shortness of breath, and dry cough. She has had a poor appetite associated with nausea, vomiting, and loose stools with some abdominal cramping. Past medical history includes hypertension, type 2 diabetes, dyslipidemia, and chronic obstructive pulmonary disease. She smokes ½ pack of cigarettes per day, drinks two glasses of wine on the weekends, and does not use drugs. Recent travel includes one short trip to the local beach last month, on the first day of summer. She denies international travel or camping. She has had one sick contact, her friend from the spa weekend, who also recently became ill. She recalls that they had different meals at lunch that day. Physical examination demonstrates scattered rales. Chest x-ray is shown in Figure 6.2 and is read as diffuse patchy infiltrates and hilar adenopathy. What is the MOST COMMONLY performed test used to rapidly identify the likely pathogen?

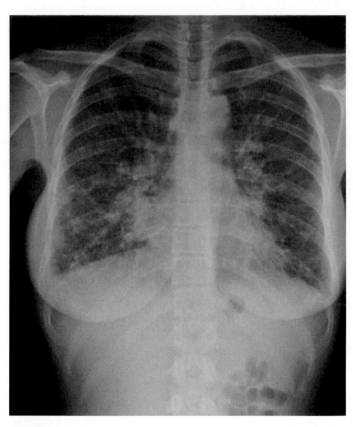

(A) Complete blood count with differential
(B) Fecal ova and parasite microscopy
(C) Sputum analysis
(D) Urinary antigen test

19. A 39-year-old alcoholic man is found down and brought to the emergency department. He is unable to give an accurate history because of his level of intoxication. His vital signs include T 101°F, HR 97, RR 14, and SpO$_2$ 92% on RA. Physical examination reveals a toxic appearing man with rigors and a wet sounding cough productive of copious, thick, blood-tinged sputum. He has coarse breath sounds in the left upper lobe. Which x-ray finding is most characteristic of the MOST LIKELY pathogen?
   (A) Abscess
   (B) Bulging fissure sign
   (C) Patchy infiltrate
   (D) Pleural effusion

20. A 42-year-old man presents to the emergency department with a fever and cough. He has had 3 days of rhinorrhea, mild sore throat, malaise, and cough. His cough was initially productive of white sputum and has become more purulent. Low-grade temperatures have now risen to 101.1°F. He is a ½ pack per day smoker with no alcohol or drug use. He has a pet parakeet. He takes no medications. There is no recent travel history. Vital signs are BP 125/79, HR 99, RR 18, and SpO$_2$ 94% on RA. On physical examination, he has inspiratory rales at the right base. Laboratory findings include a white blood cell count of 13.3 with a left shift. Chest x-ray reveals a right lower lobe pneumonia. What is the BEST treatment regimen for this patient?
   (A) Ciprofloxacin 400 mg three times a day
   (B) Clarithromycin XL 1000 mg daily
   (C) Doxycycline 100 mg twice a day
   (D) Linezolid 600 mg daily

21. Which of the following therapeutic regimens would be MOST acceptable for a 35-year-old, end-stage renal disease patient on hemodialysis, who was last admitted to the hospital and discharged 93 days prior, now presenting with fever, cough productive of green sputum, and the following chest radiograph (Figure 6.3)?

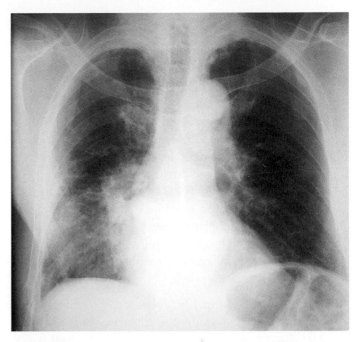

FIGURE 6.3 J.E. Tintinalli, J.S. Stapczynski, O.J. Ma, D. Yearly, G.D. Meckler, D.M. Cline: Tintinalli's Emergency Medicine: A Comprehensive Study Guide, 9th Edition: Copyright © McGraw-Hill Education. All rights reserved.

   (A) Ceftriaxone and azithromycin
   (B) Meropenem
   (C) Vancomycin and ceftriaxone
   (D) Vancomycin, cefepime, and levofloxacin

22. A 64-year-old undomiciled man presents intoxicated with fever, cough productive of rusty, brown sputum, and pleuritic chest pain. A chest x-ray is notable for a right lower lobe consolidation. Vitals are HR 110, RR 24, BP 120/58, and SpO$_2$ 97% on RA. Labs include sodium 127, potassium 4.5, chloride 105, bicarbonate 22, blood urea nitrogen 35, creatinine 1.6, glucose 126; white blood count 16 (8% bands), hemoglobin 12, hematocrit 36, platelets 245; ethanol 254. Which of the following is the MOST APPROPRIATE disposition plan?
   (A) Admit to inpatient floor
   (B) Discharge on outpatient regimen
   (C) Observation until sober, followed by discharge
   (D) Transfer to an alcohol detoxification program

23. A 75-year-old nursing home resident presents via emergency medical services with 3 days of altered mental status, cough productive of yellow sputum, respiratory distress, and fevers to 39°C. The care facility reports tachycardia and tachypnea in their transfer note. The patient is unable to provide further history, but the chart review reveals past medical history of remote breast cancer, Alzheimer's dementia, cerebrovascular accident, heart failure with preserved ejection fraction, and arthritis. Vitals include HR of 120, RR 30, BP of 102/54, and SpO$_2$ 90% on RA. Physical examination reveals a distressed, tachypneic patient, who is confused, not following commands, with coarse breath sounds, rhonchi in the right lower lobe, and 2+ peripheral edema. She has one episode of emesis during the workup.

    Labs include sodium 129, potassium 3.6, chloride 99, bicarbonate 18, blood urea nitrogen 40, creatinine 2.0, glucose 186, and hematocrit 31. A chest x-ray reveals a right lower lobe infiltrate. She has a signed Do Not Resuscitate/Do Not Intubate order. Which of the following disposition decision trees MOST accurately reflects this patient's clinical picture?
    (A) Admit to inpatient floor, her pneumonia severity index indicates high risk
    (B) Admit to inpatient floor, her pneumonia severity index indicates moderate risk
    (C) Admit to intensive care unit, her pneumonia severity index indicates high risk
    (D) Admit to intensive care unit, her pneumonia severity index indicates moderate risk, but she has a high probability of clinical decompensation

24. A 50-year-old man, managed in the medical intensive care unit after recent emergency department resuscitation for ventricular fibrillation cardiac arrest 3 days prior, complains of a cough and pleuritic, left-sided chest pain. His hospital course is as follows: return of spontaneous circulation was achieved after three rounds of cardiopulmonary resuscitation with defibrillation, epinephrine, and amiodarone; his electrocardiogram after resuscitation showed ST-segment elevations in leads V$_2$ to V$_5$ with reciprocal changes in the inferior leads. He was started on aspirin, clopidogrel, and heparin, and taken to the cardiac catheterization lab, where angioplasty and stenting were performed uneventfully. He was admitted to the medical intensive care unit for further management and was continued on the aspirin and clopidogrel, with the addition of metoprolol and atorvastatin. He now

endorses cough, productive of foul-smelling green sputum, fevers, nausea, and fatigue. His vital signs are T 39°C, HR 90, RR 24, BP 162/94, and SpO$_2$ 92% on RA. A chest x-ray shows a small, left-sided pleural effusion, and a left lower lobe infiltrate in the retrocardiac space. Which of the following is the MOST LIKELY diagnosis?
    (A) Aspiration pneumonia
    (B) Dressler syndrome
    (C) Empyema
    (D) Pneumonitis

25. A 60-year-old farmer with prior medical history of heart failure, Hodgkin's lymphoma, testicular cancer, hypertension, hyperlipidemia, and arthritis presents to the emergency department with shortness of breath. Symptoms began 3 to 6 months prior to arrival, are worse with exertion, are accompanied by nonproductive cough, and have not been relieved through the use of his wife's albuterol inhaler. He endorses occasional fevers and weight loss. He is currently undergoing active chemotherapy for his lymphoma. Bleomycin and dofetilide are on his medication list. Vital signs are T 37.4°C, HR 96, RR 20, BP 160/90, and SpO$_2$ 91% on RA. Physical examination reveals diffuse crackles and coarse breath sounds, without evidence of murmurs or peripheral edema. A bedside ultrasound reveals lung sliding, and no "B" lines. A chest x-ray reveals diffuse interstitial infiltrates and honeycombing, worse in the lower lobes. Which of the following is MOST LIKELY responsible for his current presentation?
    (A) Allergic bronchopulmonary aspergillosis
    (B) Bleomycin
    (C) Dofetilide
    (D) Heart failure

26. The majority of lung abscesses occur in which patient population?
    (A) Individuals with active malignancy
    (B) Individuals with aspiration risk
    (C) Individuals with recent thoracic surgery
    (D) Individuals with sepsis

27. A 72-year-old man complains of purulent cough and shortness of breath that has been progressive over the past several weeks despite antibiotics prescribed by his primary care physician. His vital signs are as follows: T 38.4°C, HR 146, BP 101/55, RR 36, and

SpO_2 82% on 15 L by a nonrebreathing mask. Physical examination reveals that he is using accessory muscles and in obvious respiratory distress. He has decreased breath sounds on the right with obvious dullness to percussion and a chest radiograph demonstrating opacification of the right lower lung fields with loss of the costophrenic angle and a notable meniscus. What is the MOST APPROPRIATE initial step in management?

(A) Administration of intrapleural fibrinolytics and antibiotics

(B) Echocardiogram, triple blood cultures, and antibiotics

(C) Nebulized beta-agonists, intravenous steroids, and positive pressure ventilation

(D) Thoracentesis with subsequent thoracostomy and antibiotics

28. A 46-year-old man complains of cough and pleuritic chest pain with significant weight loss and night sweats over the past several weeks. His chest CT shows a large, loculated left pleural effusion and thoracentesis results are as follows:

Pleural fluid glucose	32 mg/dL
Pleural fluid pH	7.02
Pleural fluid lactate dehydrogenase	2430 IU/L

What is the MOST LIKELY cause of this patient's symptoms?

(A) Acute exacerbation of chronic heart failure

(B) Bacterial pneumonia

(C) Esophageal perforation

(D) Renal failure

29. In a patient with a pulmonary abscess, which of the following clinical features and laboratory findings is MOST LIKELY to be present?

(A) Elevated white blood cell count

(B) Metabolic acidosis

(C) Sinus tachycardia

(D) Tachypnea

30. A 30-year-old previously healthy man with a history of alcohol abuse complains of fever and cough productive of foul-smelling sputum. His vital signs are as follows: T 38°C, HR 89, BP 131/80, and SpO_2 98% on RA. His chest radiograph is shown in Figure 6.4. Which of the following is the MOST APPROPIRATE initial antibiotic therapy?

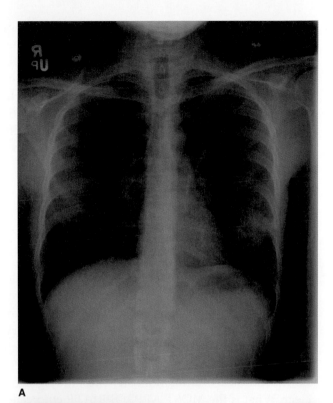

A

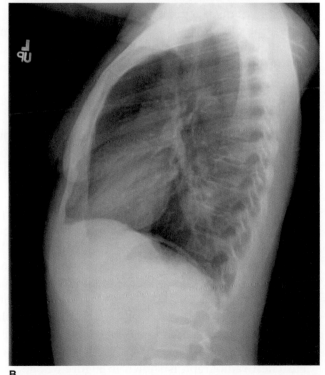

B

FIGURE 6.4 J.E. Tintinalli, J.S. Stapczynski, O.J. Ma, D. Yearly, G.D. Meckler, D.M. Cline: Tintinalli's Emergency Medicine: A Comprehensive Study Guide, 8th Edition: Copyright © McGraw-Hill Education. All rights reserved.

(A) Intravenous ceftriaxone and doxycycline

(B) Intravenous clindamycin

(C) Intravenous isoniazid and rifampin with oral ethambutol and pyrazinamide

(D) Intravenous vancomycin

31. A 3-year-old girl is brought by parents for evaluation of fever and poor oral intake. She recently immigrated to the United States from China, where she received the Bacillus Calmette-Guérin vaccine. Physical examination reveals she has cervical lymphadenopathy. Her vital signs are as follows: T 38.4°C, HR 146, BP 100/63, RR 36, and SpO$_2$ 100% on RA. Which of the following tests to evaluate for possible tuberculosis infection is MOST LIKELY to be positive in this patient?
    (A) Acid-fast smear
    (B) Chest x-ray
    (C) Mantoux skin test
    (D) Sputum cultures for acid-fast bacteria

32. A 47-year-old homeless patient presents for evaluation of screening a tuberculin skin test that was placed 48 to 72 hours previously. Upon examination of the forearm, there is a 12-mm area of mild erythema and induration. The patient denies any night sweats, cough, fevers, chills, and has an otherwise normal physical examination. Her chest radiograph is clear. What is the MOST APPROPRIATE emergency department management?
    (A) Antibiotics for pneumonia, oxygen, placement in a negative pressure room with airborne precautions, and initiation of sputum and blood cultures
    (B) Initiation of four-drug therapy after coordination with outpatient provider
    (C) Initiation of isoniazid alone after coordination with outpatient provider
    (D) No further management necessary

33. A 24-year-old man presents to the emergency department for evaluation of recent fever, weight loss, and cough. He denies any history of homelessness, IV drug use, or known immunosuppression, and has never traveled outside of the country. His vital signs are as follows: T 37.6°C, HR 93, BP 121/75, RR 23, and SpO$_2$ 94% on RA. He is cachectic and uncomfortable appearing, and has scattered rhonchi on pulmonary auscultation. His examination is otherwise normal. His chest radiograph is shown in Figure 6.5, and he has positive acid-fast bacilli present on a smear. In addition to negative pressure isolation, serial sputum cultures, and antibiotic therapy, what further diagnostic tests are MOST APPROPRIATE?

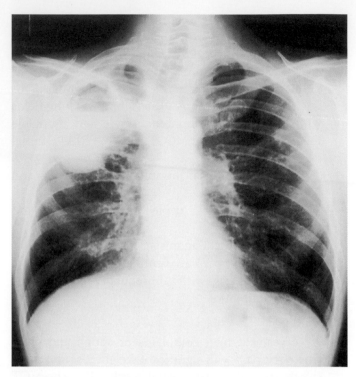

FIGURE 6.5 J.E. Tintinalli, J.S. Stapczynski, O.J. Ma, D. Yearly, G.D. Meckler, D.M. Cline: Tintinalli's Emergency Medicine: A Comprehensive Study Guide, 9th Edition: Copyright © McGraw-Hill Education. All rights reserved.

    (A) Erythrocyte sedimentation rate
    (B) Human immunodeficiency virus (HIV) testing
    (C) Lumbar puncture
    (D) Serum calcium level

34. After unknowingly caring for a patient with active tuberculosis without proper respiratory protection, which is the MOST LIKELY way for a healthcare provider to respond on future tuberculosis tests?
    (A) Negative skin screening tests both 2 weeks later and 1 year later
    (B) Negative skin screening test in 2 weeks with positive chest radiograph within the next year
    (C) Negative skin screening test in 2 weeks with positive screening test 1 year later
    (D) Positive skin screening test in 2 weeks

35. A 50-year-old man presents to the emergency department for evaluation of fever, hemoptysis, cough, and night sweats. Which of the following contributing social and/or medical history features put this patient at the highest risk for tuberculosis?
    (A) Active alcohol and IV drug use
    (B) Homelessness
    (C) Immigrant status from a high-prevalence country
    (D) Residence in a nursing home

36. What is the MOST COMMON physical examination finding in a patient presenting for evaluation and treatment of a spontaneous, atraumatic pneumothorax?
    (A) Hypoxia
    (B) Ipsilateral decreased breath sounds
    (C) Ipsilateral hyperresonance to percussion
    (D) Sinus tachycardia

37. A 50-year-old man presents for evaluation of sudden onset right-sided chest pain and shortness of breath that began spontaneously the day before. He has a history of chronic obstructive pulmonary disease but denies severe shortness of breath, infectious symptoms, associated trauma, or history of similar prior pain. His vital signs are as follows: T 37°C, HR 89, BP 113/62, RR 16, and SpO$_2$ 92% on RA. His chest radiograph shows a small right-sided pneumothorax, with less than 2 cm of space between the parietal and visceral pleura. What is the MOST APPROPRIATE initial treatment for this patient?
    (A) Catheter aspiration with immediate catheter removal after completion of aspiration and 3 hours of observation. The patient can be discharged if repeat chest radiograph shows no worsening.
    (B) Immediate needle decompression followed by chest tube insertion and admission for observation.
    (C) Observation with supplemental oxygen for 3 hours. The patient can be discharged if repeat chest radiograph demonstrates no worsening.
    (D) Small-size catheter or small-size chest tube insertion to water seal with admission for observation.

38. Which of the following is the MOST APPROPRIATE counseling to provide a patient upon discharge after a resolved pneumothorax?
    (A) High-altitude flying is not recommended until cleared by a cardiothoracic surgeon.
    (B) Pleurodesis is recommended prior to any diving activity.
    (C) Pulmonary function tests are recommended for evaluation of any recurrent pneumothorax.
    (D) Reexpansion lung injury is a serious delayed consequence of pneumothorax and may occur up to 72 hours after pneumothorax resolution.

39. Which of the following would you expect to see on pulmonary ultrasound of a pneumothorax?
    (A) B-lines
    (B) Comet tails
    (C) Loss of differentiation below and above the pleural line
    (D) Seashore sign

40. A 24-year-old man presents for sudden onset of shortness of breath following a sporting event. He reports associated right-sided pleuritic chest pain. He has never had similar symptoms and his past medical history is otherwise unremarkable. His vital signs are as follows: T 37.5°C, HR 97, BP 103/62, RR 24, and SpO$_2$ 90% on room air. His chest radiograph is shown in Figure 6.6. What is the MOST APPROPRIATE NEXT step in management or diagnosis?

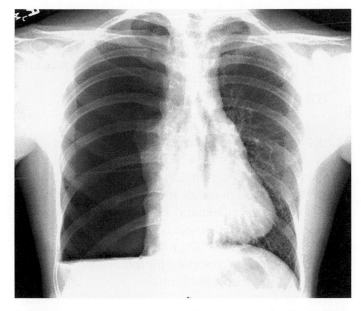

FIGURE 6.6 Reproduced with permission from Stone CK, Humphries RL (eds): Current Diagnosis & Treatment: Emergency Medicine, 8th ed. New York: McGraw-Hill Education, Inc. 2017.

    (A) Cardiothoracic consultation for video-assisted thoracic surgery and associated pleurodesis
    (B) Chest CT for evaluation of pulmonary blebs and determination of pneumothorax size
    (C) Needle aspiration with fluid analysis including cell count, Gram stain, and culture
    (D) Placement of a large bore chest tube to water seal

41. A 17-year-old adolescent girl with a history of severe asthma exacerbation presents to the emergency department for evaluation of extreme shortness of breath. Examination indicates that she has faint wheezes bilaterally and is using accessory muscles to breath. Her vital signs are as follows: T 36.5°C, HR 113, BP 132/76, RR 23, and SpO_2 90% on RA. After the administration of IV corticosteroids and inhaled albuterol, which of the following therapies is MOST LIKELY to relieve her airflow obstruction in the setting of acute exacerbation?
    (A) Heliox
    (B) Intubation and mechanical ventilation
    (C) Magnesium
    (D) Salmeterol xinafoate and formoterol

42. In the patient with severe asthma, which of the following findings is MOST sensitive for impending respiratory failure?
    (A) Decreased respiratory rate with altered mentation
    (B) Forced expiratory volume in 1 second (FEV_1) or peak expiratory flow rate (PEFR) < 40% predicted
    (C) $PaCO_2$ <42 mm Hg
    (D) Very minimal breath sounds

43. A 7-year-old boy presents for evaluation of shortness of breath that began while exercising earlier in the day. The patient endorses some mild wheezing and improvement of the shortness of breath after cessation of activity and is currently asymptomatic. His vital signs and physical examination are otherwise within normal limits. What are MOST APPROPRIATE discharge instructions and medication to be prescribed for this patient?
    (A) Daily corticosteroid inhaler
    (B) Short-acting beta-agonist to be used as needed
    (C) Short-acting beta-agonist to be used as needed with daily corticosteroid inhaler
    (D) Short-acting beta-agonist to be used as needed with short taper of oral corticosteroids

44. Which of the following is the MOST COMMON complication of patients intubated for status asthmaticus?
    (A) Barotrauma
    (B) High peak airway pressures
    (C) Pneumothorax
    (D) Ventilator-associated pneumonia

45. Which of the following is the MOST CONCERNING risk factor for mortality associated with asthma exacerbation?

(A) Associated temperature greater than 38°C
(B) Early age of onset
(C) History of corticosteroid use
(D) More than two hospitalizations for asthma within the past year

46. A 62-year-old man with a history of chronic obstructive pulmonary disease (COPD) and chronic heart failure presents for evaluation of progressive shortness of breath over several days after a viral infection. Which of the following is MOST INDICATIVE of a COPD exacerbation as the primary cause of his symptoms?
    (A) B-type natriuretic peptide level <100
    (B) Chest radiograph demonstrating flattened diaphragm and increased lucency of parenchyma
    (C) Poor R-wave progression and enlarged P wave on electrocardiogram
    (D) Wheezes on pulmonary auscultation

47. A 73-year-old woman with a history of emphysema and type 2 diabetes presents for evaluation of shortness of breath and mild confusion. Her arterial blood gas is as follows: pH 7.25, pCO_2 59, HCO_3 26, and PO_2 90. With which acid-base scenario is this MOST consistent?
    (A) Acute respiratory acidosis with compensatory metabolic alkalosis
    (B) Chronic respiratory acidosis with compensatory metabolic alkalosis
    (C) Metabolic acidosis with compensatory respiratory alkalosis
    (D) Metabolic and respiratory acidosis

48. Which of the following is the MOST LIKELY trigger of an acute exacerbation of chronic obstructive pulmonary disease?
    (A) Bacterial infection
    (B) Change in blood pressure medications
    (C) Cold weather
    (D) Pulmonary embolism

49. In the patient with an acute exacerbation of chronic obstructive pulmonary disease, which of the following interventions is MOST LIKELY to decrease emergency department length of stay prior to discharge?
    (A) Inhaled beta-agonist
    (B) Intravenous methylprednisolone
    (C) Oral doxycycline
    (D) Oral or intravenous methylxanthine

50. A 60-year-old man with a history of chronic obstructive pulmonary disease, hypertension, coronary artery disease, and paroxysmal atrial fibrillation presents for evaluation of shortness of breath and worsening cough with purulence despite taking his scheduled medications. He is sitting upright in the gurney, extremely agitated, unable to answer questions regarding orientation, and pulling away his face mask during evaluation. His vital signs are as follows: T 38°C, HR 123, BP 145/72, RR 34, and SpO_2 84% on RA, despite supplemental oxygen provided by nonrebreathing mask at 15 L/min. His chest radiograph is shown in Figure 6.7, and his electrocardiogram demonstrates sinus tachycardia. Which of the following is the MOST APPROPRIATE NEXT step in management and diagnosis?
    (A) Arterial blood gas
    (B) CT angiography
    (C) Intubation and mechanical ventilation
    (D) Noninvasive positive pressure ventilation

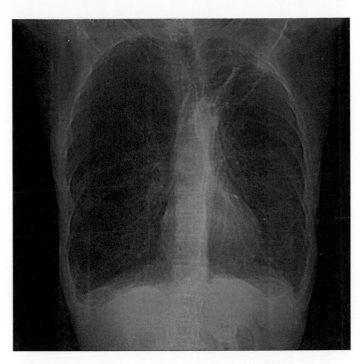

FIGURE 6.7 Reproduced with permission from J.E. Tintinalli, J.S. Stapczynski, O.J. Ma, D. Yealy, G.D. Meckler, D.M. Cline: Tintinalli's Emergency Medicine: A Comprehensive Study Guide, 9th Edition. Copyright © McGraw-Hill Education. All rights reserved.

ANSWERS

1. **The answer is A.** (Chapters 19 and 62) Amiodarone is associated with a number of serious adverse effects, including pulmonary toxicities such as pulmonary fibrosis or interstitial pneumonia. Patients on amiodarone should be monitored with pulmonary function tests (PFTs) and yearly chest x-rays. Atorvastatin is a cholesterol medication and can cause myopathy, but it would not be expected to cause the type of dyspnea this patient is experiencing. Carvedilol is a distractor; a non-specific beta-blocker could exacerbate reactive airway diseases like asthma or chronic obstructive pulmonary disease (COPD). However, the patient's symptoms and clinical history are not consistent with a COPD exacerbation, therefore the side effects of carvedilol are less likely than the side effects of amiodarone to explain his symptoms. Lisinopril can cause a chronic cough in some patients, but it would not be as likely as amiodarone pulmonary toxicity to produce the physical examination findings of crackles.

2. **The answer is D.** (Chapter 62) While any of these methods can inform volume status, a chest x-ray has limited sensitivity but better specificity for this purpose. B-type natriuretic peptide (BNP) is an excellent marker to distinguish cardiogenic versus noncardiogenic causes of dyspnea; however, in this patient with acutely elevated blood pressure in the setting of known malignant hypertension and medication nonadherence, flash pulmonary edema is most likely, especially given the absence of apparent volume overload. In the setting of flash pulmonary edema, BNP measurement is less reliable; further, this patient has a chronic and known volume overloaded state, and if a baseline BNP is not available, distinguishing the significance of her current level may challenge interpretation. Physical examination is reliable as a means of assessing volume status, though isolated pulmonary edema in the setting of increased afterload may not offer a completely specific set of symptoms to overrule the sensitivity and specificity offered by ultrasound; further, it relies on subjective provider judgement. Thoracic ultrasound of the lung is the most specific and sensitive way to distinguish decompensated heart failure from noncardiac causes with 97% sensitivity and specificity.

3. **The answer is C.** (Chapter 62) This patient has a partial but incomplete response to supplemental oxygen, which is the hallmark of shunt physiology. Patients with a right-to-left shunt, whether intracardiac, vascular, or intrapulmonary, will always transmit some percentage of deoxygenated blood from the right to left circulation, resulting in persistent desaturation since some fraction of blood never encounters pulmonary oxygen. Asphyxia

presents with desaturation, but the hypoxia resolves with increased oxygenation. Chronic obstructive pulmonary disease (COPD) can present with some degree of intrapulmonary shunting, but it generally presents as ventilation/perfusion (V/Q) mismatch, which responds completely to inhaled oxygen. Additionally, a COPD patient would be expected to present with wheezes and air trapping, while this patient presents with focal rhonchi. Pneumonia creates an intrapulmonary shunt, during which exudate fills the alveoli and prevents gas exchange. The picture is typically a mix of V/Q mismatch and shunt, depending on the degree of consolidation. In a case of pneumonia, some portions of the disease demonstrate V/Q mismatch, which leads to the partial response to oxygen but the shunt fraction remains, which prevents a complete response. Note, shunt physiology presents with either no, OR partial, response to oxygen. Pulmonary embolus typically presents with V/Q mismatch, given the obstruction to blood flow.

4. **The answer is B.** (Chapter 127) While this patient has risk factors and features of many of these conditions, his wheezing without response to albuterol plus crackles, and absence of stridor and nontoxic appearance make bronchiolitis the most likely diagnosis. Bronchiolitis presents in children younger than 2 years, with a changing clinical examination with variable features, including wheezing, rhonchi, and crackles, with variably borderline oxygen saturation. It has no specific treatment beyond supportive care, and most often the work of breathing responds to high flow oxygen by nasal cannula. Asthma is a distracting answer given the family history of asthma and the clinical picture of wheezing in the setting of a respiratory infection. Age 2 years, however, is the threshold at which asthma is diagnosed; prior to this age, reactive airway disease is the clinical diagnosis. Both asthma and reactive airway disease have a hallmark response to albuterol, and the absent response in this case argues strongly against a reactive airway component. Croup, characterized by upper airway narrowing, is typically accompanied by stridor, and an overall clinical picture with cyanosis and respiratory distress is absent in this patient. There may be a component of airway narrowing in young children due to anatomical reductions in airway caliber, which limits tolerability of swelling, but this patient has no symptoms to suggest it. Epiglottitis is characterized by upper airway swelling, and the patient has no symptoms of upper airway obstruction.

5. **The answer is B.** (Chapter 62) Chronic cough is defined as a cough lasting for more than 8 weeks (Table 6.1).

TABLE 6.1	Sequential Approach to Chronic Cough

- Obtain chest radiograph, if not already done.
- Reduce exposure to lung irritants (e.g., smoking) and discontinue angiotensin-converting enzyme inhibitors, angiotensin II receptor blockers, and β-blockers.
- Treat for postnasal discharge with an oral first-generation antihistamine/decongestant with or without an inhaled nasal steroid. If the cough improves, continue treatment and consider evaluating for sinus disease with imaging studies.
- Evaluate for bronchospasm with spirometry (include flow-volume loop to detect vocal cord dysfunction) with or without methacholine provocation; if positive, treat with inhaled bronchodilators and corticosteroids if lower source identified.
- Treat for gastroesophageal reflux with lifestyle changes, H_2 blockers, or proton pump inhibitors.
- If cough persists, obtain CT scan of the chest, especially if patient is a smoker and cough persists despite smoking cessation.
- If cough persists, consider referral to otolaryngologist for laryngoscopy, gastroenterologist for endoscopy and/or esophageal pH monitoring, or pulmonologist for bronchoscopy.

Reproduced with permission from J.E. Tintinalli, J.S. Stapczynski, O.J. Ma, D. Yealy, G.D. Meckler, D.M. Cline: Tintinalli's Emergency Medicine: A Comprehensive Study Guide, 9th Edition. McGraw-Hill Education; 2020.

The most common causes of chronic cough include smoking, postnasal drainage stimulating cough, asthma, gastroesophageal reflux, and angiotensin-converting enzyme (ACE) inhibitor usage. In this well-appearing patient presenting without a history of infectious symptoms or high-risk features for malignancy, a stepwise algorithmic approach to chronic cough is recommended. Empiric treatment with an oral antihistamine/decongestant may resolve this patient's symptoms if allergies or postnasal drainage are the culprit. Chest CT can be considered if the cough does not respond to initial treatment, but this patient is a relatively young nonsmoker with a normal two-view chest x-ray, so stepwise evaluation may spare him unnecessary radiation. Baclofen is sometimes used off-label in the treatment of intractable hiccups, but it would not be a first-line treatment for chronic cough. Patients with refractory chronic cough may benefit from referral to a pulmonologist or to an otolaryngologist for laryngoscopy, but it is unlikely that sleep apnea assessment will shed light on the cause of his chronic cough.

6. **The answer is B.** (Chapter 62) By applying Light's criteria, the pleural fluid is a transudate. In terms of overall prevalence of conditions, heart failure is the most common, and therefore causes the most transudative effusions. Cirrhosis, with less prevalence than heart failure, can also cause a transudative effusion, known as hepatic hydrothorax. Nephrotic syndrome, owing to the hypoalbuminemic state, can cause changes in oncotic pressure leading to fluid leakage from capillaries. *Streptococcus pneumoniae*, the most common pathogen in pneumonia, occasionally causes exudative pleural effusion.

7. **The answer is B.** (Chapter 63) Most patients with mild hemoptysis need no specific tests. Chest x-ray is the initial imaging modality for these patients and will yield a diagnosis up to half the time. Multidetector CT can identify and characterize bleeding from bronchial and nonbronchial arteries, as well as the pulmonary artery, and it is preferred over CT angiogram in stable patients with massive hemoptysis. There is no role for bedside ultrasound in mild hemoptysis.

8. **The answer is D.** (Chapter 63) This patient has massive hemoptysis and is unstable. Definitive bleeding control may involve surgery or interventional procedures, but the initial step is urgent bronchoscopy to identify the source of bleeding and stabilizing treatment. Unlike fiberoptic bronchoscopy, rigid bronchoscopy allows for concurrent ventilation, better suctioning, and multiple treatment options to control hemorrhage, such as passage of a Fogarty balloon catheter to tamponade bleeding, instillation of topical coagulants, and ice water lavage. Surgery is typically reserved for massive hemoptysis from leaking aortic aneurysm or fistula, iatrogenic pulmonary artery injury, or thoracic trauma.

9. **The answer is A.** (Chapter 63) Placing the patient with the affected lung in the dependent position prevents blood from spilling into the unaffected side. The other options would not offer the same advantages. Elevating the head of the bed has been shown to reduce ventilator-associated pneumonia in intubated patients, but this is not the initial priority for patients with massive hemoptysis. The prone position is indicated for select patients with severe acute respiratory distress syndrome. Trendelenburg has no role in maximizing ventilation in postintubation positioning.

10. **The answer is A.** (Chapter 64) This patient has a cough and chest pain productive of yellow sputum following an upper respiratory infection, consistent with acute bronchitis. While this patient is a smoker, putting him at risk for chronic obstructive pulmonary disease and chronic bronchitis, both present with different symptomatology. Chronic obstructive pulmonary disease, especially the emphysematous variant, typically presents with wheezing and respiratory distress, and chronic bronchitis requires at least a 2-year history for diagnosis. While the symptoms and history may represent pneumonia, the absence of fever, and otherwise normal vital signs, and benign examination make this less likely. The productive cough that clears over the day reflects a normal course of tracheobronchial inflammation that clears with increased mucociliary clearance and respiratory activity. Pneumonia would not be expected to clear in this manner, so it is not the most likely diagnosis.

11. **The answer is D.** (Chapter 64) This child presents with a prolonged cough, described as coming in "episodes," in the setting of missed vaccinations. While the diagnosis of bronchitis is probable, the potential for pertussis is elevated in this patient given the missed vaccinations and description of the history and deserves further testing. Birth in India predisposes the patient to risk of tuberculosis; however, the features of the illness are less consistent with tuberculosis, and without additional information regarding duration of life abroad, the living conditions, potential exposures, or general health status, would not warrant additional workup for this particular presentation. It is very common for bronchitis to persist for 7 to 21 days, so the duration of symptoms falls within the expected spectrum of disease. History of fever is not specific for any particular condition, and by itself may be a benign or concerning finding.

12. **The answer is C.** (Chapter 64) Differentiating pneumonia from bronchitis clinically can be difficult. Traditionally, providers do not reliably assess the likelihood of these conditions based on history and physical examination alone. This patient may have a benign respiratory infection, bronchitis, pleurisy, pneumonia, or other serious causes of chest pain and fever. Further, he demonstrates at least two criteria that increase the likelihood of pneumonia (tachycardia, fever). Obtaining a chest x-ray is the most appropriate next step. While the patient may have pneumonia, he likely does not require inpatient admission, but this cannot be fully assessed without further workup and potentially using a risk stratification scheme such as the CURB-65 score. This patient may or may not have a serious infection, so supportive care may be all that is needed but not before additional workup and imaging; therefore, discharge home is not the next best step. Infectious workup, including blood cultures and complete blood count, may be warranted in this patient, but the most useful action at this point is to obtain a chest x-ray to exclude or include pneumonia.

13. **The answer is D.** (Chapter 64) There is little evidence to suggest that any particular acute bronchitis treatment is beneficial unless there are specific symptoms to be addressed. Albuterol has been shown to be of benefit when patients are wheezing or have reactive airway disease, but this patient is not an asthmatic and has a nonfocal examination. Azithromycin has no demonstrated value in this setting unless the bronchitis is complicated by emphysema, chronic bronchitis exacerbation, or intercurrent pneumonia. Antibiotics have not been shown to reduce the duration or symptoms of bronchitis as it is most often viral. Diphenhydramine may have a role if the patient also has concurrent allergic symptoms, but this patient has no such demonstrated condition. Therefore, there is no specific reason to prescribe diphenhydramine.

14. **The answer is B.** (Chapter 64) While all of these patients meet some criteria for being at higher risk of complications from influenza, an immunocompromised patient with a low CD4 count and concomitant pulmonary disease is at the highest risk for major complications. An adult on low-dose steroids with epilepsy is still at increased risk but not as high as a patient with direct immunocompromise and known disease in a system commonly affected by influenza. The pediatric patient could benefit on the basis of age, but this child is otherwise healthy and is on the upper limit of normal for benefit. Postpartum women are at risk, especially if they are within 2 weeks of birth; this patient is outside that time window, and while her infant is at risk if she has influenza, she is likely at a lower risk level by this point.

15. **The answer is D.** (Chapter 64) This patient, if he has clinical pertussis, would be unlikely to present with any specific parenchymal lesions on the chest x-ray. He would most likely have a normal chest film. If he had pneumonia, this would represent a superimposed infection, and his symptoms are more suggestive of an upper respiratory or bronchial location. Upper lobe cavitary lesions describes the radiographic findings of tuberculosis, and while the patient has risk factors, he does not have hemoptysis, weight loss, night sweats, or other specific stigmata of tuberculosis. Ground glass infiltrates and hilar prominence are seen in sarcoidosis or infiltrative lung disease, and this patient lacks both the risk factors and the appropriate clinical history for these conditions.

16. **The answer is A.** (Chapter 65) This patient most likely has pneumonia due to aspiration. He has many risk factors for aspiration: obesity, sleep apnea, recent intubation, and hospitalization (presumably eating in a semi-recumbent position as most hospital patients do). Aspiration is the most common mechanism for developing pneumonia, although inhalation and hematogenous spread are also potential mechanisms. Hematogenous spread can be seen with *Staphylococcus aureus* and *Streptococcus pneumoniae*, but this patient was not recently ill and had no source for seeding the lungs. Pleuritic chest pain, endothelial damage, and recent surgery can be associated with pulmonary embolus, but the associated symptoms of fatigue, productive cough, and fever in the setting of his aspiration risk, all point to an infectious condition rather than a vascular condition. Healthcare-associated pneumonia risks include being hospitalized for 2 or more days within the past 90 days.

17. **The answer is D.** (Chapter 65) This patient has a classic presentation of pneumococcal pneumonia with sudden onset disease, rigors, rust-colored productive cough, high fevers, chest pain, and a lobar infiltrate on x-ray. The elderly, minorities, patients with immune suppression (splenectomy, transplant, human immunodeficiency virus, sickle cell disease), and children <2 years old, or children who attend group day care, are at highest risk for pneumococcal pneumonia. Symptoms of *Haemophilus influenzae* are typically gradual onset fever, dyspnea, and pleuritic chest pain. It can occur in any age group but most commonly occurs in the elderly or those with chronic lung disease, sickle cell disease, immunocompromise, diabetes, and alcoholism. The most frequently reported pathogens among patients with nursing home-acquired pneumonia are *Streptococcus pneumoniae* and *H. influenzae*. *Mycoplasma pneumoniae* is characterized by upper and lower respiratory tract symptoms, nonproductive cough, headache, malaise, fever, and a reticulonodular pattern or patchy infiltrates on the x-ray. *Pseudomonas* is characteristically found in recently hospitalized, debilitated, or immunocompromised patients with fever, dyspnea, and cough. X-ray reveals patchy infiltrates with frequent abscess formation.

18. **The answer is D.** (Chapter 65) This patient most likely has *Legionella pneumoniae*. Risk factors for *Legionella* include tobacco use, chronic lung disease, being a transplant recipient (especially in the first 3 months post-transplant), and immunosuppression. *Legionella* can cause a wide array of symptoms, from benign disease to multisystem organ failure and acute respiratory distress syndrome. There is no seasonality to *L. pneumoniae*, but it is observed more frequently in the summer months as the frequency of other pathogens wanes. In about half of patients with community-acquired pneumonia, no specific pathogen is identified. A complete blood count would be nonspecific. The concurrent gastrointestinal distress in the setting of the confirmed pneumonia points to *Legionella* alone, rather than both a primary intestinal source and a respiratory source of infection. With no travel history, nor ingestion of freshwater (as occurs with campers), the likelihood of a parasite is also low. The sputum of patients with *Legionella* demonstrates few neutrophils and no predominant bacterial species. Although sputum culture detects all species of legionella, it is technically difficult, requires special agar media, and takes at least 5 days to obtain results. Therefore, sputum analysis in *Legionella* is inferior to the commonly available urinary antigen test for detection, which is rapid and yields same day results.

19. **The answer is B.** (Chapter 65) This patient most likely has *Klebsiella pneumoniae*. Patients with *Klebsiella* pneumonia have sputum that is described as brown "currant jelly" and is thick, with short, plump, gram-negative, encapsulated, paired coccobacilli. This patient is an alcoholic, which puts him at higher risk for *Klebsiella*, especially with this description of the sputum as thick and bloody. Chest x-ray in *Klebsiella* typically reveals an upper lobe infiltrate, bulging fissure sign, and/or abscess formation. Abscess can be found in many types of pneumonia, such as *Staphylococcus aureus*, *Pseudomonas aeruginosa*, anaerobic organisms, and sometimes *Legionella pneumophila* pneumonia, making it less specific for *Klebsiella*. Bulging fissure is most often seen in *Klebsiella*. Patchy infiltrates are often seen with *Haemophilus influenzae*, *Moraxella catarrhalis*, *Chlamydophila pneumoniae*, and *Mycoplasma pneumoniae*. Pleural effusion is also heterogenous and can be found in *S. pneumoniae*, *H. influenzae*, and *L. pneumophila*.

20. **The answer is B.** (Chapter 65) In outpatient management of low-risk pneumonia, single drug therapy is the common first choice, using a macrolide, such as azithromycin (500 mg on the first day and 250 mg for the next 4 days) or clarithromycin (1000 mg daily for 7 days). Doxycycline is a second-line choice, and with emerging antibiotic drug resistance, the Centers for Disease Control and Prevention recommends that fluoroquinolones (e.g., levofloxacin [750 mg daily for 5 days], moxifloxacin [400 mg daily for 7–14 days], or other respiratory fluoroquinolones) be reserved for patients who cannot tolerate other agents, have documented pneumococcal resistance, or have failed other therapies. Fluoroquinolones should also be avoided in patients with myasthenia gravis. Ciprofloxacin is one part of the recommended triple drug regimen for healthcare-associated pneumonia, and it confers antipseudomonal activity. Linezolid is also part of the recommended triple drug regimen for healthcare-associated pneumonia and is usually a substitute for vancomycin for antimethicillin-resistant *Staphylococcus aureus* coverage.

21. **The answer is D.** (Chapter 65) This patient, although discharged more than 3 months ago from the hospital, should be treated for healthcare-associated pneumonia because of her hemodialysis. Other conditions that qualify patients as having healthcare-associated pneumonia include being hospitalized for 2 or more days within the past 90 days, residing in a nursing home or long-term care facility, being on home IV antibiotics, receiving chronic wound care, receiving chemotherapy, and having an immunocompromised state. Acceptable regimens for healthcare-associated pneumonia consist of three drug regimens covering methicillin-resistant *Staphylococcus aureus*, gram-negative and resistant organisms including pseudomonas, and atypical organisms. Ceftriaxone

and azithromycin would be acceptable for community-acquired pneumonia. Meropenem offers a broad-spectrum coverage, but it would not sufficiently cover all the recommended pathogens. The combination of vancomycin and ceftriaxone is a more suitable regimen for meningitis, and although it could cover many pneumonia pathogens, in this case some gram-negative pathogens (particularly pseudomonas) and atypical organisms would be not be covered.

22. **The answer is A.** (Chapter 65) This patient has pneumonia and is intoxicated. In addition, because the patient is undomiciled, there are social concerns and uncertainty how the patient will appropriately obtain care and resources outside of the hospital. Several pneumonia scoring systems help calculate risk among patients with pneumonia in the emergency department. The most well-studied tools are the pneumonia severity index (PSI) and the CURB-65 rule. This patient's data permits analysis by the CURB-65 system, and he scores a total of 3 points, 1 each for confusion (although he is intoxicated, his risk must be assumed higher since a true mental status examination either cannot be conducted or is confounded), uremia (blood urea nitrogen >7 mmol/L), and blood pressure (diastolic below 60). He does not score points for 65 years or more, or respiratory rate. Having a CURB-65 score of 3 increases his risk of mortality in the outpatient setting. Additionally, even if his risk can be adjusted down for the confounding factor of intoxication, he is still at an increased risk given his homelessness and substance abuse and should be considered for admission. Discharging the patient would be risky. Observing him and reassessing once sober is an excellent idea; however, even without the sober reevaluation, his risk for progression of pneumonia combined with his social risk factors remains intermediate to high. Transferring him to a detox center would not address the actual medical problem of pneumonia.

23. **The answer is C.** (Chapter 65) This patient has a pneumonia severity index (PSI) greater than 130 (age, nursing home resident, congestive heart failure, cerebrovascular accident, abnormal mental status, elevated blood urea nitrogen, hyponatremia, and low saturation on room air), placing her in the highest severity class, which recommends admission to an intensive care unit. Her predicted mortality is at least 29.2%. While no risk stratification tool is infallible to replace clinical judgment, this elderly patient with substantial comorbidity and clear evidence of clinical decompensation (altered mental status, tachycardia, diastolic hypotension, desaturation, tachypnea, respiratory distress, hyponatremia, pre-renal azotemia, and kidney disease) should be considered high risk on clinical grounds alone, necessitating frequent monitoring in case

noninvasive positive pressure ventilation or escalation in care is required. Although choice A correctly computes the severity index, a general medicine floor would likely not have sufficient resources for the management of this patient. Describing this patient as moderate risk is a miscalculation of her pneumonia severity index, so choice B is incorrect, as it assigns too low a level of care/severity score. Although the appropriate disposition of this patient is to the intensive care unit, choice D has flawed logic, as it also miscalculates her pneumonia severity index.

24. **The answer is A.** (Chapter 65) This patient is presenting with symptoms consistent with pneumonia, probably from aspiration during his resuscitation (risk factors from cardiopulmonary resuscitation include loss of gag/cough reflex, variant intrathoracic, gastric, and intra-abdominal pressure, and gastric distention from bag valve mask ventilation). Supine positioning during a code situation, as well as the loss of neurologic function, plus alterations in protective reflexes and pressure/distention physiology, increase the likelihood of aspiration events. Further, the description of this patient's sputum suggests an anaerobic source, commonly from oral flora. Dressler syndrome is a probable cause of chest pain and effusion after a myocardial infarction, which typically occurs 5 to 7 days or later after infarction; 3 days, while possible, would be very early for this condition. Further, Dressler's syndrome presents with pericarditis symptomatology, not a clinical picture suggestive of pneumonia with a pulmonary infiltrate. Empyema is possible, though this patient's effusion is small on chest x-ray and his early time course makes this condition less likely. It is more likely that his effusion is simple and parapneumonic. Pneumonitis is possible and probable, and it commonly occurs from chemical aspiration of gastric acid; however, the chest x-ray would not be expected to show a focal consolidation, so the most likely diagnosis is aspiration pneumonia.

25. **The answer is B.** (Chapter 65) This patient presents with chronic cough and a clinical picture consistent with interstitial lung disease—crackles, interstitial infiltrates, and honeycombing on chest x-ray, and an ultrasound without suggestive features of airspace disease or effusion. He has a history of heart failure and malignancies. Bleomycin is commonly used to treat both lymphomas and testicular cancer, and is well known for causing pulmonary fibrosis and interstitial pneumonitis. Allergic bronchopulmonary aspergillosis is certainly something for which he is at risk, given his occupation; however, it typically resolves once exposure to the antigen is eliminated. Additionally, he has a chronic picture of lung disease without a clear exposure. Dofetilide is a class III antiarrhythmic and of the same class (generally) as amiodarone; however, it is not known

for specifically causing pulmonary fibrosis, unlike amiodarone. Heart failure typically presents with volume overload, pleural effusions, and interstitial/alveolar edema, which this patient lacks.

26. **The answer is B.** (Chapter 66) The vast majority (80%) of lung abscesses are primary abscesses occurring in healthy patients or in patients with a risk of aspiration. Secondary lung abscesses, or those associated with malignancy, sepsis, or recent thoracic surgery, account for only 20% of lung abscesses.

27. **The answer is D.** (Chapter 66) The appropriate treatment for this patient is thoracentesis with subsequent thoracostomy and antibiotics. Given this patient's history of antibiotic-resistant pulmonary infection and chest radiograph, his most likely diagnosis is empyema. Treatment of empyema typically involves antibiotics in addition to tube thoracostomy followed by possible video-assisted thoracoscopic surgery for lysis of adhesions and administration of intrapleural fibrinolytics. However, this patient is too unstable for surgical intervention and requires immediate stabilization in the emergency department via thoracentesis or thoracostomy with definitive management to follow. The patient has no evidence of concomitant bronchoconstriction so there is likely little use for nebulized beta-agonists, steroids, and positive pressure ventilation. An echocardiogram could be performed in evaluation of endocarditis but would require prior stabilization.

28. **The answer is B.** (Chapter 66) Pleural effusions can be classified into two major groups – transudates and exudates, which can be determined by pleural fluid analysis. Empyemas are exudative effusions and are characterized by low pleural pH, low glucose, and elevated fluid lactate dehydrogenase. The majority (56%) of empyemas are caused by pulmonary infections, most commonly bacterial pneumonia. Esophageal perforation is a less frequent cause of empyema (4%). Heart failure exacerbation and renal failure are transudative pleural effusions and are therefore not the cause of this patient's symptoms.

29. **The answer is A.** (Chapter 66) Pulmonary abscesses are indolent processes and therefore unlikely to produce evidence of acute infections such as tachycardia, tachypnea, and fever. Hemoptysis is present in only up to 25% of cases. Most patients with pulmonary abscess do have laboratory findings consistent with infection such as elevated white blood cell count or erythrocyte sedimentation rate.

30. **The answer is B.** (Chapter 66) The patient in the above question has a lung abscess visualized on chest radiograph. Lung abscesses are typically caused by aspiration of gastric contents that contain anaerobic bacteria. Clindamycin and ampicillin/sulbactam are good first-line agents for anaerobic coverage. Ceftriaxone with doxycycline are appropriate antibiotics for community acquired pneumonia but would not offer appropriate anaerobic coverage. Vancomycin would be helpful if the infection was confirmed to be caused by methicillin-resistant *Staphylococcus aureus*. Combination therapy of ethambutol, isoniazid, pyrazinamide, and rifampin is appropriate for patients in whom there is a high concern for active tuberculosis.

31. **The answer is C.** (Chapter 67) Patients who receive Bacillus Calmette-Guérin (BCG) vaccination for tuberculosis prevention will often have a positive Mantoux skin test result even in the absence of infection. The appropriate tuberculosis blood test for use in patients with a history of BCG vaccine is an interferon-γ release assay (IGRA). Children with tuberculosis have a lower rate of pulmonary cavitary lesions, yielding lower rates of classic tuberculosis findings on the chest radiograph. Sputum cultures and acid-fast smears are also less likely to be positive in children, with positive sputum findings in only about 40% of pediatric patients ultimately treated for tuberculosis.

32. **The answer is C.** (Chapter 67) Interpretation of the tuberculin skin test requires adjustment for patient's risk factors. Induration over 10 mm is considered positive in patients who belong to high-prevalence groups such as immigrants and residents of nursing homes or homeless shelters. This patient, with an induration of greater than 10 mm, most likely has latent tuberculosis and should be started on isoniazid after discussion with an outpatient provider for follow-up. If pulmonary tuberculosis is suspected, patients should receive antibiotic coverage and be admitted for definitive testing, with subsequent initiation on four-drug therapy. However, this patient has no pulmonary symptoms and a clear chest radiograph and thus does not require this management.

33. **The answer is B.** (Chapter 67) Human immunodeficiency virus (HIV) coinfection is a major risk factor for development of active tuberculosis and tuberculosis-associated death. Approximately 20% of patients with HIV and latent tuberculosis will go on to develop active tuberculosis, in comparison to 1% to 13% of the general population. As such, HIV testing is an important risk stratification test in otherwise heathy patients with active tuberculosis. An erythrocyte sedimentation rate is likely to be elevated in this patient with active infection, but this is not specific for tuberculosis infection. A lumbar puncture for evaluation of CSF involvement is appropriate if

patients have neurologic complaints or findings but not a standard test in patients with isolated pulmonary tuberculosis. Serum calcium can often be elevated in patients with sarcoidosis or malignancy with similar chest radiographs, but these diagnoses are less likely in patients with positive for tuberculosis.

34. **The answer is A.** (Chapter 67) Only 30% of patients become infected after a single droplet exposure. Of patients who do contract tuberculosis, the tuberculin skin test is negative until 1 to 2 months after exposure. Only 1% to 13% of healthy patients with latent tuberculosis go on to develop active tuberculosis.

35. **The answer is C.** (Chapter 67) Immigrants from countries with a high prevalence of tuberculosis are at the highest risk of having tuberculosis. Other risk factors for tuberculosis, such as homelessness, active alcohol and drug use, and nursing home residence, are associated with lower prevalence of tuberculosis and are therefore less significant risk factors.

36. **The answer is D.** (Chapter 68) The most common physical examination finding in patients with pneumothoraces is sinus tachycardia. Because these pneumothoraces are small, decreased breath sounds and hyperresonance to percussion are often absent. Hypoxia can be present but is less prevalent than sinus tachycardia and more likely to be a feature of a tension pneumothorax.

37. **The answer is D.** (Chapter 68) This patient has a secondary small spontaneous pneumothorax, and as such, requires placement of catheter or tube insertion and subsequent hospitalization for observation of improvement. Both supplemental oxygen and catheter aspiration followed by 3 hours of observation are appropriate treatments for patients with stable first-time primary spontaneous small pneumothoraces, but this patient's history of chronic obstructive pulmonary disease disqualifies him from this treatment. Needle decompression followed by chest tube insertion is appropriate for the patient with tension pneumothorax, but this patient does not have features consistent with tension pneumothorax.

38. **The answer is B.** (Chapter 68) Patients who have had a pneumothorax are at high risk of recurrence and should be cautioned against diving prior to definitive management and prevention of future pneumothoraces by video assisted thorascopic surgery and pleurodesis. High-altitude flying is not recommended for at least 7 to 14 days after pneumothorax resolution but does not require cardiothoracic clearance. Pulmonary function tests are helpful

measurements of contributing disease severity but have little bearing on management or prevention of future pneumothoraces. Reexpansion lung injury is uncommon and occurs shortly after pneumothorax resolution; this is usually mild and requires no treatment more than observation and supplemental oxygen.

39. **The answer is C.** (Chapter 68) Ultrasound has an excellent sensitivity and specificity for detection of traumatic pneumothorax. On a healthy lung, the sliding visceral pleura against the stationary chest wall causes artifacts caused by sonographic reverberation such as comet tails and the sliding sign. In M-mode, the movement of the healthy lung against the chest wall is often referred to as the "seashore." The loss of differentiation below and above the pleural line in M-mode is indicative of interpleural air and associated pneumothorax. B-lines are a finding consistent with heart failure exacerbation and would not be expected in a patient with a pneumothorax.

40. **The answer is D.** (Chapter 68) Large bore chest tubes are required for appropriate resolution of hemopneumothorax, as seen on this patient's chest radiograph. Fluid analysis may be helpful in the determination of the cause of the hemopneumothorax, but needle aspiration is not sufficient for pneumothorax resolution in the setting of an existing fluid component. This patient may eventually benefit from chest CT and video-assisted thoracic surgery if there is failure to resolve the hemopneumothorax but does not need these interventions prior to chest tube placement.

41. **The answer is C.** (Chapter 69) Magnesium reduces airflow obstruction by serving as a smooth muscle relaxant; it is an important adjunctive therapy in patients with acute severe exacerbation. Long-acting beta-agonists, such as salmeterol xinafoate and formoterol, are indicated for twice-daily maintenance therapy in patients with severe asthma but should not be used in the setting of acute exacerbation. Patients with significant altered mental status or respiratory fatigue may require intubation and mechanical ventilation to eliminate work of breathing, but this does not serve to relieve airflow obstruction. Heliox may theoretically lower airway resistance but has not been demonstrated to make significant changes in the clinical setting.

42. **The answer is A.** (Chapter 69) In the patient with acute asthma exacerbation, decreased respiratory rate and altered mentation are indicative of hypercarbia with associated respiratory fatigue and thus requires immediate intervention to prevent impending respiratory failure.

Other signs of respiratory compromise or severe exacerbation include a forced expiratory volume in 1 second (FEV_1) or peak expiratory flow rate (PEFR) less than 25% of predicted or a $PaCO_2$ over 42 mm Hg. Minimal breath sounds often indicate a significant exacerbation but are not specific for impending respiratory failure.

43. The answer is B. (Chapter 69) This patient, who is experiencing exercise-related shortness of breath that improves after cessation of activity, has exercised-induced, mild intermittent asthma. These exacerbations should improve quickly with a short-acting beta-agonist and should require no other therapy. Corticosteroid inhalers should be prescribed for exacerbation prevention only in patients with mild or moderate persistent asthma. Oral corticosteroids are recommended only in the case of acute exacerbation, which this patient denies.

44. The answer is B. (Chapter 69) Mechanical ventilation is a necessary intervention for asthma patients in severe respiratory distress, but it has multiple complications. All of the above complications can occur in patients intubated for severe asthma exacerbation, but the majority of these complications, such as pneumothorax, hemodynamic impairment and barotrauma, are direct results of the elevated peak airway pressures caused by airflow obstruction. Poor airway movement can also contribute to increased mucus plugging, which in turns put patients at risk for atelectasis and pulmonary infection.

45. The answer is D. (Chapter 69) Risk factors for asthma-exacerbation-related death are as follows: more than two hospitalizations or three emergency department visits for asthma within the past year, using more than two canisters per month of short-acting beta-agonist, difficulty perceiving airway obstruction or its severity, and social features such as low socioeconomic status or illicit drug use. History of corticosteroid use, associated temperature, and early age of onset do not reliably predict mortality from asthma exacerbation.

46. The answer is A. (Chapter 70) It is important to determine the likely cause of shortness of breath in this patient as treatment will vary significantly depending on diagnosis. A B-type natriuretic peptide of less than 100 effectively rules out heart failure exacerbation as the primary cause of dyspnea. Patients can have wheezing in either heart failure or chronic obstructive pulmonary disease (COPD) exacerbations. The findings on chest radiograph and electrocardiogram (flattened diaphragm and increased lucency of pulmonary parenchyma on chest radiograph and enlarged P wave and poor R-wave progression on electrocardiogram) are chronic changes associated with COPD; however, neither help with immediate diagnosis in the setting of an exacerbation.

47. The answer is A. (Chapter 70) This patient is most likely suffering an acute exacerbation of her chronic obstructive pulmonary disease (COPD) causing acute respiratory acidosis with compensatory metabolic alkalosis. The pH of less than 7.4 and PCO_2 of greater than 40 indicate a primary respiratory acidosis. The next step is to determine whether the acidosis is acute or chronic and whether there is appropriate metabolic compensation. In acute respiratory acidosis, the serum bicarbonate rises by 1 mEq/L for each 10 mm Hg increase in PCO_2, and the pH will change by $0.008 \times (40-PCO_2)$. This patient, with her PCO_2 59, serum bicarbonate 26, and pH 7.25, fits into this category. In chronic respiratory acidosis, the bicarbonate rises by 3.5 mEq/L for each 10 mm Hg increase in PCO_2 and the pH will change by $.03^*(40-PCO_2)$. Changes outside of these ranges suggest an accompanying metabolic disorder.

48. The answer is A. (Chapter 70) More than 75% of patients with acute exacerbations have evidence of viral or bacterial infection, with up to half specifically due to bacteria. Other important triggers, such as cold weather, pulmonary irritants, and beta-blockers are less frequent. Pulmonary embolisms have been identified in 20% to 25% of patients with a severe chronic obstructive pulmonary disease (COPD) exacerbation without otherwise diagnosed precipitant but do not account for the plurality of general exacerbations.

49. The answer is A. (Chapter 70) Administration of inhaled beta-agonists and anticholinergic agents has been demonstrated to improve and decrease emergency department length of stay, especially when used together. Corticosteroids have been demonstrated to shorten the recovery time in acute exacerbations of chronic obstructive pulmonary disease (COPD) but given 6-hour delay before onset of action is unlikely to alter emergency department length of stay. Oral antibiotics are an important component of therapy if a patient's exacerbation is determined to be caused by a bacterial infection, but they are not necessary in every patient with COPD exacerbation. Methylxanthines, such as theophylline and aminophylline, serve both to improve breathing mechanics and decrease inflammation but have not been demonstrated to reliably improve patients in acute exacerbation.

50. The answer is C. (Chapter 70) This patient is clinically unstable and in respiratory distress requiring immediate airway intervention. The appropriate intervention is intubation and mechanical ventilation to stabilize the airway prior to further investigation into the cause of the patient's dyspnea. Noninvasive ventilation is an appropriate choice for many patients in respiratory distress but is contraindicated in the case of highly uncooperative or obtunded patients. An arterial blood gas would be helpful to determine the degree of the patient's respiratory distress and a CT angiogram would be an appropriate test to evaluate for possible pulmonary embolism, but emergent airway management should not be deferred for these diagnostic studies.

Abdominal and Gastrointestinal Disorders

7

QUESTIONS

1. Which of the following statements about abdominal pain in the elderly patient is TRUE?
   - (A) A low white blood cell (WBC) count has a low predictive value for surgical disease in the elderly.
   - (B) Fever is a reliable marker for disease.
   - (C) Patients older than 80 years have decreased mortality if the diagnosis is incorrect at the time of admission.
   - (D) Surgical complications are less common than in younger patient populations.

2. A 28-year-old woman presents to the emergency department with right lower quadrant pain for the past 2 days. She states the pain is constant but fluctuating in intensity. She denies any past medical history or abdominal surgeries. She is sexually active with her husband only and has no history of sexually transmitted infections. She states she has ovarian cysts. Her vital signs are BP 130/80, P 105, T 37.8°C, and SpO$_2$ 99% on RA. On palpation of her abdomen, she has mild right quadrant tenderness without Rovsing's sign, rebound or guarding. What is the NEXT BEST step in her management?
   - (A) Consult general surgery
   - (B) Order a CT abdomen and pelvis with IV contrast
   - (C) Order a transvaginal ultrasound
   - (D) Perform a pelvic examination

3. What is the treatment for epiploic appendagitis?
   - (A) Antacids
   - (B) Antibiotics
   - (C) Operative management
   - (D) Supportive care

4. What is the MOST common cause of gastroparesis?
   - (A) Bariatric surgery
   - (B) Diabetes
   - (C) Gastroesophageal reflux disease
   - (D) Idiopathic

5. An 80-year-old woman presents to the emergency department with diarrhea for the past 1 week. She states that she is currently on day 6 of cephalexin for a urinary tract infection. She reports that she is having approximately four to five episodes of loose, watery, foul-smelling, nonbloody stools per day for the past 2 days. She denies fever, nausea, vomiting, or abdominal pain. On examination her vital signs are within normal limits, she appears well hydrated, and her abdomen is soft, nontender, and nondistended with normoactive bowel sounds. You send a *Clostridium difficile* stool toxin immunoassay, and it comes back positive for toxin A. What is the NEXT BEST step?
   - (A) Administer an antiperistaltic medication
   - (B) Advise the patient to stop the cephalexin
   - (C) Consult general surgery
   - (D) Discharge the patient with metronidazole 500 mg three times a day orally

6. Which of the following statements regarding traveler's diarrhea is CORRECT?
   (A) Antibiotics shorten the duration of illness by approximately 24 hours.
   (B) Antimotility agents should be used in patients with bloody diarrhea.
   (C) Loperamide when combined with an antibiotic regimen does not shorten the duration of symptoms.
   (D) Probiotics are not safe.

7. What is the BEST way to diagnose Crohn's disease?
   (A) Abdominal x-ray series
   (B) Colonoscopy
   (C) CT abdomen/pelvis with PO and IV contrast
   (D) Stool studies

8. A 35-year-old man with history of ulcerative colitis presents to the emergency department with severe abdominal pain for the past 3 days, which acutely worsened today. His vital signs are BP 80/60, P 120, T 38.5°C, and SpO$_2$ 99% on RA. His abdomen is diffusely tender, distended, and tympanic. You obtain an x-ray (see Figure 7.1). What is your NEXT BEST step in the management of this patient?

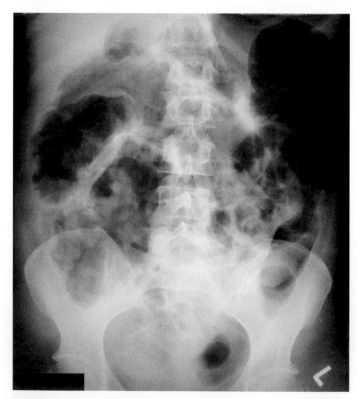

FIGURE 7.1 Reproduced with permission from Schwartz DT (ed): Emergency Radiology: Case Studies. McGraw-Hill, Inc., 2008.

   (A) Administer broad-spectrum antibiotics
   (B) Consult surgery
   (C) Order IV fluids bolus
   (D) Place a nasogastric tube

9. Which of the following statements about fecal impaction is TRUE?
   (A) A regimen of medications is not necessary after disimpaction.
   (B) Diarrhea rules out fecal impaction.
   (C) Enemas provide substantial relief.
   (D) Manual disimpaction is a painful procedure that may require sedation.

10. A 50-year-old man with history of esophageal varices, cirrhosis, alcohol abuse, and atrial fibrillation on warfarin presents to the emergency department with eight episodes of hematemesis. His vital signs are BP 70/40, P 120, RR 20, T 37°C, and SpO$_2$ 96% on RA. On physical examination he is unresponsive, not following verbal commands, not responsive to painful stimuli, and actively vomiting 1 L of bright red blood. His peripheral pulses are thready. What is the NEXT BEST step?
    (A) Administer 2 L of normal saline bolus
    (B) Order a complete blood count with differential
    (C) Order a prothrombin time/international normalized ratio (PT/INR)
    (D) Prepare to intubate the patient

11. Which of the following is TRUE regarding reversing a coagulopathy in a patient with a life-threatening active upper gastrointestinal (GI) bleed?
    (A) INR >1.5 is not a significant predictor of mortality in patients with an upper GI bleed who are receiving anticoagulants.
    (B) Endoscopy should be delayed until coagulopathy is reversed.
    (C) Reverse the coagulopathy without concern for the INR.
    (D) Tranexamic acid has shown benefit in the management of upper GI bleeding.

12. What is the MOST common cause of lower gastrointestinal (GI) bleeding?
    (A) Diverticular disease
    (B) Malignancy
    (C) Polyps
    (D) Upper GI bleeding

13. What is the MOST common cause of lower gastro-intestinal (GI) bleeding with an established source below the ligament of Treitz?
    (A) Colitis
    (B) Diverticular disease
    (C) Malignancy
    (D) Polyps

14. A 35-year-old woman presents to the emergency department with a chief complaint of bloody stools. She states that she has been having approximately two to three stools per day mixed with bright red blood for the past 5 days. She is not on any blood-thinning medications. She denies any fever, nausea, vomiting, or abdominal pain. Her vital signs in triage are all within normal limits. What is the NEXT BEST step?
    (A) Consult gastroenterology
    (B) Cross-match for packed red blood cells
    (C) Order a complete blood count with differential
    (D) Perform a rectal examination

15. Which of the following regarding diffuse esophageal spasm is TRUE?
    (A) Chest pain is not a common symptom.
    (B) Dysphagia is constant.
    (C) Dysphagia progresses over time.
    (D) Treatment involves control of acid reflux and consideration of smooth muscle relaxants.

16. What is the MOST common cause of esophageal perforation?
    (A) Boerhaave's syndrome
    (B) Foreign body ingestion
    (C) Iatrogenic
    (D) Trauma

17. What is the MOST common location of a spontaneous esophageal perforation?
    (A) Left posterolateral wall of distal esophagus
    (B) Left posterolateral wall of proximal esophagus
    (C) Right posterolateral wall of distal esophagus
    (D) Right posterolateral wall of proximal esophagus

18. A 2-year-old girl is brought into the emergency department by her mother after the mother found the girl choking after playing with a coin purse. Her mother thinks the patient may have swallowed something because she did not see her spit or vomit anything up. On examination her vital signs are within normal limits, she has no stridor or drooling, her posterior oropharynx in normal, her lungs are clear, and she is not in any respiratory distress. X-ray shows a radiopaque foreign body in the stomach. She is drinking and eating without any distress. What is the NEXT BEST step?
    (A) Admit the patient to the pediatrics service for serial abdominal examination
    (B) Consult gastroenterology for emergent endoscopic retrieval
    (C) Discharge the patient with follow-up with pediatrician in 24 to 48 hours
    (D) Order intravenous glucagon

19. Based on this x-ray, what is the foreign body and location (Figure 7.2)?

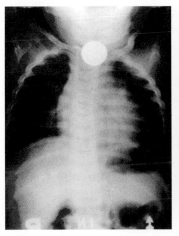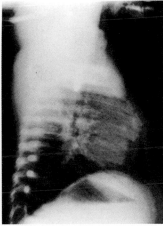

FIGURE 7.2 Reproduced with permission from Effron D (ed): Pediatric Photo and X-Ray Stimuli for Emergency Medicine, vol II. Columbus, OH, Ohio Chapter of the American College of Emergency Physicians, 1997, case 27.

    (A) Button battery located in the esophagus
    (B) Button battery located in the trachea
    (C) Coin located in the esophagus
    (D) Coin located in the trachea

20. What is the management of a swallowed button battery located in the esophagus?
    (A) Admit the patient for serial abdominal examination
    (B) Consult a specialist for emergent endoscopic retrieval
    (C) Discharge the patient with follow-up with the pediatrician in 24 to 48 hours
    (D) Order intravenous glucagon

21. Which of the following statements regarding food impaction is CORRECT?
    (A) Glucagon 1 to 2 mg intravenously can be used.
    (B) If a first dose of glucagon is unsuccessful, a second should not be attempted.
    (C) Meat tenderizer should be used.
    (D) Seafood is the most commonly identified in food impaction.

22. A 70-year-old man presents to the emergency department complaining of epigastric abdominal pain for 4 weeks. He reports unintentional weight loss (30 lb in the past 4 weeks), persistent vomiting, and dysphagia. His abdomen is soft and nontender. Labs in the emergency department, including a complete blood count with differential and comprehensive metabolic panel, are within normal limits. He is able to eat and drink and wants to go home. What is the NEXT BEST step in this patient's management?
    (A) Arrange for urgent outpatient follow-up with gastroenterology for endoscopy
    (B) Discharge the patient and prescribe an antacid
    (C) Order an abdominal CT scan
    (D) Order an abdominal x-ray

23. What is the gold standard for the diagnosis of peptic ulcer disease?
    (A) CT abdomen and pelvis with oral and intravenous contrast
    (B) Endoscopy
    (C) *Helicobacter pylori* testing
    (D) Ultrasound

24. Which of the following statements about peptic ulcer disease is TRUE?
    (A) If nonsteroidal anti-inflammatory drug (NSAID)–associated ulcers are present, the patient can continue to take NSAIDs because the damage is already done.
    (B) Patients with peptic ulcer disease are not at risk for peptic ulcer bleeding or perforation.
    (C) Traditional therapy includes proton pump inhibitors (PPIs), H_2 receptor antagonists (H2RAs), sucralfate, and antacids.
    (D) Treatment of *H. pylori* infection, when present, does not decrease recurrence rate.

25. What is the MOST COMMON complication of peptic ulcer disease?

    (A) Infection
    (B) Obstruction
    (C) Perforation
    (D) Upper gastrointestinal (GI) bleeding

26. A 43-year-old obese woman presents to the emergency department for a 2-day history of nausea, vomiting, and constant, severe epigastric abdominal pain. She states that her pain radiates to her back. She denies any medical problems. She has had an appendectomy in the past. She takes no medications. On physical examination, she is afebrile and tachycardic but otherwise hemodynamically stable. She has guarding in her right upper quadrant and epigastric region, without rebound. Her labs are remarkable for a WBC 14.9, bilirubin 2.3, alanine aminotransferase (ALT) 155, alkaline phosphatase 220, and lipase of 1100. Which of the following is the MOST APPROPRIATE NEXT step in management of this patient?
    (A) Consult gastroenterology for an endoscopic retrograde cholangiopancreatography
    (B) Consult surgery for a cholecystectomy
    (C) Discharge the patient with antiemetics and outpatient gastrointestinal (GI) follow-up.
    (D) Start 1 to 2 L of fluid resuscitation

27. The following ultrasound image is most consistent with what diagnosis, if you were also told that the common bile duct measures 4 mm (Figure 7.3)?

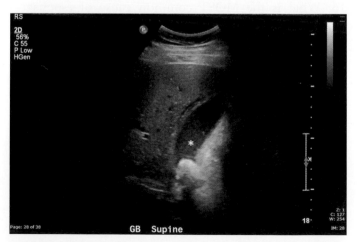

FIGURE 7.3 Image contributed by Bart Besinger, MD, FAAEM.

    (A) Acalculous cholecystitis
    (B) Cholecystitis
    (C) Choledocholithiasis
    (D) Hepatitis

28. A 60-year-old man with a history of multiple abdominal surgeries presents to the emergency department for evaluation of a "bulging mass" under his umbilicus. He states that he used to be able to "push it back in," but since yesterday he has noted that it has enlarged and is extremely painful to touch. His vitals are T 39.1°C, P 114, BP 92/68, RR 25, and SpO$_2$ 92% on RA. You attempt to reduce the bulge twice without success. You decide to obtain a CT scan of the abdomen/pelvis to evaluate this further. While you are waiting on the CT scan, the lab calls you with a critical value of lactic acid 8.0 and white blood cell (WBC) count 21,000. You start aggressive fluid resuscitation, place the patient on a cardiac monitor, and make him NPO. What is the BEST NEXT step in management?
    (A) Admit patient for pain control
    (B) Give analgesics and attempt to reduce it again
    (C) Schedule outpatient surgery
    (D) Start intravenous piperacillin/tazobactam

29. What is the leading cause of cirrhosis in the United States?
    (A) Acetaminophen toxicity
    (B) Alcohol
    (C) Hepatitis C
    (D) Nonalcoholic fatty liver disease

30. Which of the following statements is TRUE regarding hepatorenal syndrome?
    (A) Hemodialysis does not help prevent progression of the disease.
    (B) It is usually not associated with ascites formation or spontaneous bacterial peritonitis.
    (C) It only occurs in chronic liver failure patients.
    (D) Median survival is only a few weeks without treatment once patients develop progressive oliguria and doubling creatinine.

31. A 65-year-old woman presents to the emergency department with abdominal pain, nausea, and vomiting for 2 days. Her vital signs are T 39.4°C, P 115, BP 100/82, RR 20, and SpO$_2$ 95% on RA. On physical examination, she has scleral icterus, right upper quadrant tenderness with guarding, and a positive Murphy's sign. Bedside ultrasound shows a common bile duct diameter of 15 mm. Which of the following interventions is the DEFINITIVE management for this patient's diagnosis?

(A) Endoscopic retrograde cholangiopancreatography
(B) Intravenous antibiotics
(C) Oral antibiotics and follow-up with surgery for cholecystectomy
(D) Outpatient follow-up with gastroenterology

32. Which medication treats the MOST COMMON risk factor for hepatorenal syndrome?
    (A) Albumin
    (B) Cefotaxime
    (C) *N*-acetylcysteine
    (D) Octreotide

33. A 50-year-old man with alcoholic liver cirrhosis presents to the emergency department with altered mental status and worsening abdominal distention over the past week. He denies fever, chills, vomiting, or diarrhea. His examination is significant for distention and diffuse abdominal tenderness. You perform a diagnostic paracentesis that shows 400 white blood cells (WBCs) with 90% PMNs and 10% lymphocytes, high protein, and normal glucose. What is the BEST treatment for this condition?
    (A) Ampicillin and an aminoglycoside
    (B) Midodrine
    (C) Thiamine
    (D) Third-generation cephalosporin

34. What is the first-line treatment for hepatic encephalopathy?
    (A) Cephalosporins
    (B) Furosemide
    (C) Lactulose
    (D) Spironolactone

35. A 34-year-old woman with a history of heavy alcohol use presents with a 3-day history of nausea, vomiting, generalized weakness, abdominal pain, and jaundice. Her labs are remarkable for a negative pregnancy test and acute elevation of her transaminases (aspartate aminotransferase [AST] 1800 and alanine aminotransferase [ALT] 900). Which of these factors, if present, mandates admission?
    (A) Albumin >3.5
    (B) Bilirubin >4.0
    (C) Glucose <50
    (D) Prothrombin time/international normalized ratio (PT/INR) >25% above normal

36. In a patient with a small bowel obstruction, which of the following is an indication for emergent operative management?
    (A) Air-fluid levels on plain films
    (B) Closed-loop obstruction
    (C) Presence of transition point on CT scan
    (D) Prior abdominal surgery

37. Which of the following is a risk factor for the development of cecal volvulus?
    (A) Advanced age
    (B) History of constipation
    (C) Male gender
    (D) Pregnancy

38. An 18-year-old man with no significant past medical history presents with right lower quadrant abdominal pain with associated nausea and vomiting for approximately 1 day. His vitals are T 37.9°C, P 103, BP 118/84, RR 18, and SpO$_2$ 99% on RA. His examination is significant for tenderness to palpation with guarding in the right lower quadrant and reproduction of pain in the right lower quadrant with palpation of the left lower quadrant. Labs are significant for white blood cell (WBC) 13,500. Which of the following is the MOST APPROPRIATE NEXT step?
    (A) Antiemetics and trial of oral rehydration
    (B) CT scan
    (C) Surgical consultation
    (D) Ultrasound

39. A 52-year-old woman presents with left lower quadrant pain. Her vitals are T 38.1°C, P 98, BP 132/84, RR 18, and SpO$_2$ 99% on RA. On examination, she has tenderness in the left lower quadrant. Labs are significant for white blood cell (WBC) 18,200. A CT scan with IV contrast is obtained and shows evidence of sigmoid diverticulitis with adjacent tissue inflammation and infection. Which of the following is the MOST REASONABLE NEXT step in treatment?
    (A) Admission for IV metronidazole + levofloxacin
    (B) Discharge on oral metronidazole + levofloxacin for 7 days
    (C) Placement of percutaneous drain
    (D) Repeat CT scan with oral and rectal contrast

40. Which of the following is UNLIKELY to be the cause of a fever on post-op day 3 following surgery?

(A) Pneumonia
(B) Thrombophlebitis
(C) Urinary tract infection (UTI)
(D) Wound infection

41. A 32-year-old woman with a history of morbid obesity presents 6 weeks after gastric bypass surgery complaining of nausea, diarrhea, and epigastric discomfort. She describes onset of these symptoms, as well as diaphoresis and palpitations, immediately after eating any meal. She has no symptoms between episodes. On examination, the patient is well-appearing and in no distress. Her vitals are T 37.0°C, P 76, BP 122/78, RR 18, and SpO$_2$ 99% on RA. Her abdomen is soft and nontender, and her surgical wounds are healing well. Which of the following recommendations is MOST LIKELY to help this patient's symptoms?
    (A) Consumption of small, dry meals
    (B) Drinking large amounts of fluids with meals
    (C) Treatment with antiemetics
    (D) Treatment with H$_2$ blockers

42. For which of these patients is drainage in the emergency department appropriate?
    (A) A 23-year-old pregnant woman with rectal pain that is worse with defecation and associated with a tender mass in the posterior midline that is palpable on digital rectal examination
    (B) A 45-year-old healthy man with a tender, fluctuant mass palpable at the anal verge that is more painful with sitting and immediately prior to defecation
    (C) A 55-year-old woman who presents with a tender mass just lateral to the anal verge with a large area of induration and rectal discharge
    (D) A 65-year-old man with a history of diabetes with a painful mass lateral to the anal verge with associated fever and leukocytosis

43. A 35-year-old man with history of hemorrhoids presents with rectal bleeding. Which of the following historical features should prompt further evaluation for nonhemorrhoidal etiology of the bleeding?
    (A) Bright red blood on the surface of passed stool
    (B) Itching around the anus
    (C) Passage of blood clots
    (D) Sudden onset of severe pain

44. Which of the following is TRUE regarding emergency management of rectal foreign bodies?
    (A) Following removal of a large or sharp foreign body, the patient may be immediately discharged from the emergency department.
    (B) Foreign bodies in the rectal ampulla can rarely be palpated on digital examination.
    (C) Large bulbar objects frequently create a vacuum-like effect in the rectal ampulla, making removal by simple traction difficult.
    (D) When sharp objects are suspected in the rectum, digital rectal examination is preferred over anoscopy.

45. Which of the following is the MOST COMMON type of anorectal abscess?
    (A) Intersphincteric
    (B) Ischiorectal
    (C) Perianal
    (D) Supralevator

46. Which of the following is TRUE regarding the use of ultrasound in the diagnosis of appendicitis?
    (A) A normal appendix is compressible with a maximum diameter of 6 mm.
    (B) Inflammation must be seen throughout the entire length of the appendix to diagnose appendicitis.
    (C) Sensitivity of ultrasound for detection of appendicitis is highest among obese patients.
    (D) Ultrasound has been proven to be ineffective for diagnosis in pregnant women.

47. A 58-year-old woman presents to the emergency department with left lower quadrant pain. Workup reveals diverticulitis without evidence of phlegmon, perforation, or abscess. Which of the following would be a contraindication to outpatient management?
    (A) Ability to tolerate oral intake in the emergency department
    (B) Heart rate of 80 after IV fluids
    (C) History of renal transplant
    (D) White blood cell (WBC) count of 15,000

48. A 57-year-old man presents with abdominal pain and vomiting. His vital signs are T 37°C, P 110, BP 142/88, RR 18, and SpO$_2$ 99% on RA. On examination, his abdomen is distended with high-pitched bowel sounds and diffuse tenderness. Air-fluid levels are seen on plain films. He denies any prior history of abdominal surgery, and his past medical history is significant only for hypertension. Which of the following is the MOST LIKELY cause of his condition?
    (A) Carcinoma
    (B) Diverticulosis
    (C) Inflammatory bowel disease
    (D) Inguinal hernia

49. A 22-year-old man presents with rectal pain, purulent anal discharge, and lower abdominal cramping. He admits to having receptive anal intercourse with a new partner recently, and a condom was not used. Which of the following is TRUE regarding this condition?
    (A) Nearly all patients with anorectal gonorrhea will develop these symptoms.
    (B) Patients with this condition should be tested for human immunodeficiency virus.
    (C) Stool softeners will generally worsen this condition.
    (D) Treatment should not be started until results of sexually transmitted infection testing have returned.

50. Which of the following techniques may aid in reduction of rectal prolapse?
    (A) Alternating periods of pressure with "breaks" for the patient
    (B) Application of artificial sweetener to the prolapsed segment
    (C) Application of internal rolling force using the thumbs
    (D) Having an assistant hold the buttocks together while reduction is attempted

ANSWERS

1. **The answer is A.** (Chapter 71) A low WBC count has a low predictive value for surgical disease in the elderly. Among those >80 years old, mortality almost doubles if the diagnosis is incorrect at the time of admission. Fever is not a reliable marker for serious disease, and the elderly may be hypothermic in the presence of serious abdominal infection. Surgical complications are more common: perforated viscus, gangrenous gallbladder, necrotizing pancreatitis, strangulated hernia, and infarcted bowel.

2. **The answer is D.** (Chapter 71) The presence of right lower quadrant pain in a woman who has an appendix is a common diagnostic dilemma. In general, the results of pelvic examination, consideration of patient risk factors for gynecologic versus gastrointestinal (GI) disease, and the clinician's best estimate of pretest probability for gynecologic versus GI disease are the best guides for further imaging. If pretest probability favors gynecologic disease, a transvaginal ultrasound would be the next step. If pretest probability favors GI disease or appendicitis, abdomino-pelvic CT scanning would be the next step. She does not have any peritoneal signs on her abdominal examination and therefore does not warrant a surgical consult at this time.

3. **The answer is D.** (Chapter 71) Epiploic (omental) appendages are fatty pedicular structures, typically 3 cm in length, that are found on the serosal surface of the normal colon. The cardinal sign is pain, which can mimic acute diverticulitis or acute appendicitis. In general, patients do not appear systemically ill, and fever is unusual. Nausea and vomiting are infrequent, but diarrhea has been reported in up to 25% of cases. The treatment is supportive and nonoperative. Pain control should be provided. Antibiotics are not indicated. Most cases resolve spontaneously within 1 to 2 weeks.

4. **The answer is D.** (Chapter 72) The most common cause is "idiopathic," but other causes include diabetes, bariatric and gastric surgery, viral illness, gastroesophageal reflux disease, and nonulcer dyspepsia. Connective tissue or neurologic disease, and even pregnancy, can also be associated with gastroparesis.

5. **The answer is B.** (Chapter 73) The most important initial therapy is stopping the inciting antibiotic. With the exception of aminoglycosides, almost all antibiotics have been associated with *Clostridium difficile*–associated disease. Do not give antiperistaltic medications. Surgery should be consulted for suspected toxic megacolon or intestinal perforation for consideration of colectomy. While oral metronidazole is the first-line therapy for mild to moderate disease, this is not the next best step.

6. **The answer is A.** (Chapter 73) Antibiotics shorten the duration of illness by about 24 hours. Even though most cases of infectious diarrhea are self-limited, due to the inconvenient and debilitating nature of the disease, ciprofloxacin is the recommended treatment for all patients believed to have an infectious diarrhea who do not have a contraindication to the drug (e.g., children, allergy, pregnancy, or drug interaction). Loperamide shortens the duration of symptoms when combined with an antibiotic regimen. Do not use antimotility agents in the subset of patients with bloody diarrhea or suspected inflammatory diarrhea because of the possibility of prolonged fever, toxic megacolon in *Clostridium difficile* patients, and hemolytic uremic syndrome in children infected with Shiga-toxin producing *Escherichia coli*. Probiotics are safe and beneficial when used alongside rehydration therapy.

7. **The answer is B.** (Chapter 73) Diagnosis of Crohn's disease is confirmed by colonoscopy. Pain radiographs of the abdomen may demonstrate obstruction, perforation, or toxic megacolon. Abdominal CT scanning with PO and IV contrast may identify bowel wall thickening, segmental narrowing, destruction of the normal mucosal pattern, mesenteric edema, fistulas, and abscesses. Stool studies may be useful to diagnose a specific pathogen in patients with prolonged infectious diarrhea.

8. **The answer is B.** (Chapter 73) Toxic megacolon develops in advanced cases of colitis when the disease process extends through all layers of the colon. The result is a loss of muscular tone within the colon, with dilation and localized peritonitis. Plain radiography of the abdomen demonstrates a long, continuous segment of air-filled colon greater than 6 cm in diameter. Loss of colonic haustra and "thumb printing," representing bowel wall edema, may also be seen. The distended portion of the atonic colon can perforate, causing peritonitis and septicemia. Mortality is high. Medical therapy with nasogastric suction, IV prednisolone 60 mg/d, or hydrocortisone 300 mg/d, parenteral broad-spectrum antibiotics active against coliforms and anaerobes, and IV fluids should be attempted as initial therapy, although early surgical consultation is the most important initial step.

9. **The answer is D.** (Chapter 74) Manual disimpaction is a painful procedure for which patients may require sedation. Physician resistance to manual disimpaction does the

patient a disservice, as enemas provide little or no relief. Diarrhea does not rule out fecal impaction, especially in the elderly, debilitated patient, and failure to perform a rectal examination will result in misdiagnosis. After disimpaction, prescribe a regimen of medications and medical adjuncts to properly reestablish fecal flow.

10. **The answer is D.** (Chapter 75) This patient requires emergent intubation given he has unstable vital signs and is unresponsive, with clinical concern for deterioration and airway protection. While he may require massive blood transfusion and coagulopathy correction, this should not delay management of his airway.

11. **The answer is D.** (Chapter 75) In patients with life-threatening bleeding receiving anticoagulants, reverse the coagulopathy without concern for the INR unless there are contraindications to reversal, such as cardiac or vascular stents. In less severe bleeding, carefully consider the risks of reversal therapy. An international normalized ratio (INR) ≥1.5 is a significant predictor of mortality in patients with an upper gastrointestinal (GI) bleed who are receiving anticoagulants. Reversal should not delay time to endoscopy. Tranexamic acid, an antifibrinolytic agent, has shown benefit in the management of upper GI bleeding.

12. **The answer is D.** (Chapter 76) Because blood must travel through the upper gastrointestinal (GI) tract down to the lower GI system, upper GI bleeds are the most common source for all causes of blood detected in the lower GI bleeding system. Among patients with an established lower GI source of bleeding (i.e., bleeding past the ligament of Treitz), the most common cause is diverticular disease, followed by colitis, adenomatous polyps, and malignancies.

13. **The answer is B.** (Chapter 76) Among patients with an established lower gastrointestinal source of bleeding (i.e., bleeding past the ligament of Treitz), the most common cause is diverticular disease, followed by colitis, adenomatous polyps, and malignancies.

14. **The answer is D.** (Chapter 76) Thorough examination of the rectal area may reveal an obvious source of bleeding, such as a laceration, masses, trauma, anal fissures, or external hemorrhoids. A vaginal or urinary source of bleeding mistaken for a gastrointestinal source will be identified by examination and testing. Perform a digital rectal examination to detect gross blood (either bright red or maroon) and for guaiac testing. Rectal examination can also detect the presence of masses. Anoscopy may also aid in the diagnosis. While the patient may require a complete blood count, cross-match for packed red blood cells, and a

gastroenterology consult, a rectal examination should be performed first.

15. **The answer is D.** (Chapter 77) Diffuse esophageal spasm is the intermittent interruption of normal peristalsis by nonperistaltic contraction. Therapy involves control of acid reflux and consideration of smooth muscle relaxants and/or antidepressants, although effectiveness is unclear. Dysphagia is intermittent and does not progress over time. Chest pain is a common symptom in patients with esophageal spasm.

16. **The answer is C.** (Chapter 77) Iatrogenic perforation is the most common cause of esophageal perforation. The perforation rate from endoscopy is lower in an esophagus free of disease than in a diseased esophagus. Dilation of strictures increases the risk of perforation greatly. Other intraluminal procedures, such as variceal therapy and palliative laser treatment for cancer, are also associated with perforation. Boerhaave's syndrome is full-thickness perforation of the esophagus after a sudden rise in intraesophageal pressure. The mechanism is sudden, forceful emesis in about three fourths of the cases; coughing, straining, seizures, and childbirth have been reported as causing perforations as well. Blunt or penetrating neck trauma can cause esophageal perforation. Foreign body ingestion or food impaction may result in perforation of the esophagus as well.

17. **The answer is A.** (Chapter 77) Most spontaneous perforations occur through the left posterolateral wall of the distal esophagus. Proximal perforation, seen mostly with instrumentation, tends to be less severe than distal perforation and can form a periesophageal abscess with minimal systemic toxicity.

18. **The answer is C.** (Chapter 77) If the object is distal to the pylorus, has a benign shape and nature, and the patient is comfortable and tolerating intake by mouth, treatment is expectant with outpatient follow-up. Circumstances that warrant urgent endoscopy retrieval of esophageal foreign bodies are ingestion of sharp or elongated objects (toothpicks, aluminum soda can tabs, multiple foreign body ingestion, button battery ingestion, evidence of perforation, coin at the level of the cricopharyngeus muscle in a child, airway compromise, presence of a foreign body for >24 hours).

19. **The answer is C.** (Chapter 77) Plain films are used to screen for radiopaque objects. Coins in the esophagus generally present their circular face on anteroposterior films (coronal alignment), as opposed to coins in the trachea, which show that face on lateral films.

20. **The answer is B.** (Chapter 77) A button battery lodged in the esophagus is a true emergency requiring prompt removal because the battery may quickly induce mucosal injury and necrosis. Perforation can occur within 6 hours of ingestion. Morbidity caused by the battery is likely related to the flow of electricity through a locally formed external circuit.

21. **The answer is A.** (Chapter 77) If glucagon therapy is attempted, an initial dose of 1 to 2 milligrams IV is given (for adults). If the food bolus is not passed in 20 minutes, an additional dose can be given. The use of proteolytic enzymes (e.g., Adolph's Meat Tenderizer®, which contains papain) to dissolve a meat bolus is contraindicated because of the potential for severe mucosal damage and esophageal perforation and the availability of superior alternatives. Meat is the food most commonly identified in food impaction.

22. **The answer is A.** (Chapter 77) Although not all patients with undiagnosed dyspepsia require endoscopy, those with "alarm features" do. Alarm features include age >50 years with new-onset symptoms, unexplained weight loss, persistent vomiting, dysphagia or odynophagia, iron deficiency anemia or gastrointestinal (GI) bleeding, abdominal mass or lymphadenopathy, and family history of upper GI malignancy. Alarm features raise the index of suspicion for gastric or esophageal cancer, as well as other potentially serious conditions, but the features are not specific. X-ray and CT are not reliable diagnostic tests to rule out esophageal or gastric malignancy.

23. **The answer is B.** (Chapter 78) The gold standard for the diagnosis of peptic ulcer disease is visualization of an ulcer by upper endoscopy. It is important to know how to diagnose an *Helicobacter pylori* infection because it causes most peptic ulcers, but *H. pylori* infection alone does not properly diagnose peptic ulcer disease. A CT scan or ultrasound is not sensitive for peptic ulcer disease.

24. **The answer is C.** (Chapter 78) After peptic ulcer disease is diagnosed, the goal of treatment is to heal the ulcer while relieving pain and preventing complications and recurrence. Traditional therapy includes proton pump inhibitors (PPIs), H₂ receptor antagonists (H2RAs), sucralfate, and antacids. Treatment of *Helicobacter pylori* infection, when present, dramatically decreases the recurrence rate. If nonsteroidal anti-inflammatory drug associated ulcers are present, the offending agent should be stopped whenever possible. A patient with peptic ulcer disease is at risk for bleeding or perforation.

25. **The answer is D.** (Chapter 78) Bleeding is the most common complication of peptic ulcer disease. About 400,000 patients per year are admitted to the hospital in the United States due to nonvariceal upper gastrointestinal bleeding, and peptic ulcer disease is the most common cause. Perforation and obstruction are complications of peptic ulcer disease but are not the most common.

26. **The answer is D.** (Chapter 79) This patient has gallstone pancreatitis, which generally is more common in women. Risk factors for pancreatitis include smoking, obesity, and diabetes. Excessive alcohol consumption can also lead to pancreatitis and is more common in men. Patients often present with epigastric pain radiating to the back, chest, or flanks. An elevated alanine aminotransferase (ALT) >150 U/L within 48 hours of symptoms has a >85% positive predictive value for gallstone pancreatitis. The definitive treatment for gallstone pancreatitis is an endoscopic retrograde cholangiopancreatography; however, the initial treatment for all patients with pancreatitis is fluid resuscitation. Early aggressive hydration decreases morbidity and mortality. In this patient who is septic from pancreatitis, fluid resuscitation should not be delayed for imaging studies.

27. **The answer is B.** (Chapter 79) This is an abdominal ultrasound image of the gallbladder-liver interface. This image is diagnostic for acute cholecystitis. The arrowhead is pointing to a gallstone. The asterisk shows gallbladder sludge, and the arrow shows pericholecystic fluid. If the common bile duct is >5 mm, that is consistent with common bile duct dilation, which is seen in choledocholithiasis.

28. **The answer is D.** (Chapter 84) This patient's presentation is suspicious for an incarcerated and strangulated umbilical hernia. He is in septic shock secondary to strangulation. This is a surgical emergency and requires emergent surgical consultation. Initial management includes making the patient NPO, IV fluid resuscitation, and broad-spectrum IV antibiotics, such as cefoxitin or piperacillin/tazobactam. Administration of antibiotics should not be delayed while awaiting surgical consultation.

29. **The answer is C.** (Chapter 80) Cirrhosis is the 12th leading cause of death in the United States, and hepatitis C is the leading cause of hepatic cirrhosis, followed by alcoholic liver disease. Acute liver failure is rare and most commonly caused by acetaminophen toxicity (46%). Hepatitis B as the most common infectious cause of acute liver failure.

30. **The answer is D.** (Chapter 80) Hepatorenal syndrome is a complication of cirrhosis that often accompanies spontaneous bacterial peritonitis. It can occur during acute or

chronic liver failure. There are two types of hepatorenal syndrome. Type 1 carries the worst prognosis with a median survival of 2 weeks without treatment. Type 1 hepatorenal syndrome is defined as progressive oliguria and doubling of serum creatinine over 2 weeks. Type 2 hepatorenal syndrome is characterized by a gradual renal impairment. Dialysis can be used to bridge patients to liver transplant, if they fail medical therapy.

31. **The answer is A.** (Chapter 79) This patient's presentation is most consistent with ascending cholangitis. Ascending cholangitis is a life-threatening condition associated with a high mortality. It is the result of biliary obstruction with a bacterial superinfection. Patients classically present with fevers, jaundice, and right upper quadrant pain (Charcot's triad). The patient's symptoms can progress to confusion and shock (Reynolds Pentad). The initial treatment for these patients includes inpatient admission, fluid resuscitation, early antibiotics, and emergent surgical consultation. The definitive management is endoscopic retrograde cholangiopancreatography for biliary decompression.

32. **The answer is B.** (Chapter 80) Hepatorenal syndrome is a complication of cirrhosis that accompanies spontaneous bacterial peritonitis (SBP). A diagnostic paracentesis should be performed if SBP is suspected. The recommended treatment for SBP is cefotaxime. Correcting the underlying cause of hepatorenal syndrome may reverse the process, but the definitive treatment is liver transplant. *N*-acetylcysteine is recommended for acute hepatitis from toxic causes including acetaminophen as well as non-acetaminophen medications and mushroom toxicity. Octreitide may be used for upper gastrointestinal bleeding.

33. **The answer is D.** (Chapter 80) Spontaneous bacterial peritonitis (SBP) is associated with high mortality rates. Cirrhotic patients who present with fever, chills, and abdominal pain with ascites should undergo a diagnostic paracentesis to rule out SBP. The current treatment recommendation for SBP is cefotaxime 2 g every 8 hours. Antibiotics should not be delayed for a positive culture. A PMN count >250 cells/mm^3 is diagnostic for SBP. Ampicillin in combination with an aminoglycoside is an alternative treatment; this regimen is associated with significant side effects, however, and therefore should not be considered first line. Thiamine is used to prevent Wernicke-Korsakoff encephalopathy in alcoholic cirrhosis but is not the treatment for SBP.

34. **The answer is C.** (Chapter 80) Lactulose is the current mainstay of therapy for hepatic encephalopathy. In an acidified environment, it binds to ammonia and excretes

it into the stool. It can be given orally or rectally. Spironolactone is used to treat ascites. Furosemide use does not treat hepatic encephalopathy. Antibiotics are used to treat spontaneous bacterial peritonitis but are not the first-line treatment in hepatic encephalopathy.

35. **The answer is C.** (Chapter 80) In patients with acute hepatitis, the decision for inpatient versus outpatient management can be complicated. Patients should initially be treated with fluid resuscitation, antiemetics, and pain management. Careful consideration is given to admission for pregnant women and elderly patients. In cases of acute hepatitis, patients with elevated bilirubin ≥20 mg/dL, prothrombin time (PT) of 50% above normal, hypoglycemia, low albumin, or active gastrointestinal bleeding should be admitted to the hospital for further management.

36. **The answer is B.** (Chapter 83) In general, small bowel obstruction can be managed nonoperatively, often with a nasogastric tube and intravenous fluids. In a closed-loop obstruction, however, obstruction is present on both ends of a segment of bowel, leading to a "closed loop" of bowel. In this situation, bowel contents cannot escape distally or proximally, increasing the risk of bowel necrosis and shock. Emergent surgery is necessary to relieve this obstruction.

37. **The answer is D.** (Chapter 83) Cecal volvulus, rotation of the cecum and ascending colon, is distinct from a sigmoid volvulus, which involves the sigmoid colon. This condition is found more commonly in young, thin females, and there is a higher incidence in pregnant patients. A sigmoid volvulus, in contrast, is found more frequently in patients who are elderly, bedridden, or have a psychiatric history. Although sigmoid volvulus is more common, early identification of a cecal volvulus is important as this represents a surgical emergency.

38. **The answer is C.** (Chapter 81) Based on this patient's clinical presentation, there is a high suspicion for appendicitis. In these straightforward cases, surgical consultation should be obtained early to expedite management. If imaging is recommended by the surgeon, early consultation can also provide guidance regarding the most appropriate imaging to obtain. As this patient's presentation is consistent with appendicitis, it is important that he not take in anything by mouth in anticipation of likely surgery.

39. **The answer is A.** (Chapter 82) The CT scan in this case demonstrates diverticulitis with phlegmon, making this a case of complicated diverticulitis. Although uncomplicated diverticulitis can be managed in the outpatient

setting, in diverticulitis with complications (such as phlegmon development or abscess), inpatient management is generally recommended. In cases of a phlegmon or small (<4 cm) abscess, IV antibiotics are often all that is required. For a larger abscess, percutaneous drain can be effective. Oral and rectal contrast would not provide any additional diagnostic information in this case.

40. **The answer is D.** (Chapter 87) The common causes of fever are often remembered with the mnemonic "five Ws": wind (atelectasis or pneumonia), water (urine), wound, walking (venous thrombosis), and wonder drugs (drug fever). Of these, respiratory-related issues, urinary tract infection (UTI), and thrombophlebitis are all common in the first 72 hours following surgery. In contrast, wound infections usually take longer to develop (typically 7–10 days).

41. **The answer is A.** (Chapter 87) The symptoms described in this case are consistent with dumping syndrome, a common complication after surgery in which the pylorus is removed or bypassed. Symptoms occur when stomach contents (which are hyperosmolar) are dumped into the jejunum. This leads to a rapid influx of extracellular fluid and autonomic response. The most effective treatment for this is dietary modification with separation of solids and liquids. Patients should eat small, dry meals and avoid drinking too much fluid with these meals.

42. **The answer is B.** (Chapter 85) Anorectal abscesses are common, and it is critical to distinguish between simple perianal abscesses and a more complicated perirectal abscess. A perianal abscess is superficial, easily palpable at the anal verge, and typically not associated with systemic symptoms. Perirectal abscesses, in contrast, are often extensive and complicated due to the large potential space around the rectum and communicating to the deep postanal space. This category includes ischiorectal, submucosal, intersphincteric, and supralevator abscesses. All perirectal abscesses require surgical drainage in the operating room.

43. **The answer is C.** (Chapter 85) Hemorrhoids are the most common cause of rectal bleeding. Itching and visible blood on the surface of stool are typical symptoms. Sudden severe pain is indicative of an acutely thrombosed external hemorrhoid. Passage of blood clots is extremely unusual for hemorrhoidal bleeding, so this should prompt evaluation for alternative etiology.

44. **The answer is C.** (Chapter 85) A variety of rectal foreign bodies may be encountered in the emergency department,

and proper management is important. Removal of large bulbar objects can be complicated by a vacuum-like effect in the rectal ampulla. One strategy for dealing with this is passage of a Foley catheter past the object, then filling the balloon with air. Foreign bodies in the rectum typically can be palpated on digital examination, but bodies above the rectosigmoid junction are usually not palpable. When a sharp object is suspected, anoscopy is preferred over digital exam. Following removal of a large or sharp object, the risk of laceration or perforation should be considered. Following removal, patients should undergo careful examination and x-rays to evaluate for free air. Observation for up to 12 hours to monitor for signs of perforation is suggested after removal of large or sharp foreign bodies.

45. **The answer is C.** (Chapter 85) Perianal abscess is the most common type of anorectal abscess and the only one that can be drained in the emergency department. Patients typically complain of pain that becomes worse immediately before defecation and is better after defecation. The pain may also be worsened after sitting. The abscess is palpated at the anal verge as a superficial tender mass. In contrast, perirectal abscesses, such as supralevator, ischiorectal, or intersphincteric, require drainage in the operating room. In contrast to the superficial perianal abscess, these are deeper and more complicated, and are often associated with systemic symptoms.

46. **The answer is A.** (Chapter 81) The use of ultrasound for diagnosis of appendicitis has become more common, especially in populations in which radiation should be avoided. For this reason, it is considered to be the first-line imaging study in children and pregnant women. In obese patients, this examination can be extremely challenging. When looking at ultrasound evaluation of the appendix, it is important that entire appendix be visualized as inflammation may be seen only at the distal end.

47. **The answer is C.** (Chapter 82) The majority of cases of diverticulitis are uncomplicated, and outpatient management is often appropriate. Contraindications to outpatient management include ill appearance, unstable vital signs, immunosuppression, intractable vomiting, uncontrolled pain, or severe comorbidities.

48. **The answer is D.** (Chapter 83) Adhesions following prior abdominal surgery are the most common cause of small bowel obstruction, with incarcerated groin hernias as the second most common cause. Other hernias, such as umbilical or femoral, are occasionally sites of incarceration, though this is uncommon. Diverticulitis can occasionally lead to large bowel obstruction.

49. **The answer is B.** (Chapter 85) The patient in this question is presenting with proctitis, likely due to a sexually transmitted infection. Proctitis is caused by inflammation of the rectal mucosa due to prior radiation, infection, autoimmune disorders, vasculitis, or ischemia. Infectious etiologies commonly include gonorrhea, chlamydia, syphilis, herpes simplex virus 2 (HSV-2), and human immunodeficiency virus (HIV). The majority of patients with gonococcal proctitis, however, are asymptomatic. As with most sexually transmitted infections in the emergency department, patients should be treated empirically rather than delaying treatment for confirmatory tests. Patients with HIV are at higher risk for developing proctitis, so HIV testing (with appropriate outpatient follow-up) is an important part of emergency department evaluation. Treatment of proctitis includes stool softeners, sitz baths, hygiene, and pain medication.

50. **The answer is C.** (Chapter 85) Rectal prolapse occurs when there is circumferential protrusion of the rectum through the anal canal. The prolapse can involve the mucosa only or all layers of the rectum. Prolapse can often be reduced in the emergency department with the application of gentle, continuous pressure. Internal rolling force with the fingers may aid in reduction. Taping the buttocks apart for this procedure can also help with reduction. If the rectal walls have become edematous, granulated sugar can be applied for approximately 15 minutes to reduce edema. Artificial sweeteners are not effective.

Renal and Genitourinary Disorders

8

QUESTIONS

1. An 88-year-old man presents to the emergency department with severe abdominal pain. He reports difficulty urinating over the past few weeks and has not been able to void since last night. What is MOST COMMON etiology of acute urinary retention in this demographic?
   (A) Adverse medication effect
   (B) Benign prostatic hypertrophy
   (C) Neurogenic bladder
   (D) Tumor

2. What is the clinical syndrome that results from irreversible loss of renal function?
   (A) Azotemia
   (B) End stage renal disease
   (C) Hyperammonemia
   (D) Uremia

3. A 72-year-old man with a past medical history of end-stage renal disease (ESRD) on hemodialysis presents with discomfort and discoloration over his right upper extremity fistula site. The absence of a bruit or thrill on examination should prompt what NEXT step in management?
   (A) Obtain coagulation studies
   (B) Ultrasound of fistula
   (C) Heparin administration
   (D) Local tissue plasminogen activator (tPA) injected promptly into the hemodialysis catheter

4. An 84-year-old woman with a past medical history of end-stage renal disease (ESRD) on dialysis presents from hemodialysis with brisk bleeding from her fistula. Her vitals are within normal limits. What is the MOST APPROPRIATE NEXT step in management?
   (A) Absorbable gelatin sponges or 1% zeolite (QuikClot) applied to bleeding site
   (B) Direct pressure held for at least 5 to 10 minutes
   (C) Give protamine IV, consult nephrology
   (D) Tourniquet, deep suture placement

5. What is cited as the MOST COMMON complication during hemodialysis?
   (A) Bleeding from fistula or graft site
   (B) Hyperkalemia
   (C) Hypokalemia
   (D) Hypotension

6. A 55-year-old man with a past medical history of end-stage renal disease (ESRD) on dialysis is thought to display characteristic features of dialysis dysequilibrium. Which of the following BEST describes this diagnosis?
   (A) Clinical syndrome following dialysis that presents with variable symptoms but typically headache, vomiting, ataxia that can progress to altered mental status, seizures, and death
   (B) Dizziness and hypotension during the dialysis session
   (C) Metabolic derangements following dialysis leading to nausea, vomiting, ataxia
   (D) Self-limiting gait ataxia and vertigo following dialysis

7. A 33-year-old woman G3P2 at 7 months' gestation presents to the emergency department after twisting her ankle. Her x-rays are unremarkable. A urine analysis sent from triage reveals + white blood cell (WBCs), moderate bacteria, and is positive for leukocyte esterase. The patient denies any urinary symptoms. What is the APPROPRIATE management?
   (A) Antibiotics and admission
   (B) Antibiotics, urine culture and OB follow-up
   (C) No antibiotics, discharge with OB follow-up
   (D) No antibiotics, order a urine culture

8. A 74-year-old man with a past medical history of spinal cord injury from a prior motor vehicle collision (MVC) with consequent neurogenic bladder with chronic Foley catheter presents with fatigue. His workup in the emergency department is unremarkable except for a urinalysis which reveals 90 white blood cell (WBCs), 20 red blood cells (RBCs), and leukocyte esterase positive. Does this patient have a urinary tract infection (UTI)?
   (A) Yes, he should be treated with antibiotics.
   (B) No, he should not be treated with antibiotics.
   (C) Unclear, he should be empirically treated if no other cause for his symptoms is found.
   (D) Unclear, treatment should be deferred until a urine culture returns positive.

9. Acute kidney injury is defined best by which of the following?
   (A) Decrease in renal function defined by a glomerular filtration rate (GFR) <60
   (B) Decrease in renal function defined by creatinine greater than 1.5
   (C) Decrease in renal function with need for renal replacement therapy
   (D) Decrease in renal function over hours to days resulting in accumulation of toxic metabolic waste.

10. Which of the following BEST defines an uncomplicated urinary tract infection (UTI)?
    (A) UTI in a patient with normal anatomy and genitourinary (GU) function, without significant comorbidities or recent GU tract instrumentation
    (B) UTI in nonpregnant patients
    (C) UTI in a patient with normal vitals
    (D) UTI without fever

11. An ambulance brings in an unresponsive young patient who was "found down" in his apartment by his roommate after a night of binge drinking. His serum creatine kinase level returns at nearly 12,000 IU/L. CT of the brain shows no acute findings. ECG reveals normal sinus rhythm. Which of the following evidence-based treatments should the patient definitely receive?
    (A) Aggressive hydration with isotonic saline solution IV
    (B) Alkalinization of the urine with an infusion of isotonic saline solution with sodium bicarbonate at 100 mL/h, titrate for pH >7.0
    (C) Diuresis with a loop diuretic such as furosemide 40 mg IV
    (D) Mannitol and Ringer's lactate infusion IV

12. What BEST characterizes a complicated urinary tract infection (UTI)?
    (A) UTI in adults over the age of 65
    (B) UTI with significant dysuria and frequency
    (C) UTI with fever
    (D) UTI in a patient with abnormal anatomy or function of GU tract with comorbidities that increase the risk of adverse outcomes

13. A 24-year-old man with no past medical history presents with intermittent severe right-sided flank pain. He denies any trauma. The pain radiates to his right groin. On examination his abdomen is nontender, and his urogenital examination is normal. Which is the MOST LIKELY diagnosis?
    (A) Abdominal aortic aneurysm
    (B) Nephrolithiasis
    (C) Pyelonephritis
    (D) Testicular torsion

14. What is the primary treatment for urologic stone disease within the emergency department?
    (A) Foley placement
    (B) Hydration
    (C) Pain control
    (D) Tamsulosin

15. A healthy 33-year-old woman is diagnosed in the emergency department with a 2-mm nonobstructive stone at the ureteropelvic junction. Her urine analysis shows 57 red blood cells (RBCs) but is otherwise normal. Her pain is controlled with 15 mg of Toradol. Which of the following are the MOST APPROPRIATE discharge instructions?
    (A) Pain medication as directed, strain urine and drink plenty of fluids. Follow-up with urology electively.
    (B) Pain medication as directed, strain urine and follow up with urology or primary care within 1 week. Return for high fevers, severe pain unresponsive to analgesics, or persistent nausea and vomiting.
    (C) Pain medication as directed, strain urine, urgent next day urology follow-up
    (D) Pain medication as directed, strain urine, urgent next day urology follow-up, return to emergency department if stone has not passed in 2 days.

16. A 90-year-old man with a past medical history of benign prostatic hypertrophy presents with abdominal pain and inability to urinate for the past 24 hours. A Foley catheter is placed in the emergency department. His blood chemistries reveal blood urea nitrogen (BUN) of 52 and creatinine of 2.1. His urine output has been about 350 mL/h during the first 4 hours of his emergency department stay. What is the BEST NEXT step in management?
    (A) Admit for obstructive acute kidney injury (AKI) and postobstructive diuresis
    (B) Foley to leg bag and discharge home with urology follow-up
    (C) Remove Foley catheter and discharge with urology follow-up
    (D) Remove Foley catheter, voiding trial, follow-up with urology

17. What level of elevation of creatine kinase (CK) levels is diagnostic for rhabdomyolysis?
    (A) Above 5,000 U/L
    (B) Fivefold or more elevation above the upper range of normal
    (C) Above 10,000 U/L
    (D) Any elevation above the upper range of normal

18. A 40-year-old man presents with a painful erection that has lasted for several hours. Which medication is MOST LIKELY to have caused this condition?
    (A) Metoprolol
    (B) Ranitidine
    (C) Trazodone
    (D) Zolpidem

19. You are evaluating a 67-year-old patient with no known medical history who reports a fever, shaking chills, and scrotal pain and redness that is spreading rapidly. Inspection of the area reveals the following findings (Figure 8.1). His fingerstick glucose is 354 mg/dL. A point-of-care lactate is 4.1 mmol/L. Vital signs are notable for BP 88/57, HR 105, RR 20, and T 101.7°F. In addition to broad-spectrum antibiotics and IV fluids, what is the MOST APPROPRIATE initial step in management?
    (A) Administer tetanus toxoid
    (B) Bedside ultrasound
    (C) Hyperbaric oxygen therapy
    (D) Surgical consultation

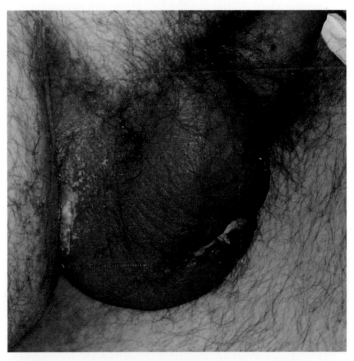

FIGURE 8.1 Reproduced with permission from J.E. Tintinalli, J.S. Stapczynski, O.J. Ma, D. Yealy, G.D. Meckler, D.M. Cline: Tintinalli's Emergency Medicine: A Comprehensive Study Guide, 9th Edition. Copyright © McGraw-Hill Education. All rights reserved.

20. A 57-year-old patient with a history of nephrolithiasis and recent ureteral stent placement presents due to lightheadedness. Vitals: T 98.7°F, HR 94, BP 112/56, RR 18, SpO$_2$ 96% on RA. Laboratory results include hemoglobin of 6.7, and a microscopic urinalysis shows 5 white blood cells (WBCs), 15 red blood cells (RBCs), and few squamous cells. What is the MOST APPROPRIATE NEXT step in management?
    (A) Admit to urology
    (B) Obtain a noncontrast CT of the abdomen and pelvis
    (C) Place three-way catheter and start continuous bladder irrigation
    (D) Send serum iron studies

21. An elderly diabetic patient with a history of chronic obstructive pulmonary disease (COPD), hypertension, chronic kidney disease, and erectile dysfunction status post placement of penile prosthesis 1 week ago presents with altered mental status and complaints of penile pain. Vital signs as follows: T 102.5°F, HR 108, BP 96/58, RR 22, SpO$_2$ 93% on RA. Inspection and palpation of the area reveals tenderness along the penile shaft. What are the key elements necessary for management of this condition?
    (A) Broad-spectrum IV antibiotics and urologic consultation for removal of device
    (B) Foley catheter placement and urologic consultation for admission
    (C) Pain management and urologic consultation for removal of device
    (D) Urologic consultation for admission and IV ceftriaxone

22. How can mumps orchitis be differentiated from testicular torsion?
    (A) Imaging
    (B) Pain
    (C) Swelling
    (D) Unilateral

23. A young boy presents with the following injury to his penis (Figure 8.2). What are the BEST potential treatments for this problem?

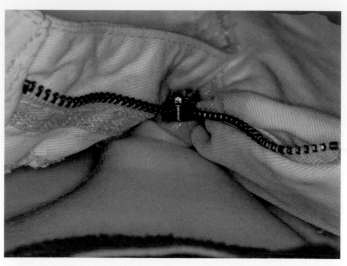

FIGURE 8.2 Photo contributor: Kevin J. Knoop, MD, MS

    (A) Analgesics, application of ice pack, transfer for urologic evaluation
    (B) Injection of lidocaine 1% plus epinephrine, use of a Kelly clamp to remove entrapped tissue
    (C) Local anesthetic, application of mineral oil or surgical lubricant, use of a wire cutter
    (D) Oral narcotic analgesia, use of a scalpel to free the affected tissue from entrapment

24. An uncircumcised male presents with penile pain for several hours that began after sexual intercourse. Examination reveals marked edema and venous engorgement of the glans penis with an inability to reduce the foreskin. What is the NEXT BEST step in emergency department management of this condition?
    (A) Urology consultation for operative intervention
    (B) Corporal aspiration of 5 mL of blood with an 18G needle at the 3 and 9 o'clock positions
    (C) IV antibiotics, analgesics, and urologic consultation for admission
    (D) Tightly wrapping the edematous glans with a 2-in elastic bandage

25. What organisms cause the majority of cases of urethritis?
    (A) *Chlamydia trachomatis* and *Neisseria gonorrhoeae*
    (B) Herpes simplex virus and human papillomavirus
    (C) *Staphylococcus aureus* and *Streptococcus pyogenes*
    (D) *Trichomonas vaginalis* and *Ureaplasma urealyticum*

ANSWERS

1. The answer is B. (Chapter 92) Although benign prostatic hypertrophy (BPH) is the most common reason for acute urinary retention in the emergency department, it is important to tease out possible factors in the history and physical examination which could point to alternative etiologies. Relevant historical factors could include a history of prostatism, nocturia, or terminal dribbling. Incontinence may be associated with BPH secondary to overflow, but symptoms like urgency, frequency, and hesitancy may occur with infectious causes as well. Infectious sources may cause accompanying fever and chills. If the patient has a history of trauma, bladder calculi, surgery, or radiation to the prostate or bladder, these facts may steer the physician toward alternative diagnostic possibilities. Common pharmacologic causes of urinary retention include anticholinergics, opiates, anesthetics, and decongestants.

2. The answer is D. (Chapter 90) The irreversible loss of renal function is called end stage renal disease (ESRD). Uremia is the clinical syndrome resulting from loss of ESRD. It is a multifaceted syndrome comprised of signs and symptoms resulting from end organ dysfunction. Azotemia is simply defined as the build-up of nitrogenous waste in the blood stream but does not imply a clinical manifestation of renal dysfunction. A broad array of signs and symptoms occur in uremia. Neurologic manifestations include, but are not limited to, altered mental status, slurred speech, seizures, paresthesias, and headaches. Common gastrointestinal features are nausea, vomiting, diarrhea, abdominal pain, and distention secondary to ascites. Anemia secondary to decreased erythropoietin levels or decreased red blood cell (RBC) count survival can manifest as chest pain, shortness of breath, fatigue. Chest pain, dyspnea, hypoxia may result from fluid overload, accelerated coronary artery disease (CAD), uremic cardiomyopathy, pericardial disease, and tamponade physiology. Excretory failure, resulting in inability to remove metabolic waste through the urine and buildup of toxins within the plasma, is the leading hypothesis behind the pathophysiology of uremia. Over 70 toxins are reported. Many of these are protein bound, are not removed through dialysis and thought to play on causal role in end organ system dysfunction. The loss of renally produced hormones plays an additional role in production of the clinical syndrome of uremia. Lack of erythropoietin, which stimulates RBC production, results in anemia. Kidneys also synthesize and release 1 alpha hydroxylase. Without this hormone, the active form of vitamin D is not available. This decrease gut calcium absorption consequently elevates parathyroid hormone and causes renal

bone disease. Free radical formation increases in the uremic state, which has been linked to development of atherosclerosis and amyloid formation.

3. The answer is B. (Chapter 90) Doppler ultrasound should be the first diagnostic step when evaluating a fistula site with absent bruit or thrill. Complications of vascular access in patients with end-stage renal disease (ESRD) account for the most inpatient hospital days. The most common complications within this subset of patients is infection and vascular pathology. Inadequate flow within the vascular access is frequently due to stenosis or thrombosis. Both complications clinically present with loss of a bruit or thrill on examination. Treatment options if thrombosis or significant stenosis is present include clot removal, angioplasty, or local tPA injection. Management of the above complications should involve consultation with vascular surgery. While laboratory results may help guide decisions, they should not be solely relied upon for diagnosis. Coagulation studies would not be the first step in management in this case. Anticoagulation with heparin or local alteplase is not indicated without first establishing the diagnosis. If local tissue plasminogen activator (tPA) is to be given for acute fistula thrombosis, it should be discussed and given after consultation with vascular surgery.

4. The answer is B. (Chapter 90) Manual direct pressure is the first step in management of acute hemorrhage of a vascular access site. Acute bleeding from a fistula site can be life threatening. Anticoagulation, aneurysmal bleeding, and anastomosis rupture are common causes of hemorrhage. When presented with acute hemorrhage, direct pressure should first be held for 5 to 10 minutes. Some emergency departments have clips designed to apply direct pressure. Additional treatments include application of sponges soaked in reconstituted thrombin or chemical thrombotics to the hemorrhage site. Protamine administration can be given to reverse heparin given during dialysis. Local lidocaine with epinephrine can be administered to be site. A deep suture can be placed. A tourniquet can be applied proximally to the vascular access if the above methods have failed. If a tourniquet has been placed, vascular surgery should be emergently consulted as this is a temporizing method.

5. The answer is D. (Chapter 90) Hypotension is the most common complication to occur during dialysis. It can occur in approximately 50% of dialysis sessions. During dialysis, through the process of ultrafiltration, 1 to 3 L of fluid is typically removed. Rates of fluid removal can vary; however, it can occur as quickly as 2 L/h. As fluid is dialyzed from the patient, blood pressure maintenance is managed by compensatory action of the cardiovascular system and fluid shifts to the intravascular space from the interstitial and intracellular compartments. Excessive extrafiltration, secondary to inaccurate dry weight estimation is the most common etiology of hypotension during dialysis. Bleeding from the vascular access site also occurs and is a known complication of dialysis. Heparin is administered during dialysis to keep the access patent. Electrolyte derangements such as hypercalcemia and hypermagnesemia are an additional complication that can arise. Typically, electrolyte abnormalities stem from improper dialysate concentrations.

6. **The answer is A.** (Chapter 90) Dialysis dysequilibrium syndrome is a clinical entity occurring at the end of dialysis. If large solute clearances occur during dialysis, cerebral edema can develop as a result of osmolar imbalance between the blood-brain barrier. This manifests clinically as a wide array of symptoms and signs but typical symptoms include nausea, headaches, dizziness, and confusion. Signs include vomiting, altered mental status, seizures, hypertension. Seizures and death can result. Treatment includes stopping dialysis and administration of IV mannitol.

7. **The answer is B.** (Chapters 91 and 99) The patient has asymptomatic bacteriuria. Despite lack of symptoms, in a pregnant patient it is recommended to treat with antibiotics and send the urine for culture. Treatment with antibiotics is suggested in order to prevent low birth weight and pyelonephritis, which can theoretically result in preterm labor or sepsis. Pregnancy increases the inherent risk of urinary tract infection (UTI) due to the physiologic changes of the genitourinary (GU) tract leading to urinary stasis. Organisms responsible for most UTIs in pregnancy are similar to the general population. Asymptomatic bacteriuria can be treated with a cephalosporin, nitrofurantoin, or trimethoprim sulfamethoxazole. It is recommended that nitrofurantoin and trimethoprim sulfamethoxazole be used as first line in the second and third trimesters.

8. **The answer is C.** (Chapter 95) Catheter-associated urinary tract infections (UTIs) are a common nosocomial infection. Bacteriuria is near universal by 30 days of catheter placement. The urinary tract is exposed to pathogens by bacteria that build up within the lumen of the catheter or along the outer surface. Biofilm formation is the first step to infection. Once formed, pathogenic bacteria in the biofilm are protected from elimination by the flow of urine and the immune system. Catheter-associated UTI should be suspected not only in cases of classic symptoms

of fever, dysuria, hematuria, pelvic discomfort, or flank pain but also in cases of atypical and nonspecific symptoms such as altered mental status, weakness, malaise, and fatigue or lethargy. Guidelines suggest such patients should be treated with antibiotics if no other cause for the symptoms is identified in the workup. Patients who have suffered a spinal cord injury may present with increased spasticity or autonomic dysreflexia as well. Treatment includes removal and replacement of the Foley if necessary and antibiotics.

9. **The answer is D.** (Chapter 88) Acute kidney injury (AKI) is the loss of renal function over time resulting in the loss of internal homeostasis and build-up of metabolic waste. The Acute Kidney Injury Network (AKIN) and Risk, Injury, Failure, Loss, Endstage (RIFLE) are two classification systems that have numerical definitions of AKI. However, these established criteria are relative to the patient's baseline, rather than specific laboratory value definitions.

10. **The answer is A.** (Chapter 91) An uncomplicated urinary tract infection (UTI) is an infection of the urinary tract in a patient with normal genitourinary anatomy and physiology. In addition, the patient must not have significant comorbidities that would increase the risk of adverse outcomes. There must be no recent history of instrumentation of the genitourinary tract. Pyelonephritis in and of itself does not automatically define a UTI as complicated. The presence or absence of a fever alone is not within the strict definition of complicated or uncomplicated UTI. A complicated UTI can exist in a patient with normal vitals.

11. **The answer is A.** (Chapter 89) Aggressive hydration with saline solution is the mainstay of treatment for rhabdomyolysis. There are no prospective controlled trials showing a benefit for the use of bicarbonate for alkalinization of the urine, and mannitol may be harmful due to forced osmotic diuresis in hypovolemic patients. Ringer's lactate contains potassium, and patients with rhabdomyolysis typically are hyperkalemic due to release of intracellular potassium into the bloodstream with muscle injury. Normal saline infusion should be titrated for urine output of greater than 200 mL/h.

12. **The answer is D.** (Chapter 91) A complicated urinary tract infection (UTI) is defined as an infection of genitourinary (GU) tract in a patient with abnormal anatomy or physiology of the renal system and with comorbidities that place the patient at risk of adverse outcomes. Complicated UTI is not defined by clinical symptoms. Advanced age is a risk factor for complicated UTI but does not define it.

13. **The answer is D.** (Chapter 94) Nephrolithiasis is the most likely diagnosis. The typical constellation of symptoms includes intermittent flank pain that radiates to the groin. Pain is usually acute in onset. Of note, patients may present with tenderness, guarding or rigidity on abdominal examination. Patients appear uncomfortable and may writhe in discomfort. Nausea and vomiting are commonly associated with bouts of pain. The location of the pain may correlate with the location of the stone with upper ureter stones referring to the flank, mid-ureter to the left lower abdominal quadrant and distal ureter to the groin. Testicular torsion is on the differential; however, this would classically be associated with abnormal testicular lie, loss of cremasteric reflex, and lack of flank pain. An abdominal aortic aneurysm would be unusual in a 24-year-old. This diagnosis can present with flank or abdominal pain mimicking nephrolithiasis but typically in patients older than 50 years. Risk factors for AAA include age >50, smoking, hypertension, family history, and connective tissue disorders. Pyelonephritis should be suspected in a patient presenting with urinary symptoms plus associated symptoms such as fevers, nausea, vomiting, or flank pain.

14. **The answer is C.** (Chapter 94) Pain control is the mainstay of treatment for nephrolithiasis. Supportive care also includes antiemetics for nausea and vomiting. Nonsteroidal anti-inflammatory drugs (NSAIDs) are the recommended first-line treatment in those without contraindications because of their direct effect on the ureter. By inhibiting prostaglandin synthesis, NSAIDs target the source of pain. Additional pain control, including narcotics, may be required in the emergency department. Fluids have not been shown to result in any difference in stone passage or pain control. Consider fluid administration to correct a fluid deficit if the patient experienced significant vomiting. A Foley catheter does not play a role in the acute management of nephrolithiasis. Medical expulsive therapy with tamsulosin can be considered as adjunctive treatment. The literature is mixed regarding efficacy, but it may have an effect on stone passage depending on stone size.

15. **The answer is B.** (Chapter 94) Discharging patients with nephrolithiasis is appropriate if the stone is small enough to likely pass spontaneously, pain is controlled by oral analgesics and there are no signs of significant infection. After discharge, patients can strain their urine in order to capture a stone for potential analysis. Prescriptions for oral analgesics and medical expulsive therapy should be given. Return precautions should include severe unrelenting pain, fevers, and persistent vomiting. Urology or primary care follow-up within 1 week is appropriate.

Patient education is important. They should be aware that stone passage rates are variable depending on stone size and the location. Larger kidney stones may take up to 30 days to pass.

16. **The answer is A.** (Chapter 92) The patient in this scenario should be admitted for two reasons. First, patients with acute kidney injury secondary to obstruction should be hospitalized to trend renal function. In addition, the patient is this scenario is displaying evidence of postobstructive diuresis. After Foley catheter placement, urine output should be measured for 4 hours. If urine output exceeds 200 mL/h, the patient should be admitted for volume replacement matching urinary loss. A majority of patients with acute urinary retention relieved by Foley catheter placement can be discharged. If no significant acute kidney injury (AKI) or postobstructive diuresis is present, a leg bag can be placed and the patient can go home and follow up with urology in the next 3 to 7 days. If the patient is able to be discharged, they should be educated on Foley catheter care and given strict return precautions including returning to the emergency department for abdominal pain, penile pain, fevers, or catheter dysfunction.

17. **The answer is B.** (Chapter 89) Creatine kinase levels are the most sensitive assay for muscle injury that causing rhabdomyolysis. The normal range of creatine kinase levels goes up to approximately 200 U/L. Mild elevations of creatine kinase levels do not meet the definition for rhabdomyolysis and do not require treatment as such. Levels fivefold or greater warrant treatment.

18. **The answer is C.** (Chapter 93) The antidepressant trazodone, also commonly used to treat insomnia, is known to cause low-flow priapism. Metoprolol is not one of the antihypertensives that is typically associated with priapism; hydralazine, prazosin, and calcium channel blockers. Likewise, zolpidem is not one of the neuroleptic medications that are most associated with priapism; however, other similar medications such as sertraline and hydroxyzine are. Aside from medications, priapism can also be caused by drugs of abuse, spinal cord tumors, toxic exposures such as rabies or black widow bites, penile trauma, sickle cell disease, or leukemia.

19. **The answer is D.** (Chapter 93) In Fournier's gangrene, urgent surgical consultation is of critical importance in the treatment plan. The other key elements are aggressive fluid resuscitation and broad-spectrum antibiotics. The diagnosis of Fournier's gangrene is typically made clinically, and computed tomography or other imaging

should not delay operative intervention, since any delay potentially allows for worsening of the rapid progression of necrosis.

20. **The answer is B.** (Chapter 95) Acute anemia in the setting of a recent ureteral stent placement procedure should prompt concern for a retroperitoneal hematoma, which can be evaluated by CT scan. Admission to urology without a definitive diagnosis of this complication would not be optimal for management. Iron studies are not typically useful in the emergency department setting. The number of red blood cells noted on this urinalysis do not suggest gross hematuria that would necessitate continuous bladder irrigation.

21. **The answer is A.** (Chapter 95) This patient has evidence of sepsis secondary to the placement of a penile prosthetic device. The definitive treatment is removal of the device. The most common organisms including gram-positive organisms such as *Staphylococcus aureus* and gram-negative bacilli. Broad-spectrum antibiotic coverage is appropriate. Ceftriaxone will cover gram-negative organisms but is not adequate coverage in sepsis potentially caused by *S. aureus*. Foley catheter placement is not necessary in this patient based on the information provided. Urologic consultation is necessary as patients with a prosthetic device as the cause of serious infection will require device removal. Admission with pain management only and no antibiotic treatment would not be adequate.

22. **The answer is A.** (Chapter 93) Mumps orchitis and testicular torsion can present in a very similar fashion, with unilateral testicular pain, tenderness, and swelling. Both can be quite painful. Imaging can aid in the diagnosis of testicular torsion. Decreased vascular flow to the testicle can be seen on ultrasound.

23. **The answer is C.** (Chapter 93) Zipper entrapment of the penis or scrotum is the most common genital injury in male pediatric patients. Local anesthetic can be used, and then it is recommended to attempt application of a non-toxic lubricant to ease removal of the zipper. If this alone is not effective, a wire cutter can be used to cut the median bar of the zipper, which is easily accessible in the case of the image provided. If only the zipper teeth are involved, a cut can be made to the cloth in between the teeth to release the zipper. Use of a scalpel on the entrapped tissue should not be necessary. Lidocaine with epinephrine is generally avoided in penile injuries.

24. **The answer is D.** (Chapter 93) A paraphimosis is a true urologic emergency, and an EM physician must be prepared to address this without assistance from a urologist if one is not immediately available. Wrapping the glans with a 2-in bandage can reduce edema, allowing the foreskin to become reducible. Other methods that can be tried include manual pressure to reduce glans edema, local anesthetic injection, and, as a final measure if the initial attempts are unsuccessful, superficial dorsal incision of the constricting band to prevent tissue necrosis. Urologic referral is necessary even if the foreskin is reduced, as the paraphimosis can recur unless surgically addressed. Corporal aspiration is the treatment for priapism.

25. **The answer is A.** (Chapter 93) The diagnosis of urethritis is clinically made, through presentation with purulent discharge from the urethra. Most cases are secondary to gonorrhea and chlamydia, and as such, the best empiric treatment is ceftriaxone 250 mg intramuscular (IM) and 1 g azithromycin orally or 100 mg doxycycline twice daily for 10 days. The other sexually transmitted diseases listed are less common causes of urethritis. Staph and strep are not common causes of urethritis.

Obstetrics and Gynecology

9

QUESTIONS

1. A 45-year-old woman presents with 5 days of lower abdominal pain and vaginal bleeding. She has a recent history of irregular, heavy menstrual bleeding and went through 5 tampons today. Her vital signs are BP 100/55, HR 95, RR 18, and T 98.7°F. Her hemoglobin is 11.2 g/dL. What is the NEXT BEST step in her management plan?
   (A) Order a factor VIII clotting activity, and if normal, discharge with outpatient gynecology follow-up
   (B) Obtain a pelvic ultrasound, and if negative, discharge with oral progestin and gynecology follow-up
   (C) Order a pregnancy test, and if negative and nothing seen on pelvic examination, discharge with gynecology follow-up for an endometrial biopsy
   (D) Perform a pelvic examination, and if she isn't passing clots, discharge with oral progestin

2. A 27-year-old nonpregnant, healthy woman presents with 2 days of light-headedness and heavy vaginal bleeding, soaking through two pads per hour for the past 4 to 5 hours. Her menstrual periods are usually regular. Her vital signs are BP 90/40, HR 120, RR 20, and T 98.2°F. On pelvic examination she has bleeding from her cervical os and is passing clots. You initiate fluid resuscitation and blood transfusion. What is recommended as the NEXT BEST therapy?
   (A) Estrogen
   (B) Tranexamic acid
   (C) Vaginal packing
   (D) Vasopressin

3. A 16-year-old young woman presents with 2 days of vaginal bleeding and discharge without abdominal pain. Her last menstrual period was 3 weeks ago, and her menses are typically every 28 days. Her vital signs are unremarkable, and her urine pregnancy test is negative. Which of the following is TRUE about managing this patient?
   (A) A speculum examination is contraindicated in adolescents with intact hymen.
   (B) Bleeding disorders are the most common cause of abnormal uterine bleeding in adolescents.
   (C) Consider sexual abuse in an adolescent patient with suspected sexually transmitted infection.
   (D) Pelvic infections are the most common cause of abnormal uterine bleeding in adolescents.

4. A 37-year-old woman who was started on Clomid last week for infertility presents with diffuse abdominal pain, abdominal distension, and shortness of breath. No prior surgical history. She is hemodynamically stable. Her urine pregnancy test is positive. What is the NEXT BEST test in her management plan?
   (A) Abdominal CT
   (B) Beta-human chorionic gonadotropin (β-hCG) level
   (C) Chest CT
   (D) Focused assessment sonography in trauma (FAST)

5. A 25-year-old woman presents with diffuse abdominal pain, nausea, fatigue, and malaise. No dysuria or vaginal discharge. This is her third emergency department visit for similar symptoms in 3 weeks. She is concerned that she may be pregnant. Her urine pregnancy test is negative. and she has mild diffuse abdominal tenderness on examination. After controlling her pain, which of the following is the NEXT BEST step in her management plan?
   (A) Assess for potential physical or sexual abuse
   (B) Discharge the patient with primary care doctor follow-up
   (C) Order a pelvic ultrasound
   (D) Order an abdominal-pelvic CT

6. A 38-year-old woman presents with 2 days of constant right lower abdominal pain, which started after returning home from the gym. On examination she has right lower quadrant tenderness and no adnexal or cervical motion tenderness. Her urine pregnancy test is negative. Which of the following is TRUE about her presentation and management?
   (A) Positive urinalysis indicates they pain is from a urinary tract infection.
   (B) Presence of ovarian arterial flow alone on transvaginal pelvic ultrasound excludes ovarian torsion.
   (C) Risk factors for ovarian torsion include pregnancy, infertility treatments, and history of ovarian cysts.
   (D) Unremarkable pelvic examination excludes ovarian torsion as the cause of her pain.

7. A 42-year-old woman, G1P0, estimated gestational age 6 weeks by last menstrual period, presents with sudden-onset, right-sided, lower abdominal pain and vaginal bleeding. She has been treated with Clomid for infertility. Her vital signs and pelvic examination are unremarkable. Her beta-human chorionic gonadotropin (β-hCG) is 5580. Her bedside transabdominal ultrasound shows an intrauterine pregnancy with a small subchorionic hemorrhage. What is the NEXT BEST in your management plan?
   (A) Discharge home with instructions to return in 2 days for repeat β-hCG
   (B) Discharge home with obstetrics clinic follow-up within the week
   (C) Immediate obstetrics consultation for laparoscopy
   (D) Perform a bedside transvaginal ultrasound

8. A 32-year-old woman, G4P3, estimated gestational age 10 weeks based on last menstrual period, who presents with heavy vaginal bleeding, passing clots, and crampy lower abdominal pain for 3 days. Her vital signs are stable, she is afebrile, and her pelvic examination shows some mild bleeding from a closed cervical os. Her hemoglobin is 11 g/dL and her beta-human chorionic gonadotropin (β-hCG) is 560 mIU/mL. Her bedside transvaginal ultrasound shows a thickened uterine stripe without any heterogeneous material. What is her MOST LIKELY diagnosis?
   (A) Complete abortion
   (B) Incomplete abortion
   (C) Inevitable abortion
   (D) Septic abortion

9. A 29-year-old woman had a syncopal episode and presents with severe lower abdominal pain. Her vital signs are BP 95/57, HR 65, RR 20, and T 98.2°F. Her beta-human chorionic gonadotropin (β-hCG) is 1575 mIU/mL (Figure 9.1). She is Rh positive. Bedside ultrasound was performed. Which management plan is MOST APPROPRIATE?

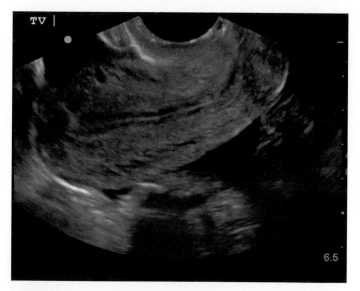

FIGURE 9.1 Photo contributor: Lauren Oliveira, DO.

   (A) Administer methotrexate
   (B) Consult OB/GYN immediately
   (C) Discharge with outpatient obstetrics follow-up in 1 week for repeat ultrasound
   (D) Discharge with outpatient obstetrics follow-up in 2 days for repeat β-hCG level

10. A 35-year-old woman with history of irregular menses presents with left lower abdominal pain and spotting on the toilet paper with wiping. She has no prior history of sexually transmitted infections or prior surgeries. Her vital signs are BP 117/75, HR 78, RR 16, and T 98.4°F. Her examination shows mild left adnexal tenderness, no masses. Serum beta-human chorionic gonadotropin (β-hCG) is 5780 mIU/mL. She is Rh positive. Which ultrasound finding would make you comfortable discharging her with outpatient OB/GYN follow-up?
    (A) A yolk sac within a larger sac surrounded by 5 mm of myometrium
    (B) An empty intrauterine sac without a yolk sac or fetal pole
    (C) An intrauterine mass with solid and cystic components, with a snowstorm appearance
    (D) Thickened uterine stripe without a gestational sac

11. A 27-year-old woman presents with vaginal bleeding and lower abdominal pain. Her last menstrual period is unknown. Her urine human chorionic gonadotropin (hCG) is positive. Which of the following features increase her risk of ectopic pregnancy?
    (A) Alcohol use
    (B) History of ovarian cyst
    (C) Multiple sexual partners
    (D) Young maternal age

12. A 30-year-old pregnant woman in her third trimester presents to the emergency department for care. Which of the following treatments for the paired condition should you avoid because of her pregnancy?
    (A) Epinephrine—status asthmaticus
    (B) Insulin drip—diabetic ketoacidosis
    (C) Low molecular weight heparin—pulmonary embolism
    (D) Synchronized cardioversion—unstable atrial fibrillation with rapid ventricular response

13. A 35-year-old woman who delivered a healthy baby 2 weeks ago presents after having a seizure and complaining of a severe right-sided headache. She has a history of migraine headaches. She has no prenatal or delivery complications. Her vital signs are BP 150/90, HR 87, RR 20, and T 98.7°F. She is sleepy, but wakes to voice, follows commands appropriately, and moves all extremities symmetrically. Which of the following would be the BEST INITIAL treatment for her symptoms?

(A) Labetalol
(B) Low-molecular-weight heparin (LMWH)
(C) Magnesium
(D) Metoclopramide

14. A 28-year-old woman, G1P0 at 35 5/7 weeks' gestation presents with leakage of clear fluid down her legs. She has no abdominal pain, vaginal bleeding, or fever. She is hemodynamically stable and has no abdominal tenderness. On speculum examination you see a closed cervical os, no vaginal bleeding, with scant pooling of fluid. Which of the following findings on microscopy will make you obtain an emergent obstetrics consultation?
    (A) Arborization pattern
    (B) Uniflagellar motile organism
    (C) Pseudohyphae
    (D) Rod-shaped bacteria

15. A 37-year-old woman, G2P1, estimated gestational age at 30 weeks, presents with acute shortness of breath and chest pain. Her chest pain is right sided, worse with deep breathing. She has bilateral leg edema. She is otherwise healthy. Her vital signs are BP 130/75, HR 104, RR 24, and SpO$_2$ 100% on RA. She has a normal pulmonary examination, no abdominal tenderness, bilateral lower extremity edema (right more than left), but no calf tenderness. Which of the following is the BEST initial test to help guide her management?
    (A) Chest CT pulmonary angiography
    (B) D-dimer assay
    (C) Pulmonary perfusion scan
    (D) Ultrasonography of the lower extremities

16. A 38-year-old woman in her third trimester presents with diffuse abdominal pain and no vaginal bleeding or gush of fluid. Her vital signs are BP 106/70, HR 95, RR 22, and T 98.4°F. Which of the following statements is TRUE?
    (A) Digital and speculum examination should be a routine part of her initial examination
    (B) HELLP (hemolysis, elevated liver enzymes, and low platelets) syndrome may present initially without high blood pressure
    (C) Placental abruption is excluded by the absence of vaginal bleeding
    (D) Premature rupture of membranes is excluded if her examination shows no leakage of fluid from the cervix or pooling of fluid in the vagina

17. What is the correct sequence of the cardinal movements of a normal vaginal delivery?
    (A) Engagement, extension, descent, external rotation, flexion, and internal rotation
    (B) Engagement, flexion, descent, internal rotation, extension, and external rotation
    (C) Flexion, engagement, internal rotation, descent, extension, and external rotation
    (D) Descent, flexion, engagement, external rotation, extension, and internal rotation

18. A 28-year-old woman, G1P0, estimated gestational age 37 weeks, presents with irregular abdominal contractions and no vaginal bleeding or gush of fluid. Which of the following fetal heart tracings is MOST reassuring?
    (A) Consistent fetal heart rate around 140 to 150, with a drop in heart rate near the end of a uterine contraction, then a slow return to baseline
    (B) Drops in fetal heart rate that occur just after uterine contractions, with a return to baseline heart rate
    (C) Fetal heart rate drops to 60 after a contraction without a return to baseline after contraction ends
    (D) Fetal heart rate fluctuates between 120 and 170 with brief accelerations in heart rate

19. A 30-year-old woman delivered a healthy baby vaginally. You deliver the placenta easily, and within about 5 minutes, you notice active bleeding from the vagina. Which of the following is the MOST APPROPRIATE first step?
    (A) Administer oxytocin
    (B) Massage the uterine fundus
    (C) Pack the vaginal vault
    (D) Suture the perineal laceration immediately

20. A 20-year-old healthy woman presents with vaginal discharge and itching. She has a red, inflamed cervix and malodorous, frothy vaginal discharge. Her vaginal fluid on microscopy shows the following organism (Figure 9.2). Which of the following historical features increases her risk for significant adverse health outcomes if this condition is untreated?

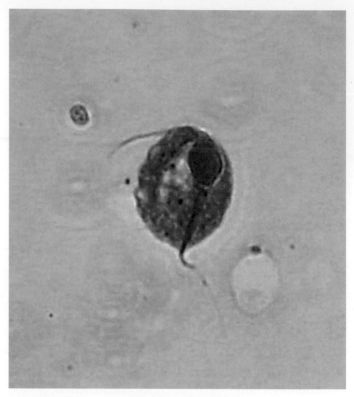

FIGURE 9.2 Reprinted with permission of Piotr Rotkiewicz.

    (A) Concurrent gonorrhea or chlamydia infection
    (B) Diabetes
    (C) History of multiple sexual partners
    (D) Pregnancy

21. A 20-year-old woman presents with vaginal discharge and itching for 3 days. On examination, she has thick white "cottage cheese" discharge, some of which adheres to the vaginal walls. Her last menstrual period was 3 weeks ago. Her pregnancy test is negative. On microscopy, you see vaginal epithelial cells and some bacteria, but no budding yeast or pseudohyphae. What is the BEST NEXT step in her management?
    (A) Ceftriaxone IM and azithromycin PO
    (B) Fluconazole PO
    (C) Metronidazole PO
    (D) Send and wait for *Candida* cultures and treat only if positive

22. A 25-year-old woman presents with perineal pain. She has no fever and no history of trauma. The patient has one sexual partner. Her external vaginal examination is shown in Figure 9.3. How would you best manage this patient?

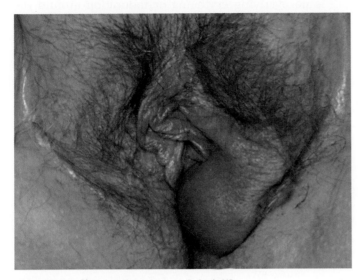

FIGURE 9.3 Photo contributor: Lawrence B. Stack, MD.

(A) Antibiotic treatment targeting chlamydia and gonorrhea, then refer to gynecology for marsupialization
(B) Broad-spectrum antibiotics treatment and sitz baths
(C) Incision and drainage, followed by packing placement
(D) Incision and drainage, followed by Word catheter placement, and oral antibiotics

23. A 32-year-old woman presents with lower abdominal pain, right upper quadrant (RUQ) abdominal pain, and abnormal vaginal discharge. She has a negative pregnancy test. On examination she has tenderness in the right upper quadrant and cervical motion tenderness, but no adnexal tenderness. Which of the following management plans is controversial?
(A) Empiric treatment with antibiotics prior to culture results
(B) Immediate intrauterine device (IUD) removal
(C) Perform bedside RUQ ultrasound to exclude biliary disease causing her symptoms
(D) Testing for concurrent human immunodeficiency virus (HIV), syphilis, and bacterial vaginosis infections

24. A 20-year-old woman presents with copious vaginal discharge and lower abdominal pain. She has cervical motion tenderness and lower abdominal tenderness on examination. You treat her with ceftriaxone IM and doxycycline for 2 weeks. She asks you how she may decrease her risk of this infection. What is your recommendation?
(A) Avoid getting pregnant
(B) Ask her gynecologist to insert an intrauterine device
(C) Have her sexual partner be treated for urethritis
(D) Use vaginal douching more frequently

25. A 29-year-old woman presents with lower abdominal pain, mild postcoital vaginal bleeding, and dysuria. Her vital signs are normal. She has suprapubic abdominal tenderness, left adnexal tenderness, and cervical motion tenderness. Her last menstrual period was 3 weeks ago. Which diagnostic test would be MOST helpful for prioritizing her differential diagnosis?
(A) No testing necessary, begin empiric treatment for pelvic inflammatory disease
(B) Obtain pelvic ultrasound
(C) Order a urinalysis
(D) Order a urine beta-human chorionic gonadotropin (β-hCG)

26. A 28-year-old woman, G1P1, presents with 1 week of bilateral breast pain, worse during breastfeeding, worse on the right breast. She is afebrile, and her right breast shows a well-circumscribed, indurated area of erythema around her areola. An ultrasound of her breast shows a cobblestone appearance of the subcutaneous tissue but no fluid collection. Which of the following statements is TRUE about her management plan?
(A) She may be discharged with directions to use warm compresses and continue to breastfeed.
(B) She may be discharged with cephalexin for 7 days and continue to breastfeed.
(C) She may be discharged with lanolin cream and breast shields.
(D) She should start using a breast pump to improve breast emptying.

27. A 31-year-old woman presents with 1 week of right breast pain, swelling, and redness. There is no discharge from the nipple. She is not breastfeeding. On examination her vital signs are normal, and she has a well-circumscribed, tender, indurated, area of erythema just underneath her right nipple. No discharge is noted. Her bedside ultrasound shows a heterogenous hypoechoic area in the subcutaneous tissue. Which of the following statements is TRUE about her management?
    (A) Admit for IV antibiotics and immediate surgical consultation
    (B) If no improvement with oral antibiotics, refer for a breast biopsy
    (C) Incision and drainage followed by antibiotics for 7 days
    (D) US-guided needle aspiration

28. A 34-year-old woman presents with lower abdominal pain and vaginal spotting. She has recently undergone a gynecologic procedure. In which of these patients should you defer the pelvic examination until after consulting with a gynecologist?
    (A) In the patient who just had an abdominal hysterectomy
    (B) In the patient who just had a vaginal hysterectomy
    (C) In the patient who just had a dilatation and curettage
    (D) In the patient who is undergoing fertility treatment

29. A 48-year-old woman presents with diffuse severe abdominal pain, vomiting, and subjective fever. She had a laparoscopic myomectomy 3 days prior. On examination, she is febrile with predominant, diffuse abdominal pain, and guarding with palpation. There is no overlying erythema or induration around the incision sites. Which of the following complications of the laparoscopic surgery should be highest on your differential diagnosis?
    (A) Bowel injury
    (B) Bowel obstruction
    (C) Postoperative surgical infection
    (D) Vascular injury with postoperative hematoma

30. A 58-year-old woman presents with lower abdominal pain after an abdominal total hysterectomy and bilateral oophorectomy. Which of the following statements is TRUE about the complications of her surgery?
    (A) Genitourinary injuries are uncommon and often go unrecognized until several weeks after surgery.
    (B) Pelvic pathology is uncommon after a hysterectomy, so a pelvic examination is not helpful for diagnosis.
    (C) Wound dehiscence occurs most commonly after 2 postoperative weeks and presents with a tearing sensation, followed by serosanguineous discharge from the incision.
    (D) Wound infections occur within the first 2 postoperative weeks and may require hospital admission and IV antibiotics.

ANSWERS

1. **The answer is C.** (Chapter 96) The best initial test in a woman of reproductive age with vaginal bleeding is a pregnancy test to exclude pregnancy-related causes of bleeding. This patient is hemodynamically stable, with mild anemia that would not require transfusion. If she's not pregnant, she could be discharged with outpatient gynecology clinic follow-up. With her recent history of irregular menstrual bleeding, she may be perimenopausal or at higher risk of endometrial hyperplasia or adenocarcinoma, so she should receive an endometrial biopsy to exclude malignancy prior to starting any oral contraceptives to control the bleeding. Pelvic examination would be appropriate for a nonpregnant woman with stable menstrual bleeding. Checking factor VIII clotting activity would be more relevant if the patient were a young adult. While 20% of young women with heavy menstrual bleeding have an underlying coagulation disorder, with von Willebrand's disease being most common, it would be unusual for a 45-year-old woman not to have experienced some complication of the disease prior to this episode. Imaging to exclude structural uterine diseases that may cause abnormal, heavy bleeding or other etiologies for abdominal pain would be most appropriate after excluding pregnancy.

2. **The answer is A.** (Chapter 96) This patient has unstable vital signs and heavy vaginal bleeding. In addition to blood transfusion, IV conjugated estrogen is the first-line medical management for acute uterine bleeding in patients without an underlying coagulopathy. Vasopressin may be given to patients with von Willebrand's disease who have uterine bleeding but is not considered first-line therapy for patients without underlying coagulopathy. Vaginal packing is not recommended for uterine bleeding, because it increases the risk of infection and may hide ongoing blood loss. Tranexamic acid (a lysine derivative that prevents fibrin degradation) has been shown to decrease uterine bleeding. However, it is primarily used for intraoperative bleeding and is not yet considered first-line therapy.

3. **The answer is C.** (Chapter 96) In an adolescent patient with suspected sexually transmitted infection or abnormal vaginal bleeding, sexual abuse and sexual trauma should be considered, by taking a private, detailed sexual history. A pediatric speculum examination can usually be tolerated even in adolescents with intact hymen. Bleeding disorders and pelvic infections need to be considered in the differential diagnosis for adolescents with abnormal uterine bleeding, but anovulatory bleeding is still the most common cause of bleeding in this age group.

4. **The answer is D.** (Chapter 97) The next best test is a focused assessment sonography in trauma (FAST) to look for pleural effusion, pericardial effusion, and intra-abdominal free fluid suggestive of ovarian hyperstimulation syndrome or ruptured ectopic pregnancy. The findings can help with risk stratification, consultant management plan, and disposition. An abdominal CT may be a helpful diagnostic test in the evaluation of a nonpregnant woman with abdominal pain and exclude vascular thrombosis, which is a known complication of infertility treatments. It is usually not considered the next best test in a pregnant woman because of the risk of ionizing radiation exposure. A serum beta-human chorionic gonadotropin (β-hCG) level may be helpful in guiding the management of patients in early pregnancy but does not help as much in diagnosing ovarian hyperstimulation syndrome. A chest CT may be helpful in excluding pulmonary embolism, another complication of infertility treatments but is not the next best test in this patient's management.

5. **The answer is A.** (Chapter 97) In patients with multiple emergency department visits for similar complaints, it is important to consider the possibility of physical or sexual abuse and screen for intimate partner violence. A stable, nonpregnant patient without an acute abdomen may ultimately be discharged with close outpatient follow-up, but her return visits for nonspecific symptoms should raise the suspicion for possible intimate partner violence or depression prior to discharge. Diagnostic imaging may be used to evaluate a nonpregnant woman with abdominal pain; guide your testing using a good history and examination.

6. **The answer is C.** (Chapter 97) Risk factors for ovarian torsion include pregnancy, infertility treatments, and history of ovarian cysts. An unremarkable pelvic examination cannot be used solely to exclude ovarian torsion as a potential etiology for this patient's pain. Be careful using a urinary tract infection as the definitive diagnosis of a patient's symptoms. For example, an acute appendicitis may cause inflammation of the urinary tract, which would result in a positive urinalysis. Keep your differential diagnosis broad. Loss of arterial blood flow to the ovary is a late finding for ovarian torsion and should not be used as the only ultrasound finding to exclude torsion. The most common ultrasound finding is edema around the ovary or fallopian tube. Up to 26% of ultrasounds may even show normal adnexa.

7. **The answer is D.** (Chapter 98) This patient has a higher risk for a heterotopic pregnancy because of her infertility

treatments, so a transvaginal ultrasound is the best next test to visualize the adnexae and exclude a concurrent ectopic pregnancy. Discharging home with obstetrics follow-up may be the correct answer for the majority of pregnant women with an ultrasound documenting an intrauterine pregnancy. Be very careful with women who have taken ovulation-inducing drugs because of their higher than normal risk of a heterotopic pregnancy. Immediate laparotomy is unlikely the next step in management for a patient with an intrauterine pregnancy, even for a patient at risk of a heterotopic pregnancy. Repeat beta-human chorionic gonadotropin (β-hCG) may be appropriate for patients with suspected ectopic pregnancy and an indeterminate ultrasound. The serum β-hCG should double every 2 days in a normal pregnancy.

8. **The answer is A.** (Chapter 98) This patient most likely had a spontaneous, complete abortion, based on her history, physical examination, and bedside ultrasound. Her beta-human chorionic gonadotropin (β-hCG) level is low relative to her estimated gestational age. A septic abortion is less likely because she doesn't have any obvious signs of infection. An inevitable abortion is defined as vaginal bleeding and cervical dilatation. This patient's cervical os is closed. An incomplete abortion is defined as passage of only parts of conception with retained material within the uterus that may be seen on ultrasound.

9. **The answer is B.** (Chapter 98) This patient has signs and symptoms of a ruptured ectopic pregnancy, and after initial resuscitation with crystalloid, an emergent obstetrics consultation is indicated. Her bedside transvaginal ultrasound shows a thickened enometrial stripe but no early signs of intrauterine pregnancy: gestational sac, yolk sac, or fetal pole and her beta-human chorionic gonadotropin (β-hCG) is in the discriminatory zone for transvaginal ultrasound. Her ultrasound also shows a small amount of free fluid in her pelvis. Methotrexate is a medical treatment for unruptured ectopic pregnancy in hemodynamically stable women. This patient is hypotensive, although not tachycardic, probably because of her vagal response to the bleeding. In the hemodynamically stable pregnant woman with suspected ectopic pregnancy and β-hCG levels lower than the discriminatory zone for a transvaginal ultrasound, discharge with follow-up in 2 days for repeat β-hCG level and ultrasound may be appropriate.

10. **The answer is A.** (Chapter 98) A yolk sac within a larger sac surrounded by at least 5 mm of myometrium is an early sign of an intrauterine pregnancy. Since the patient is hemodynamically stable and has an intrauterine pregnancy, she may be discharged with outpatient follow-up. A thickened uterine stripe with no other signs

of an intrauterine pregnancy is an ectopic pregnancy until proven otherwise in this setting. If this is a desired pregnancy, the patient needs to follow up in 2 days for serial beta-human chorionic gonadotropin (β-hCG) testing in addition to a repeat ultrasound in 1 week. A snow storm appearance is the ultrasound description of a molar pregnancy. This patient needs urgent obstetrics consultation. An empty intrauterine sac could be an anembryonic pregnancy or possible ectopic pregnancy. Her β-hCG is high enough that one should see a yolk sac or fetal pole within the gestational sac.

11. **The answer is C.** (Chapter 98) A patient with a history of multiple sexual partners has a higher risk of sexually transmitted infections, which is a risk factor for ectopic pregnancy. Other major risk factors include history of tubal sterilization, conception with an intrauterine device in place, advanced maternal age, prior ectopic pregnancy, cigarette smoking, and assisted reproduction techniques.

12. **The answer is A.** (Chapter 99) Avoid epinephrine in pregnant patients with status asthmaticus because of concerns about potential vasoconstriction of the uteroplacental circulation. All the other treatments are safe and appropriate in pregnancy.

13. **The answer is C.** (Chapters 99 and 100) It's important to remember that postpartum patients may also have eclampsia. This patient with headache, seizure, and hypertension should be treated with IV magnesium. Metoclopramide may be used to treat migraine headaches, which is on the differential for a patient with headache but usually is not associated with seizures. Low-molecular-weight heparin (LMWH) may be used to treat central venous thrombosis, which may occur up to 4 weeks postpartum, and can present with headache and seizure. CT imaging is required for diagnosis and for excluding intracranial hemorrhage. Diagnostic imaging should be obtained prior to starting treatment. Labetalol may be used to treat hypertension and severe preeclampsia but is an adjunctive therapy for a patient with eclampsia.

14. **The answer is A.** (Chapter 100) An arborization pattern that occurs when a drop of amniotic fluid is allowed to air-dry on a microscope slide is called *ferning*. The presence of amniotic fluid in a pregnant patient less than 37 weeks of gestation indicates premature rupture of membranes. This requires emergent obstetrics consultation for possible expedited delivery. Uniflagellar motile organism describes sperm or trichomonas. Pseudohypha describes *Candida albicans*, from a patient with vaginal yeast infection. Rod-shaped bacteria is likely lactobacilli in normal vaginal fluid.

15. The answer is D. (Chapter 99) The differential diagnosis of shortness of breath and chest pain in a pregnant patient in her third trimester is broad, but this patient has symptoms suggestive of acute pulmonary embolism (pleuritic chest pain, shortness of breath, tachycardia, leg swelling) and is at increased risk because of her late pregnancy. An ultrasound to exclude deep venous thrombosis is the best initial test to help guide her management because if it shows a clot, she would require anticoagulation without having to expose her or her fetus to ionizing radiation. A D-dimer may be a good adjunctive test in the diagnostic workup of a patient with chest pain and shortness of breath, but this patient already has a moderate to high pretest probability of venous thromboembolism, so a D-dimer assay is less helpful. CT pulmonary angiogram and pulmonary perfusion scan are both acceptable diagnostic tests for diagnosing pulmonary embolism in a pregnant patient. CT-PA has high sensitivity and specificity, exposes the patient to higher breast radiation but lower fetal radiation than a pulmonary perfusion scan. A pulmonary perfusion scan may be inconclusive (especially in patients who may have chronic pulmonary disease or abnormal chest radiograph) and patients who are breastfeeding need to discard breast milk for 12 hours after the scan.

16. The answer is B. (Chapter 100) HELLP syndrome (hemolysis, elevated liver enzymes, and low platelets) is a clinical variant of preeclampsia that may present without elevated blood pressure. Patients usually present with epigastric or upper abdominal pain and may be misdiagnosed for other causes of pain, such as gastritis, biliary disease, or hepatitis. Mild placental abruption is characterized by abdominal or uterine tenderness, no or mild vaginal bleeding, and fetal distress. Always consider abruption in the patient with either acute abdominal pain OR vaginal bleeding. Be careful with routine vaginal digital and speculum examinations when evaluating the patient in late pregnancy with abdominal pain or vaginal bleeding. In the patient with placenta previa, a digital or speculum examination may precipitate severe hemorrhage. If the patient has premature rupture of membranes, a digital examination may decrease the latent period and increase the risk of infection. Premature rupture of membranes may present with a leakage of fluid from the cervical os, but diagnosis requires a combination of history and examination, nitrazine paper testing, and fern testing for vaginal amniotic fluid. Ultrasound can also be used to estimate amniotic fluid volume.

17. The answer is B. (Chapter 101) The cardinal movements made by the fetus during a normal vaginal delivery is engagement in the pelvis, flexion, descent, internal rotation, extension, and external rotation.

18. The answer is D. (Chapter 101) Fetal heart rates fluctuating between 120 and 170 with brief accelerations in rate is a reassuring fetal heart tracing. Consistent fetal heart rate around 140 to 150 with a drop in heart rate near the end of a uterine contraction then a slow return to baseline describes late decelerations in heart rate (relative to uterine contractions). Late decelerations indicate fetal distress, usually caused by processes that cause maternal hypotension, excessive uterine activity, or placental dysfunction. Fetal heart rate drops to 60 after a contraction without a return to baseline after contraction ends describes prolonged fetal bradycardia, which suggests fetal distress. Drops in fetal heart rate that occur just after uterine contractions, with a return to baseline heart rate, describes decelerations that may be seen in umbilical cord occlusion during a contraction.

19. The answer is B. (Chapter 101) After placenta delivery, massage the uterine fundus to promote contraction. Oxytocin may be given in addition to uterine massage to sustain the uterine contraction. Repair of a perineal laceration should be performed after careful examination for involvement of the anal sphincter. This is a less common cause of significant postpartum hemorrhage, and bleeding may be controlled with direct pressure.

20. The answer is D. (Chapter 102) Flagellated protozoan is shown on microscopy, which indicates *Trichomonas vaginalis* and produces a local inflammation of the vaginal and cervical mucosa. Pregnant patients are at risk for adverse health outcomes, including preterm delivery and delivery of low-birth-weight babies. Reinfection is very common and may necessitate multiple courses of antibiotics. Patients with trichomoniasis are at risk for developing pelvic inflammatory disease, and because it's a sexually transmitted infection, patients may be concurrently infected with gonorrhea or chlamydia. Concurrent infection does not necessarily lead to worse health outcomes. *Trichomonas* infection is associated with increased transmission of other infections, such as human immunodeficiency virus (HIV), herpesvirus, and human papillomavirus. Patients with a history of multiple sexual partners are at increased risk for these other viral infections.

21. The answer is B. (Chapter 102) This patient has signs and symptoms of candida vaginitis. Even though her microscopy did not show budding yeast and pseudohyphae, she is symptomatic, so empiric treatment is recommended. The topical and oral therapies for vaginal candidiasis are effecting in treating >80% of cases. Because the patient is symptomatic with signs and symptoms suggestive of *Candida*, she should be treated empirically without waiting for cultures. Metronidazole is the treatment for bacterial vaginosis, which typically presents with foul-smelling vaginal discharge. On examination, the classic description of the discharge is thin and gray, with a fishy odor. Other than the discharge, diagnosis requires visualization of >20% clue cells on a wet mount. Ceftriaxone and azithromycin are used to treat cervicitis in a patient with possible gonorrhea or chlamydia exposure.

22. **The answer is D.** (Chapter 102) This picture shows a Bartholin gland abscess. Bartholin glands are located in the labia minora, at the 4 and 8 o'clock positions. They tend to be polymicrobial, so broad-spectrum antibiotics are recommended after incision and drainage of the abscess. A Word catheter is inserted after a small incision is performed and left in place for 4 to 6 weeks to avoid recurrence. Antibiotics and sitz baths are used to treat very early abscesses that are not well defined and walled off. Routine incision and drainage with packing placement is the treatment for many abscesses. However, the packing could not be left in place for 4 to 6 weeks, which may result in recurrence. While chlamydia and gonorrhea have been implicated in Bartholin abscesses, most are polymicrobial, so broad-spectrum antibiotics are recommended. Patients may be referred to gynecology as an outpatient for marsupialization of the gland as definitive treatment.

23. **The answer is B.** (Chapter 103) In the past, intrauterine devices (IUDs) were generally removed in the setting of pelvic inflammatory disease, based on the belief that removal would allow the treatment to be more effective. However, the device is usually not the source of infection, so there is insufficient evidence to recommend immediate IUD removal prior to initiating treatment. Empiric treatment with antibiotics is recommended if the clinical picture suggests pelvic inflammatory disease. Diagnosis can be challenging, because culture results are usually not available to the emergency department at the time of initial evaluation. Overtreatment is preferred to delayed or no treatment because of the potential for serious sequelae, such as infertility. Because a patient may have multiple sexually transmitted infections, consider testing for concurrent disease, such as human immunodeficiency virus (HIV), syphilis, bacterial vaginosis, and hepatitis. Although this patient may have perihepatic inflammation from her pelvic infection, consider other diagnostic testing to narrow her differential diagnosis, such as point of care ultrasound.

24. **The answer is C.** (Chapter 103) This patient has signs and symptoms of pelvic inflammatory disease (PID), which is a complication of sexually transmitted infections of the lower genital tract. The patient's sexual partner should be treated as well to prevent reinfection. Recent intrauterine device (IUD) insertion, frequent vaginal douching, and multiple sexual partners increase the risk for PID. Pregnancy decreases the risk of PID because the cervical os is protected by the mucous plug.

25. **The answer is D.** (Chapter 103) The differential diagnosis for abdominal and pelvic pain in a young woman of reproductive age should always include possible ectopic pregnancy. A urine pregnancy test to exclude pregnancy should be obtained in patients with abdominal pain and/or pelvic or urinary symptoms. While a urinalysis may be helpful in diagnosing a urinary tract infection, be very careful attributing the patient's symptoms to a simple cystitis. Patients with cervicitis or pelvic inflammatory disease may present with similar symptoms. A pelvic ultrasound may be obtained to exclude tubo-ovarian abscess, a complication of pelvic inflammatory disease, and may show thickened, fluid filled fallopian tubes or pelvic free fluid suggesting severe pelvic inflammatory disease. It may also exclude ovarian cyst, ovarian torsion, and ectopic pregnancy. However, many patients do not require diagnostic imaging for diagnosis. This patient meets the minimum criteria for diagnosing pelvic inflammatory disease, and as long as her pregnancy test is negative (to exclude other causes of her pain), she could be treated empirically with antibiotics and outpatient follow-up.

26. **The answer is B.** (Chapter 104) This patient has a clinical picture and ultrasound finding for puerperal mastitis. The ultrasound shows cobblestoning but no drainable collection so the patient may be treated with cephalexin for 7 days. She may continue to breastfeed. Lanolin cream and breast shields are an appropriate treatment for nipple irritation or soreness from breastfeeding. Pumping may be used to improve breast emptying if there are problems with breast engorgement and inadequate milk removal from the breast. Warm compresses alone will not treat the infection.

27. **The answer is C.** (Chapter 104) This patient has symptoms, signs, and an ultrasound image suggestive of a breast abscess. Breast abscesses are treated with a 7-day course of antibiotics with activity against methicillin-resistant *Staphylococcus aureus* and anaerobes, followed by outpatient referral to a breast surgeon for needle aspiration if antibiotics alone are ineffective. Unlike soft tissue infections in other areas of the body, the initial treatment of breast abscesses is not incision and drainage of the fluid collection, but a course of oral antibiotics. The differential diagnosis of an inflamed, painful breast does include an inflammatory malignancy, which could be excluded with a biopsy. However, a needle aspiration to sample or remove the fluid collection would likely be performed prior to a

biopsy. Admission criteria for parenteral antibiotics and immediate surgical consultation are similar to any other soft tissue infection: sepsis or hemodynamic compromise, immunosuppression, rapidly progressive infection, and failure of outpatient antibiotic therapy.

28. **The answer is D.** (Chapter 105) Be very careful performing the pelvic examination in a patient who is undergoing fertility treatment because there is possibility of rupturing enlarged ovarian follicles during the examination. Consult with a gynecologist prior to performing the pelvic examination. In all the other patients, a speculum and bimanual examination should be a routine part of the physical examination.

29. **The answer is A.** (Chapter 105) Bowel injury is a major complication of laparoscopic surgery and should be considered in patients with greater than expected pain after the procedure. Bowel obstruction may develop in patients with incisional hernias, which may develop in the first postoperative week. However, this is not common after a laparoscopic myomectomy. Vascular injury is uncommon and usually recognized during the operation. Postoperatively patients may present with a hematoma that requires wound exploration by the surgeon. Postoperative surgical

infection after laparoscopy is also uncommon and rarely a serious complication. Deep pelvic infections are even more uncommon and require parenteral antibiotics and urgent surgical consultation.

30. **The answer is D.** (Chapter 105) Wound infections usually occur within the first 2 postoperative weeks; however, they can present several months after surgery. If an incisional abscess is diagnosed, the wound needs to be opened up, probed with a sterile cotton swab to confirm an intact fascia, irrigated with normal saline, and then packed with wet to dry dressings. Invasive wound infections require IV antibiotics and hospital admission. Pelvic pathology such as vaginal cuff cellulitis and pelvic infections usually occur early after surgery. A pelvic examination may show tenderness and induration of the vaginal cuff, purulent discharge, from the cuff, or a tender or fluctuant mass near the cuff. Wound dehiscence occurs between postoperative days 5 and 8 for abdominal surgeries. Patients may describe a tearing sensation, followed by bleeding or discharge from the incision. Genitourinary injuries occur more often after abdominal hysterectomy than any other surgery. Some ureteral injuries may go unrecognized. Vesiculovaginal fistulas may be seen about 10 to 14 days after surgery.

Pediatrics

10

QUESTIONS

1. What is the leading cause of mortality in children aged 1 to 24 years in the United States?
   (A) Congenital anomalies
   (B) Heart disease
   (C) Malignancy
   (D) Unintentional injuries

2. You are called to the resuscitation bay where you find a 17-year-old girl who delivered a newborn en route to the emergency department. She was unaware of her pregnancy. The newborn appears premature, is not crying, and has poor tone. After warming, drying, and stimulating the newborn, you notice gasping respirations and a heart rate of 90. What is the NEXT STEP in the resuscitation of the newborn?
   (A) Chest compressions
   (B) Endotracheal intubation
   (C) Intravenous epinephrine
   (D) Positive pressure ventilation

3. A 12-month-old boy without significant medical history is brought to the emergency department for fussiness and poor feeding for 1 day. The triage nurse notices tachycardia and is worried about septic shock. After being transported to the resuscitation bay, the infant becomes mottled and limp, with a blood pressure of 60/30 and poor perfusion of the extremities. Electrocardiogram demonstrates a narrow, complex tachycardia at 260, without noticeable p waves. What is the initial treatment?
   (A) Application of ice over the face
   (B) Adenosine (0.1 mg/kg) rapid bolus

   (C) Defibrillation (2 J/kg)
   (D) Synchronized cardioversion (0.5–1.0 J/kg)

4. A 5-year-old girl is brought to the emergency department with respiratory arrest. She becomes asystolic shortly after arrival to your resuscitation bay. The child is intubated and placed on the mechanical ventilator. Despite adequate chest wall movement and chest compressions, the child remains in asystole. What is the NEXT STEP in the resuscitation of the child?
   (A) Atropine
   (B) Defibrillation
   (C) Epinephrine
   (D) Termination of resuscitation efforts

5. A 10-year-old boy is transported to your emergency department after being struck by an automobile as he was walking home from school. His Glasgow Coma Score is 7 (Eye opening response [no response], Best verbal response [incomprehensible words], and Best motor response [flexion withdrawal from pain]). His heart rate is 120 and blood pressure is 110/67. He has obvious contusions to his head, chest and abdomen, and an open deformity to his left thigh. What is the NEXT STEP in the resuscitation of this child?
   (A) Bolus of intravenous saline
   (B) Endotracheal intubation
   (C) Intravenous antibiotics for the suspected open femur fracture
   (D) Reduction of the suspected open femur fracture

6. According to the Pediatric Emergency Care Applied Research Network prediction rules to identify children at very low risk for a clinically important intra-abdominal injury following blunt abdominal trauma, which of the following factors was identified as being associated with low risk, and therefore obviating a CT scan as part of the initial emergency department evaluation?
   (A) Absence of bowel sounds
   (B) No abdominal distention
   (C) No pelvic instability
   (D) No seat belt sign

7. A 6-year-old girl with a history of severe asthma presents to the emergency department with short-ness of breath. Despite several doses of albuterol/ipratropium bromide, intravenous methylprednisolone, and intravenous magnesium sulfate, she continues to be tachypneic and hypoxic. You decide to perform an endotracheal intubation due to her worsening mental status and inability to maintain her airway. Which of the following airway equipment combinations is MOST APPROPRIATE?
   (A) 4.0 uncuffed ETT and 1.5 straight laryngoscope blade
   (B) 4.0 cuffed ETT and 2.0 straight laryngoscope blade
   (C) 5.0 cuffed ETT and 2.0 curved laryngoscope blade
   (D) 7.0 cuffed ETT and 3.0 straight laryngoscope blade

8. A 3-month-old male infant presents to your emergency department with fever, depressed mental status, and poor perfusion. You suspect septic shock. Despite several attempts, you are unable to obtain vascular access. Which of the following is the MOST DESIRABLE location to obtain intraosseous access?
   (A) Distal tibia
   (B) Distal femur
   (C) Proximal tibia
   (D) Sternum

9. A 5-year-old boy presents to your emergency department after falling from monkey bars onto an outstretched right arm. He has an obvious closed deformity to his right distal forearm. His right arm is neurovascularly intact. A radiograph of his right forearm demonstrates a significantly angulated and displaced right distal radius and ulna fracture. Orthopedics has requested procedural sedation for reduction and casting of his right forearm fracture. Which of the following agents is MOST APPROPRIATE?
   (A) Etomidate alone
   (B) Ketamine alone
   (C) Midazolam alone
   (D) Propofol alone

10. A 2-week-old girl, born at 38 weeks' gestation, is brought to the emergency department with a reported temperature of 101.3°F at home and poor feeding for 48 hours. Physical examination reveals a newborn with poor tone and decreased perfusion of the extremities. Heart rate is 186 and respiratory rate is 80 with an oxygen saturation of 95% on room air. Bedside glucose is 90 mg/dL. After obtaining intra-venous access, which of the following is the NEXT BEST step?
   (A) Bolus of intravenous dextrose
   (B) Catheterized urinalysis and culture, followed by intravenous antibiotics
   (C) Catheterized urinalysis and culture, lumbar puncture for cerebrospinal fluid for diagnostics and culture, followed by intravenous antibiotics
   (D) Endotracheal intubation

11. A 2-week-old boy is brought to the emergency department with a chief complaint of vomiting and poor feeding. The vomitus is described as "green." There has been no fever. On physical examination, the infant is afebrile, heart rate is 140, respiratory rate is 40, and blood pressure is 90/45. Newborn appears unwell and has a taut, distended abdomen. An IV is placed and a normal saline bolus is started, blood and urine cultures are sent, and intravenous antibiotics are given for thoughts of sepsis. Which of the following should be performed NEXT in the evaluation of this newborn?
   (A) Abdominal ultrasound
   (B) Barium enema
   (C) Lumbar puncture
   (D) Upper gastrointestinal series

12. A 5-week-old male infant presents to the emergency department after having an "unresponsive" event. The mother says that the infant became limp and unresponsive shortly after feeding, stopped breathing, and turned blue. The mother gave rescue breaths and started cardiopulmonary resuscitation. Fever, congestion, or cough was not reported. The infant has

been feeding well and wetting diapers normally. On physical examination, temperature is 100.3°F (rectal), heart rate 180, respiratory rate 58, with an oxygen saturation of 99% on room air. The infant is crying without evidence of respiratory distress or dehydration. The examination is otherwise normal. What is the MOST LIKELY cause of this event?
(A) Hypoglycemia
(B) Gastroesophageal reflux
(C) Nonaccidental brain injury
(D) Urinary tract infection

13. A 39-day-old male infant (born at 36 weeks' gestation via C-section) presents to your emergency department with a tactile fever at home for 2 days and increase in "spitting" up. The infant has had nasal congestion and mild cough without evidence of shortness of breath and has been feeding well with normal number of wet diapers. On physical examination the temperature is 101.5°F (rectally), heart rate 170, respiratory rate 66, blood pressure 76/40, and oxygen saturation of 95% on room air. The infant is well appearing without respiratory distress. There is evidence of nasal congestion with crusting of the nares. What should the workup of fever in this infant include?
(A) Complete blood cell (CBC) count with differential, blood culture, urinalysis, urine culture, cerebrospinal fluid (CSF) cell count/gram stain/culture, chest radiograph, intravenous antibiotics, and hospitalization
(B) CBC with differential, blood culture, urinalysis, urine culture, CSF cell count/gram stain/culture, chest radiograph; risk stratify based on initial evaluation to high risk (intravenous antibiotics and hospitalization), or low risk (discharge home without antibiotics)
(C) Discharge home since this infant clearly has a viral upper respiratory infection
(D) Urinalysis and urine culture; discharge home with oral antibiotics if urinalysis is abnormal

14. What is the MOST COMMON serious bacterial infection in infants younger than 3 months?
(A) Bacteremia
(B) Bacterial meningitis
(C) Pneumonia
(D) Urinary tract infection

15. What is the MOST COMMON cause of meningitis in school aged children?
(A) Arboviruses
(B) Enterovirus
(C) *Streptococcus pneumoniae*
(D) *Neisseria meningitides*

16. A 3-year-old, fully vaccinated boy, with no medical history, presents to the emergency department with complaints of fevers that began late last night, waking him up from sleep. Nobody else at home is sick; however, he does attend daycare. His initial vitals reveal a temperature of 101.5°F, heart rate of 140, respiratory rate of 20, and oxygen saturation of 98% on room air. His physical examination is significant for yellow rhinorrhea and bilateral dull, erythematous but non-bulging tympanic membranes. There is no tenderness to palpation or erythema of the auricle or posterior to the auricle, and no other signs of infection. The MOST APPROPRIATE course of treatment includes:
(A) Ibuprofen and acetaminophen as needed for pain and fever control
(B) Ibuprofen and acetaminophen as needed for pain and fever control and oral Amoxicillin
(C) Ibuprofen and acetaminophen as needed for pain and fever control, oral amoxicillin, and topical ciprofloxacin drops
(D) Ibuprofen and acetaminophen as needed for pain and fever control and topical ciprofloxacin drops

17. A 4-year-old girl, with a history of nephrotic syndrome, presents with bilateral swelling of her eyes for the last 5 days. The clinician is considering periorbital and orbital cellulitis in the differential. How can the difference between the two be easily determined?
(A) Detailed physical examination demonstrating changes in visual acuity
(B) Ophthalmology consultation for a dilated eye examination
(C) Orbital and sinus CT scan
(D) Positive blood culture

18. Parents bring their 12-day-old baby boy to the emergency department for evaluation. They report he was born at 39 weeks' gestation via spontaneous vaginal delivery to a G1P0 mother with no known complications during the pregnancy or delivery; however, the mother did have limited prenatal care due to financial constraints. The newborn received all of his routine medications after birth and was discharged home on day 3 of life. They describe that 2 days ago they noticed his eyes began to appear red and swollen with purulent discharge from both eyes. The review of systems is negative for any additional symptoms. What is the MOST APPROPRIATE treatment for his child?
    (A) Admission to the hospital for intravenous antibiotics
    (B) Admission to the hospital for intravenous antivirals
    (C) Discharge home with oral antibiotics
    (D) Reassurance and discharge home with parents

19. A 14-year-old boy presents with new onset epistaxis from his right nares. He reports he was sitting in an air conditioned classroom when it started bleeding and denies any known trauma. Although he has been applying strict pressure for 20 minutes en route to the emergency department, it continues to bleed and requires nasal packing. He denies any previous excessive bleeding or bruising. Which of the following should be on the differential for his nose bleed?
    (A) Juvenile nasal angiofibroma
    (B) Rhinitis sicca
    (C) Simple epistaxis
    (D) Von Willebrand disease type 1

20. A 17-year-old boy comes to the emergency department with persistent oral bleeding after having lost a tooth playing hockey approximately 20 minutes ago. They bring the avulsed tooth with them. What is the MOST IMPORTANT NEXT step in management?
    (A) Apply pressure over the bleeding gum to achieve hemostasis and attempt to reimplant the tooth as quickly as possible
    (B) Apply pressure over the bleeding gum to achieve hemostasis, store the tooth in saline, and consult the hospital dentist on call
    (C) Scrub debris off the tooth prior to attempting to reimplant
    (D) The tooth has been avulsed for too long, so focus on stopping the oral bleeding and pain control

21. A 4-year-old girl presents to the emergency department with fever, runny nose, and cough for the last week and new onset of swelling to her neck. On examination she has a midline, nontender, neck mass that moves when she swallows and with protrusion of her tongue (Figure 10.1). What is the MOST LIKELY diagnosis?

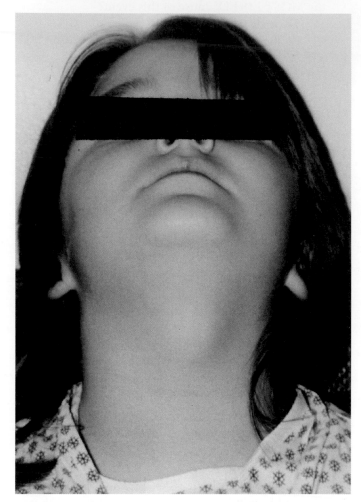

FIGURE 10.1 Reproduced with permission from J.E. Tintinalli, J.S. Stapczynski, O.J. Ma, D. Yealy, G.D. Meckler, D.M. Cline: Tintinalli's Emergency Medicine: A Comprehensive Study Guide, 9th Edition. Copyright © McGraw-Hill Education. All rights reserved.

    (A) Brachial cleft cyst
    (B) Dermoid cyst
    (C) Thyroglossal duct cyst
    (D) Thyroid cancer

22. Parents bring their 2-month-old female infant to the emergency department for evaluation of "noisy breathing." They report that the noisy breathing has been intermittent over the past few weeks, but more persistent over the past day. The infant was born at full-term gestation, did not require any respiratory support after birth, and was discharged home on day 2 of life. Physical examination is significant for biphasic stridor that does not change with prone

positioning, without any associated fever, rhinorrhea, or cough. There is no change in the severity of stridor after the administration of nebulized racemic epinephrine. What is the MOST LIKELY cause of this infant's stridor?

(A) Hemangioma
(B) Laryngomalacia
(C) Subglottic stenosis
(D) Viral croup

23. A 3-year-old fully immunized boy presents to the emergency department for evaluation of "drooling." His family reports that he had an upper respiratory infection roughly 1 week ago, associated with intermittent fever. On examination he is found to be drooling and have a muffled, "hot potato"-like voice without any stridor. He has difficulty turning his head. Neck radiographs obtained are MOST LIKELY to show what finding?

(A) Irregular tracheal margins
(B) Retropharyngeal swelling
(C) Steeple sign
(D) Thumbprint sign

24. When caring for a 6-week-old who has respiratory syncytial virus (RSV) bronchiolitis and is maintaining an oxygen saturation of 91% on room air, which of the following treatments may be considered per recommendation by the American Academy of Pediatrics?

(A) Albuterol
(B) Heliox
(C) Nebulized epinephrine
(D) Nebulized hypertonic saline

25. A known asthmatic presents to the emergency department with chest tightness, shortness of breath, and wheezing that has worsened over the last few days. After initial assessment he is found to have an oxygen saturation of 93% on room air. After administration of nebulized albuterol, what is the NEXT MOST important medication to administer is?

(A) Inhaled corticosteroids
(B) Inhaled ipratropium bromide
(C) Systemic corticosteroids
(D) Systemic magnesium sulfate

26. Which of the following factors is known to increase the likelihood of a positive chest radiograph in a child presenting to the emergency department with bacterial pneumonia?

(A) Age <1 year
(B) Fevers >39°C
(C) History of congenital anomaly
(D) White blood cell count >20,000

27. An 18-month-old child, who recently immigrated to the country, presents with increased work of breathing. Physical examination is significant for perioral cyanosis, tachypnea, a single loud S_2, and a 3/6 systolic ejection murmur heard best at the lower left sternal border. ECG shows right axis deviation and right ventricular hypertrophy. Chest radiograph obtained is shown in Figure 10.2.

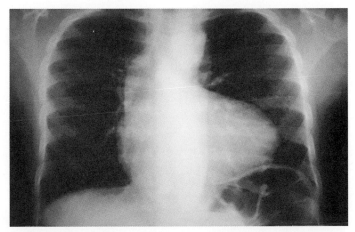

FIGURE 10.2 Reproduced with permission from Shah BR, Lucchesi M (eds): Atlas of Pediatric Emergency Medicine. New York, NY: McGraw-Hill, Inc.; 2006

What is the MOST LIKELY diagnosis is?

(A) Tetralogy of Fallot
(B) Tricuspid atresia
(C) Total anomalous pulmonary venous return
(D) Ventricular septal defect

28. A previously healthy 16-month-old boy is brought to the emergency department via ambulance after parents report he "passed out" at home. Prior to passing out, he was visibly upset and turned pale. They deny any abnormal movements of his extremities or any known trauma. No interventions were needed, and he began breathing on his own spontaneously. He is now back to his baseline per his parents. His examination is unremarkable. What is the MOST IMPORTANT diagnostic test to obtain in the emergency department as part of his workup?

(A) Electrocardiogram
(B) Electroencephalogram
(C) Serum electrolytes
(D) No testing is required

29. A patient is found to have long QT syndrome with electrolytes all within normal ranges. Which of the following medications should be initially used to treat this patient?
    (A) Class Ia antiarrhythmic agents (i.e., procainamide)
    (B) Class Ib antiarrhythmic agents (i.e., phenytoin)
    (C) Class II antiarrhythmic agents (i.e., propranolol)
    (D) Class III antiarrhythmic agents (i.e., amiodarone)

30. A 5-week-old infant is brought in by parents for vomiting. Parents state the vomiting has been increasingly forceful over the last week and most commonly occurs 15 minutes after feeding. Between episodes, the infant continues to appear hungry. There has been no associated fever, diarrhea, or apparent abdominal pain. What is the MOST LIKELY diagnosis?
    (A) Intussusception
    (B) Malrotation with volvulus
    (C) Pyloric stenosis
    (D) Viral gastroenteritis

31. Which is the BEST first-line medication for persistent vomiting associated with acute gastroenteritis in children?
    (A) Metoclopramide
    (B) Ondansetron
    (C) Prochlorperazine
    (D) Promethazine

32. A 3-year-old boy presents to the emergency department for abdominal pain. Parents report that the child has had intermittent abdominal pain, occurring several times an hour, associated with drawing his legs to his chest. He has had several episodes of nonbilious vomiting. He has not had a fever. Palpation of his abdomen produces crying, without focal tenderness. An abdominal ultrasound is performed, as shown in Figure 10.3. What is the MOST LIKELY diagnosis?
    (A) Appendicitis
    (B) Constipation
    (C) Intussusception
    (D) Meckel's diverticulum

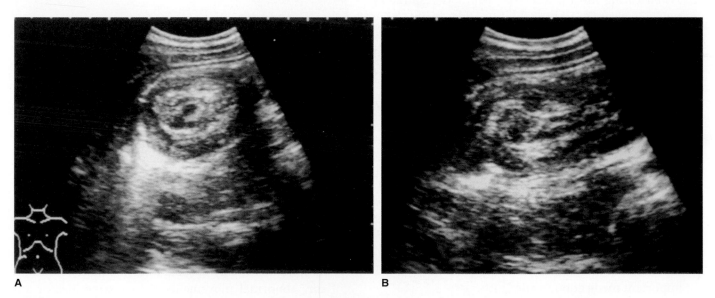

A   B

FIGURE 10.3 Reproduced with permission from Ma OJ, Mateer JR, Blaivas M: Emergency Ultrasound, 2nd ed. © New York, NY: McGraw-Hill, Inc.; 2008.

33. A 5-month-old previously healthy infant presents to the emergency department with hematemesis. She has been breastfeeding without difficulty, until today, when she had one episode of blood-streaked, nonbilious emesis. The infant is smiling, with a benign abdominal examination, and immediate capillary refill. What is the NEXT BEST step in evaluation?
    (A) Examine the patient's stool for presence of occult blood
    (B) Obtain labs, including complete blood count
    (C) Perform nasogastric lavage for evaluation of further bleeding
    (D) Take further history and examine the mother if available

34. A 13-month-old female infant is brought into the emergency department with fever for 2 days, associated with vomiting. Parents report fever has been as high as 104°F (40°C), and resolves with antipyretics. All episodes of emesis have been nonbloody and nonbilious. She has not had any diarrhea. She previously had a urinary tract infection that was culture positive for E. coli. What is the NEXT BEST step in management of this patient?
    (A) Blood and urine cultures for bacterial identification given recurrence
    (B) Empiric treatment with antibiotics to prevent pyelonephritis
    (C) Renal ultrasound for evaluation of renal abscess
    (D) Urinalysis on a specimen obtained sterilely by catheterization

35. A 5-year-old boy is brought to the emergency department by his parents for testicular pain. He has had 1 day of left testicular pain, swelling, and erythema, as seen in Figure 10.4. A urinalysis is done, without evidence of infection. Scrotal ultrasound shows vascular flow to bilateral testes with increased flow to the left epididymis. What is the BEST choice for treatment of this condition?

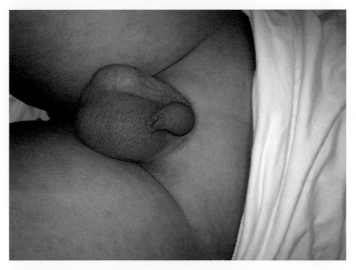

FIGURE 10.4 J.E. Tintinalli, J.S. Stapczynski, O.J. Ma, D. Yearly, G.D. Meckler, D.M. Cline: Tintinalli's Emergency Medicine: A Comprehensive Study Guide, 9th Edition: Copyright © McGraw-Hill Education. All rights reserved

(A) Analgesics and supportive measures with primary care follow-up
(B) Attempt manual detorsion in the emergency department
(C) Consult urology for delayed surgical management
(D) Intravenous antibiotics while awaiting urine culture

36. A 2-year-old girl is brought into the emergency department by parents for spotting on her underwear. Parents deny any fevers or dysuria. On examination, you see a purplish-colored, doughnut-shaped, fleshy mass just above the vaginal introitus. What is the NEXT BEST step in management of this condition?
    (A) Oral antibiotics and referral to surgery for drainage
    (B) Referral to child protective services for abuse concerns
    (C) Topical estrogen cream and sitz baths
    (D) Urgent gynecological consultation for repair

37. An 8-year-old boy is brought in by his parents for scrotal swelling. He told his parents that it started 3 days ago. He denies pain or tenderness and has not had a fever or abdominal pain. His parents brought him in today because they also noticed facial swelling, without erythema. His examination is consistent with parental findings, and also notes 2+ pitting edema to his lower extremities and swelling to his hands. His testicular ultrasound shows normal Doppler flow. A urinalysis is significant for 300 mg/dL of protein. A complete metabolic panel is obtained, with a normal creatinine, sodium, and potassium for age, and an albumin of 0.7 g/dL. Vitals are within normal limits for age. What is the BEST first treatment in the emergency department?
    (A) Administer a dose of intravenous steroids
    (B) Administer intravenous albumin followed by furosemide
    (C) Arrange admission to the intensive care unit for renal biopsy
    (D) Prepare for initiation of renal replacement therapy

38. A 6-year-old girl with known epilepsy is brought to the emergency department for a seizure. According to paramedics, the seizure began 20 minutes prior to their arrival. Relatives describe the seizure as stiffening of the entire body with leftward eye deviation, followed by generalized clonic movements. She has been taking levetiracetam and has not missed a dose. Her last seizure was 1 year ago, when she had a urinary tract infection. Paramedics gave intranasal midazolam at 0.2 mg/kg en route to your facility without resolution of the seizure. They were able to place a peripheral IV catheter, and you have given intravenous lorazepam at 0.1 mg/kg. What is the NEXT BEST medication to administer if the seizure does not resolve?
    (A) Intravenous fosphenytoin at 20 phenytoin equivalents/kg
    (B) Intravenous ketamine at 1 mg/kg
    (C) Intravenous lorazepam at 0.2 mg/kg
    (D) Intravenous propofol at 1 mg/kg

39. A 16-month-old girl is brought in by ambulance for seizure. Parents report that she had a 3-minute generalized seizure at home, which had resolved by the time EMS arrived. She was postictal for 10 minutes and is now back to her baseline. She has been febrile to 104°F (40°C) today but has not had vomiting or diarrhea. Parents report that they requested she be brought to your facility, as she had another seizure

8 hours previously and the last hospital "Did nothing." What is the BEST choice for workup of this patient?
    (A) Complete blood count and complete metabolic panel.
    (B) MRI of the brain and electroencephalogram.
    (C) No workup is indicated.
    (D) Urinalysis and culture by catheterization.

40. A 15-year-old girl presents to the emergency department for headache. She has been having headaches for the past year, which have progressed to daily. They are unrelieved by ibuprofen or acetaminophen. Her primary doctor previously ordered an MRI, which was normal, and she has those results with her. She has been describing blurry vision for a month, which prompted a visit to an optometrist. She was sent to the emergency department from the clinic, as they noted papilledema on her examination. What is the NEXT BEST step to diagnose the cause of her headaches?
    (A) Lumbar puncture with opening pressure
    (B) Repeat MRI of the brain
    (C) Urgent ophthalmology consultation
    (D) Urine drug screen and psychiatry evaluation

41. A 7-year-old boy is brought to the emergency department for "lethargy" per parents. They state that he started having nausea and vomiting today, and then became progressively less responsive. He has not had fevers. They state he was "breathing funny" today. On your examination, you see a thin boy who is diaphoretic. His vitals include HR 140, BP 110/70, RR 28, and T 99.0°F (37.2°C). The patient moans to painful stimuli, and moves all extremities. His pupils are sluggish, but equal. What is the BEST immediate test to determine the etiology of his symptoms?
    (A) CT of the head
    (B) Lumbar puncture
    (C) Serum glucose
    (D) Ultrasound of the abdomen

42. An 18-month-old girl is brought in by parents after a fall from a chair at home. She cried immediately, has not had any loss of consciousness, and has not had any vomiting. Per parents, she is acting like her normal self. On examination, you see a playful, interactive girl with a 3-cm frontal hematoma. What is the BEST course of management for this patient?
    (A) Admit for observation overnight
    (B) Head CT and observation for 6 hours
    (C) Neurosurgical consultation for clearance
    (D) Reassure parents and discharge home

43. A 15-year-old boy is sent in to the emergency department by the team doctor after a head-to-head collision with another player during a football game. The player had loss of consciousness for 15 seconds after the event, followed by confusion for about 15 minutes. At the time of your examination, the patient is slow to respond to questions and is amnestic to the event. A full neurologic examination is performed without focal findings. There are no external signs of trauma, and the patient denies pain. A head CT is done and read as normal. What is the BEST anticipatory guidance to give the patient and his parents?

   (A) Memory of the event should return fully in the next 24 hours.
   (B) Recurrent concussions are more common in the next 10 days.
   (C) Return to play immediately is advised to prevent deconditioning.
   (D) Teenagers with this condition tend to recover faster than adults.

44. A 4-year-old girl is brought in by ambulance after a motor vehicle collision. She has been placed in a cervical collar by paramedics. She is crying but moving all extremities. The following cross-table x-ray is done, due to the inability of the patient to cooperate with a neurologic examination. What is the BEST management of the findings shown in Figure 10.5?

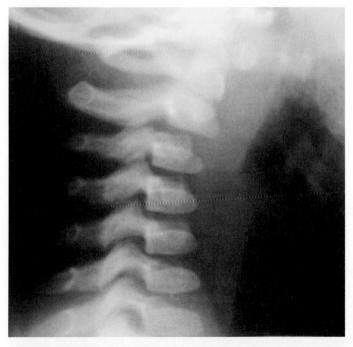

FIGURE 10.5 Reprinted with permission from Yamamoto LG: Cervical spine malalignment—true or pseudosubluxation? In: Yamamoto LG, Inaba AS, DiMauro R (eds): Radiology Cases in Pediatric Emergency Medicine, Vol. 1, Case 5. Honolulu, HI: University of Hawaii John A. Burns School of Medicine, Department of Pediatrics, 1994. http://www.hawaii.edu/medicine/pediatrics/pemxray/v1c05.html.

   (A) Emergent MRI of the cervical spine due to likelihood of ligamentous injury
   (B) No intervention needed, clear the cervical spine when clinically able
   (C) Urgent neurosurgical consultation for unstable cervical spine finding
   (D) X-ray with flexion and extension views of the c-spine to confirm findings

45. An 18-month-old boy is brought in by parents for refusal to walk. Per parents, he was acting normally until the afternoon. Mom states he was playing in the living room and she heard him crying. Since then, he has refused to bear weight on his right leg. On examination, you find no focal swelling of the limb, and full range of motion at the hip and knee. Palpation of the distal leg elicits crying. An x-ray shows a nondisplaced spiral fracture of the distal third of the tibial shaft. What is the BEST management of this condition?

   (A) Immobilization in a long leg cast and referral to child protective services
   (B) Immobilization in a long leg splint and discharge home
   (C) Immobilization in a spica cast and discharge home
   (D) No immobilization needed, refer to child protective services

46. A 5-year-old girl is brought into the emergency department for a left arm injury. Per parents, she was jumping on a trampoline and fell, landing on her outstretched left hand. She cried immediately, and parents noted significant swelling to the left elbow. She is refusing to move the arm but can move her fingers, and her distal pulses are intact. Which of the following statements regarding her injury is TRUE?

   (A) Imaging of the entire arm and shoulder should be performed, given the severity of the mechanism of injury.
   (B) Medial epicondyle fractures are the most common elbow injury found in children after a fall onto an outstretched hand.
   (C) Type 1 supracondylar fractures are flexion-type injuries usually caused by falling directly on the flexed elbow.
   (D) Type 2 supracondylar fractures may require surgical management and require urgent orthopedic consultation.

47. A 6-year-old boy is brought in by parents for limping. He states that his right hip started hurting this morning, and has become progressively worse. He has had no recent fevers. On examination, he is holding his right hip flexed and slightly abducted and complains of pain with passive range of motion of the hip, though he is able to move the joint. Laboratory examinations are performed, with pertinent findings of a normal white blood cell count and a C-reactive protein of 1.6 mg/L. Ultrasound of the hip is performed and does not show an effusion. Which of the following BEST describes management of this condition?
    (A) Complete resolution is expected, as it is a self-limited condition.
    (B) Intravenous antibiotics and admission are indicated.
    (C) Legg-Calvé-Perthes disease is an emergent complication of this condition.
    (D) Orthopedics should be consulted for a washout of the joint.

48. A 7-year-old boy is brought in by parents for rash. Mom first noticed the rash yesterday on his feet, and it has spread up his legs to his buttocks since then. He has also been complaining of intermittent abdominal pain, without nausea or vomiting. No fevers have been reported. The patient states the rash is painful, not pruritic. His ankles have had some swelling today, and he states they are slightly painful with ambulation. Pictures of the rash are shown in Figures 10.6A and B. Which of the following investigations are the MOST APPROPRIATE for this condition?

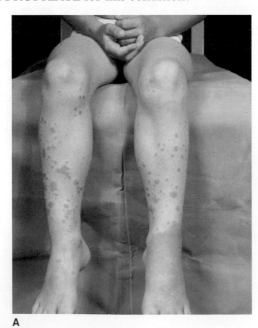

A

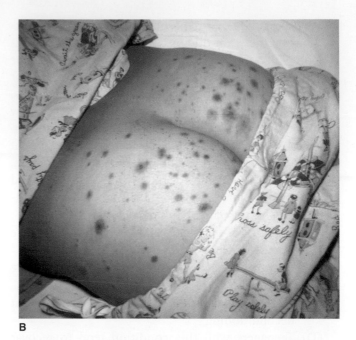

B

    (A) Complete blood count
    (B) Prothrombin time
    (C) Ultrasound of the ankles
    (D) Urinalysis

49. A 3-year-old girl is brought in by parents for fever. They state that she has had 5 days of fevers to 104°F (40°C) and has been acting more tired than normal. They saw the pediatrician 2 days ago because of the fever and a generalized rash and were told that she had a virus. Parents became concerned when the skin of her fingers started peeling today. On examination, you note the peeling skin on her fingers, along with chapped lips, mild conjunctivitis and left sided cervical chain lymphadenopathy. The BEST management of this condition is:
    (A) Admission for high-dose aspirin and intravenous immunoglobulin
    (B) Blood culture prior to the administration of intravenous antibiotics
    (C) Intravenous steroids and dermatology referral for biopsy
    (D) Supportive management of the viral illness with oral rehydration

50. A 10-day-old infant is brought in by parents for a rash. The baby has not had any fevers, is eating well, and has regained her birth weight. There were no complications with the delivery. Which of the following is TRUE about neonatal rashes?

(A) Atopic dermatitis initially presents in the days immediately after birth.

(B) Diagnosis of neonatal pustular melanosis requires microscopic evaluation.

(C) Erythema toxicum is a self-limited disease that occurs in up to 50% of infants.

(D) Seborrheic dermatitis is a fungal infection associated with candidal diaper dermatitis.

51. A 4-year-old boy with known sickle cell disease is brought in by parents for fever. Parents report fever to 102.2°F (39°C) at home, improved with acetaminophen. He is up to date on vaccines and is on prophylactic penicillin, which parents have been compliant with. Which of the following BEST describes an emergent complication of fever in this child?

(A) Acute chest crisis is frequently a complication of pneumonia.

(B) Bacteremia risk is reduced to that of the general population with prophylaxis.

(C) Parvovirus can present as recurrent severe anemia after fevers.

(D) *Streptococcus pneumoniae* is the most common cause of bacteremia in this age group.

52. A 2-year-old boy with known hemophilia B is brought to the emergency room after a fall. He gets prophylactic factor replacement two times a week. Parents report he was sitting in a booster chair at the table and fell forward, hitting his forehead on the table. He had no loss of consciousness and has not had vomiting. He complains of a headache and has an ecchymosis to his forehead. What is the NEXT BEST step in management of the patient?

(A) Order 50% factor correction and a head CT

(B) Order 50% factor correction, no indication for a head CT

(C) Order 100% factor correction and a head CT

(D) Order 100% factor correction, no indication for a head CT

53. A 7-year-old girl is sent to your facility from the pediatrician's office for abnormal labs. Per the report parents have with them, white blood cell count is 234,000 cells/mm^3, hemoglobin is 8.1 g/dL, and platelet count is 23,000 cells/mm^3. After repeating a complete blood count with peripheral smear to

confirm these findings, what is the NEXT BEST step in management?

(A) Transfusion with 10 mL/kg of irradiated packed red blood cells

(B) Transfusion with 0.1 units/kg of platelets

(C) Ultrasound-guided placement of a catheter for immediate leukapheresis

(D) Urgent consultation with hematology/oncology for initiation of chemotherapy

54. A 7-month-old boy with known ornithine transcarbamylase deficiency presents to the emergency department with lethargy. Parents state that he started having vomiting and diarrhea today, with poor oral intake. On your examination, the infant is pale, with dry mucous membranes, and only responds to painful stimuli. He has tachycardia and has a sluggish pupillary response. What is the MOST IMPORTANT laboratory examination for the resuscitation?

(A) Blood ammonia level

(B) Blood glucose level

(C) Blood lactate level

(D) Urine ketone level

55. A 4-year-old girl with known type 1 diabetes presents to the emergency department for dehydration. Her brother was recently diagnosed with acute gastroenteritis, and she has now had vomiting and diarrhea for the last day. Her mom has been checking her blood sugar and urine ketones, and both most recently read as high, despite prior correction with insulin at home, so she brought her to the emergency department. Initial pH on a venous blood gas was 7.05 with a bicarbonate of 5 mEq/L. You diagnose diabetic ketoacidosis, start intravenous rehydration and an insulin drip, and arrange for transfer to the closest children's hospital with an intensive care unit. The patient appears to be improving as she awaits transfer, with glucose levels dropping and her bicarbonate level improving. Three hours after initiation of the insulin drip, she complains of a headache and becomes more somnolent. What is the BEST first intervention for this condition?

(A) Emergent head CT

(B) Immediate intubation and hyperventilation

(C) Intravenous bolus of sodium bicarbonate

(D) Intravenous mannitol 0.5 g/kg

56. A 10-year-old developmentally delayed boy with a ventriculoperitoneal shunt is brought to the emergency department for vomiting and headache for 1 day. His mother reports no recent fevers, and his last shunt revision was 18 months ago, at which time he had presented with similar symptoms. A shunt series x-ray and a head CT show no changes from the prior imaging done. Which of the following statements BEST describes the emergency management of this patient?
    (A) Administration of IV antibiotics as this patient is high risk for shunt infection
    (B) Aspiration of the shunt by the emergency physician to reduce intracranial pressure
    (C) Consultation to neurosurgery as neuroimaging cannot rule out shunt malfunction
    (D) Observation in the emergency department for 6 hours to see if symptoms improve

57. A 12-year-old girl is brought to the emergency department by family members for behavioral concerns. She has previously lived in a group home and recently moved back in with her maternal aunt. The aunt reports that the patient is often hostile, refuses to follow directions, runs away from home several times a month, and is easily angered. She has never been arrested and has not been known to be physically aggressive. What is the BEST diagnosis for this behavior?
    (A) Attention-deficit/hyperactivity disorder
    (B) Bipolar disorder
    (C) Conduct disorder
    (D) Oppositional defiant disorder

58. Which of the following injuries is the MOST CONCERNING for abuse?
    (A) A bruise on the outer ear of a 9-month-old after falling off a couch
    (B) A femur fracture in a 3-year-old after falling off a jungle gym
    (C) A linear skull fracture in a 4-month-old after mom fell while carrying her
    (D) A nondisplaced spiral tibia fracture in a 2-year-old after falling in a playroom

59. A 2-year-old girl is brought in by her mother after telling her that an "uncle touched her down there." The last time the patient was in contact with that uncle was 1 week ago. You take an appropriate history and perform a physical examination including inspection of the genitourinary area, which does not demonstrate any evidence of injury. What is the NEXT BEST step to take in this case?
    (A) Discharge home, as a normal physical examination rules out sexual abuse
    (B) Inform the mother that you have to report this incident to child protective services
    (C) Perform a speculum examination with swabs for gonorrhea and chlamydia testing
    (D) Refer the patient for forensic collection by a trained sexual assault team

ANSWERS

1. **The answer is D.** (Chapters 106 and 110) The most common cause of mortality in children aged 1 to 24 years in the United States is unintentional injuries. In infants <1 year, the most common cause of mortality is congenital anomalies, followed by short gestation, sudden infant death syndrome, maternal complications of pregnancy, and unintentional injuries. Worldwide, the most common cause of mortality in infants and children up to the age of 9 years is malaria, in children aged 10 to 14 years is human immunodeficiency virus, and in children aged 15 to 19 years is suicide.

2. **The answer is D.** (Chapter 108) Positive pressure ventilation is indicated in a newborn who has a heart rate less than 100, is having gasping respirations, or apnea in the first 60 seconds of the resuscitation. Endotracheal intubation is indicated in the absence of improvement with bag-mask ventilation, concomitant need for chest compressions, administration of endotracheal medications, known or suspected congenital diaphragmatic hernia, or extremely low birth weight (<1000 g). Chest compressions are indicated if, despite assisted ventilation for 30 seconds, the newborn remains severely bradycardic with a heart rate <60. Intravenous epinephrine is indicated if bradycardia persists despite bag-mask ventilation followed by endotracheal intubation, adequate ventilation with 100% oxygen, and chest compressions for 45 to 60 seconds.

3. **The answer is D.** (Chapter 109) Paroxysmal atrial tachycardia (supraventricular tachycardia) is seen most often in infants presenting with narrow complex tachycardia, with a heart rate between 250 and 350. Treatment of unstable supraventricular tachycardia is immediate administration of synchronized cardioversion (0.5–1.0 J/kg). Adenosine, vagal maneuvers, and cardioversion are used to treat stable supraventricular tachycardia. Defibrillation (2 J/kg initial dose) is indicated for ventricular fibrillation or pulseless ventricular tachycardia.

4. **The answer is C.** (Chapter 109) In a child with asystole, following cardiopulmonary resuscitation (CPR), the initial treatment of choice is epinephrine. Atropine is indicated in children with symptomatic bradycardia associated with increased vagal tone or first-degree heart block in the absence of reversible causes. Defibrillation is indicated for ventricular fibrillation or pulseless ventricular tachycardia. Termination of resuscitation efforts should be considered in pediatric cardiopulmonary arrest lasting >20 minutes.

5. **The answer is B.** (Chapter 110) The most important step in trauma care for children is the assessment, stabilization, and management of the airway while maintaining inline cervical spine immobilization. Indications for endotracheal intubation in the trauma patient includes Glasgow Coma Score <8 or inability to maintain or protect the airway, inadequate oxygenation or ventilation, inability to ventilate or oxygenate with bag-valve mask, potential for clinical deterioration (facial burns, inhalation injury, etc.), flail chest, decompensated shock resistant to fluid resuscitation, or anticipated surgical intervention or need for radiologic investigation outside of the emergency department in an unstable patient.

6. **The answer is D.** (Chapter 110) In an effort to create a prediction rule to identify children at very low risk for clinically important intra-abdominal injury following blunt abdominal trauma, the Pediatric Emergency Care Applied Research Network conducted a large, multicenter study, using only history and physical examination findings. Children were included if they presented to the emergency department with blunt torso (thorax and abdomen) trauma within 24 hours of the injury. Clinically important intra-abdominal injuries were defined as injuries associated with an acute intervention, such as: death caused by the IAI, a therapeutic intervention (laparotomy, angiographic embolization to treat bleeding), a blood transfusion for anemia as a result of hemorrhage, or administration of intravenous fluids for two or more nights in patients with pancreatic or gastrointestinal injury. Children with blunt abdominal trauma were classified as very low risk if they met the following criteria: (1) no evidence of abdominal wall trauma/ seat belt sign, (2) Glasgow Coma Score >13, (3) no abdominal tenderness on examination, (4) no thoracic wall trauma, (5) no complaints of abdominal pain, (6) normal breath sounds, and (7) no vomiting.

7. **The answer is C.** (Chapter 113) Cuffed endotracheal tubes are preferred for term newborns through older children. Endotracheal tube size, measured by the internal diameter, can be estimated by the following formula in children >2 years of age: (age +16)/3.5. Although endotracheal tubes with <5.5-mm internal diameter were traditionally recommended to be uncuffed, more recent data suggest that cuffed tubes in younger children is safe, as long as cuff inflation pressures are closely monitored. Furthermore, cuffed tubes are beneficial in cases when high airway pressures or changing compliance are anticipated, such as asthma, pneumonia, or acute respiratory distress syndrome. Use of a cuffed endotracheal tube decreases the number of tracheal tube changes required to obtain a reliably sealed airway. Straight laryngoscope blades are indicated in all ages, while curved laryngoscope blades can

TABLE 10.1	Age-Based Airway Equipment Size	
Age	Internal Diameter (mm)	Blade Size
Premature	3.0 Uncuffed	0 Straight
0–6 mo	3.5 Cuffed	1 Straight
6–12 mo	4.0 Cuffed	1–1.5 Straight
1–2 y	4.5 Cuffed	1.5 Straight
3–4 y	4.5 Cuffed	1.5–2 Straight or curved
5–6 y	5.0 Cuffed	2.0 Curved
7–8 y	5.5 Cuffed	2.0 Curved
9–10 y	6.0 Cuffed	2.0 Curved
≥11 y	6.5 Cuffed	3.0 Curved

Reproduced with permission from J.E. Tintinalli, J.S. Stapczynski, O.J. Ma, D. Yealy, G.D. Meckler, D.M. Cline: Tintinalli's Emergency Medicine: A Comprehensive Study Guide, 9th Edition. McGraw-Hill Education; 2020.

be used in children 3 years and older. Suggested laryngoscope blade sizes are noted in Table 10.1.

8. **The answer is C.** (Chapter 114) Intraosseous access cannulates a noncollapsible structure that connects to the central circulation, and is indicated when there is an emergent need for vascular access and other sites are difficult, high risk, or time consuming. Access if often obtained using battery-powered cordless drills with a specialized needle, such as the EZ-IO device. Medications and fluids may be infused through the intraosseous route, and diagnostic laboratory tests may be performed on blood samples taken from the intraosseous route. The ideal location for intraosseous access is a large bone with easily palpable landmarks, a thin cortex and limited proximity to vital structures, such as the proximal and distal tibia, distal femur, and sternum. The flat surface of the anteromedial proximal tibia is easily accessible given the paucity of overlying tissue, and often the primary location for initial intraosseous attempts.

9. **The answer is B.** (Chapter 115) Procedural sedation is often required in the management of injured infants and children (Table 10.2). Depending on the indications for procedural sedation (anxiolysis, sedation, and/or analgesia), the emergency medicine physician should choose a medication, or combination of medications, to attain success in the performance of the procedure while limiting potential morbidity and mortality. In the reduction and casting of a closed forearm fracture, procedural sedation should provide anesthetic, analgesic, and amnestic effects; therefore, ketamine is often used for procedural sedation in children requiring orthopedic manipulation. Etomidate, midazolam, and propofol do not have analgesic effects, and therefore are not appropriate alone for procedures that potentially involve discomfort and pain.

10. **The answer is B.** (Chapter 116) Overwhelming neonatal sepsis is the most common cause of neonatal cardiorespiratory distress. Neonates may present with temperature instability (fever, hypothermia), central nervous system (CNS) dysfunction (lethargy, irritability, seizures), respiratory distress (apnea, tachypnea, grunting), feeding difficulty (vomiting, poor feeding, gastric distention, diarrhea), jaundice, or rashes. Management of neonatal sepsis begins with attention to airway, breathing and circulation, immediately followed by the administration of intravenous antibiotics (ampicillin, an aminoglycoside, and acyclovir). The practitioner should attempt to obtain blood, urine, and cerebrospinal fluid cultures if possible, but the administration of antibiotics should not be delayed. A lumbar puncture should not be performed on a newborn who potentially could lose their airway during the procedure. Intravenous dextrose should be given to a newborn if their bedside glucose is <40 mg/dL. The newborn in the scenario is maintaining their airway, so endotracheal intubation should be deferred.

11. **The answer is D.** (Chapter 116) An abdominal catastrophe, such as congenital malrotation with midgut volvulus or necrotizing enterocolitis, should be considered in a critically ill neonate with abdominal symptoms. Malrotation with midgut volvulus may present with bilious vomiting, irritability or lethargy, abdominal distension and discomfort, and bloody stool or heme-positive stool. If volvulus is present, the newborn may present with shock (35% mortality rate). Diagnostic test of choice is an upper gastrointestinal series, demonstrating a displaced duodenal-jejunal junction (to the right of the spine) with the jejunum on the right side of the abdomen (corkscrew appearance). Treatment is intravenous fluids and antibiotics, and emergency surgery.

12. **The answer is B.** (Chapter 117) The scenario describes a brief resolved unexplained event (BRUE), or an brief episode (less than 1 minute) that is frightening to a caregiver and involves some combination of change in breathing (absent, decreased or irregular), color change (cyanosis, pallor or plethora), changes in muscle tone (limp or stiff) and/or altered level of consciousness. The most common identifiable cause for a BRUE is gastroesophageal reflux, although other causes include bronchiolitis, seizures, nonaccidental brain injury, pertussis, and serious bacterial infections. A thorough history and physical examination should categorize the infant into low or high risk categories and thus indicate which infant requires additional evaluation, diagnostic imaging, or monitoring (Figure 10.7).

TABLE 10.2 Medications for Procedural Sedation

Class	Drug	Route	Dose	Onset	Duration	Advantages	Disadvantages	Examples	Comments
Nonpainful Procedures									
Anxiolytic	Midazolam	PO, PR, IV, IM, IN	PO/PR 0.5 mg/kg; IV/IM 0.05–0.1 mg/kg; IN 0.3–0.5 mg/kg	PO/PR 20–30 min; IV 3–5 min; IM 10–20 min; IN 5–10 min	1–4 h	Flexible route of administration	No analgesia, paradoxical reaction	CT scan; ultrasound; echocardiography	Acidic, nasal administration stings, may cause increased secretions; oral/rectal slow onset; less predictable
Sedative	Pentobarbital	PO	3–5 mg/kg	30 min	Variable	Relatively safe in oral doses	No analgesia	CT scan	Variable efficacy; long recovery times
Minor Painful Procedures									
Dissociative	Nitrous oxide	Inhaled	Titrate to effect (30%–70%)	Minutes	Minutes	Self-dosing	Not readily available	Laceration repair; LP; dental procedures	Scavenger system recommended
Analgesic	Fentanyl	IN	1.5 mcg/kg (maximum, 0.5 mL per nare)	10 min	20 min	Little to no adverse effects	Short lived	Laceration repair; suspected clavicle fracture	Equivalent to IV morphine
Analgesic and mild sedative	Subdissociative dose ketamine	IV/IN	0.3 mg/kg IV; 1 mg/kg IN	Variable	60 min	Few adverse effects		Laceration repair; abscess drainage	Paucity of pediatric data
Hypnotic/sedative	Dexmedetomidine	IN	0.5–2 mcg/kg	25 min	85 min	No respiratory/hemodynamic compromise	Long time to onset	Laceration repair; LP; abscess drainage	Paucity of data for ED procedures
Major Painful Procedures									
Hypnotic/sedative	Propofol	IV	1–2 mg/kg, followed by 0.5 mg/kg; repeat doses as needed	Seconds	Minutes	Rapid onset and short duration, motionlessness, muscle relaxant	No analgesia, respiratory and cardiovascular depressant	CT scan, LP with topical analgesic, laceration repair, reduction of dislocation	Nonanalgesic, increased requirement for younger patients, painful injection
	Etomidate	IV	0.2–0.3 mg/kg	Seconds	Minutes	Rapid onset, short duration	No analgesia, myoclonus, respiratory depressant	CT scan, short procedures requiring motionlessness	Avoid in patients with increased tone (e.g., CP) due to myoclonic jerks, painful injection
Dissociative	Ketamine	IV, IM	IV 1–1.5 mg/kg; IM 4–5 mg/kg	IV 1–2 min; IM 3–5 min	IV 15 min; IM 30–45 min	Analgesic, anesthetic, motionlessness, respiratory and cardiovascular stimulant, bronchodilator	Increased intraocular pressure, intracranial pressure, salivation; emetogenic; laryngospasm	Painful procedures requiring motionlessness (complex lacerations, fracture reductions, I&D), no reversal agent	Consider pretreatment with ondansetron; atropine and midazolam coadministration unnecessary
	Propofol + ketamine	IV	Propofol 1 mg/kg, ketamine 0.5 mg/kg	1 min	Propofol (minutes); ketamine 15–45 min	Decreased dosing for both agents, complementary side effects (lessens respiratory and cardiovascular depression, emesis)	Increased risk of serious adverse events such as oxygen desaturation (compared to ketamine alone)	Fracture reduction, I&D, complex laceration	Recent evidence suggests coadministration is associated with greater risk of adverse events

Abbreviations: CP = cerebral palsy; I&D = incision and drainage; IN = intranasally.

Reproduced with permission from J.E. Tintinalli, J.S. Stapczynski, O.J. Ma D. Yealy, G.D. Meckler, D.M. Cline: Tintinalli's Emergency Medicine: A Comprehensive Study Guide, 9th Edition. McGraw-Hill Education; 2020.

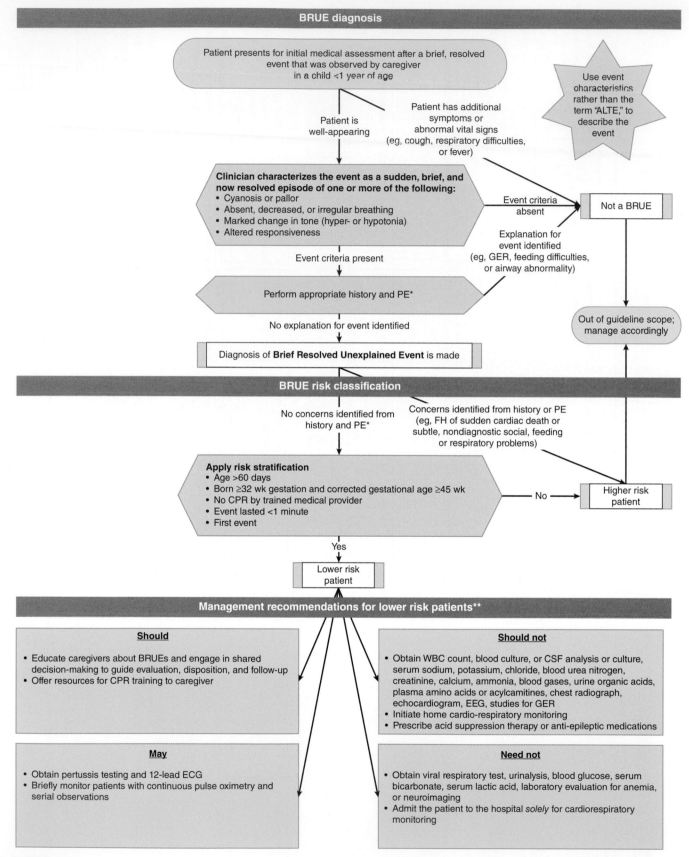

FIGURE 10.7

TABLE 10.3	Comparison of Low-Risk Rochester Criteria, Philadelphia Protocol, and Boston Criteria for Assessment of Fever in Well-Appearing Neonates and Infants[*]		
Low-Risk Criteria for Serious Bacterial Infection[*]	**Rochester Criteria**	**Philadelphia Protocol**	**Boston Criteria**
Fever	T ≥38°C (100.4°F)	T ≥38.2°C (100.8°F)	T ≥38°C (100.4°F)
Age	≤60 d	29–56 d	28–89 d
Past medical history	Term infant ≥37 wk gestation No perinatal or postnatal antibiotics No treatment for jaundice No chronic illnesses or admissions Not hospitalized longer than mother	No immunodeficiency syndrome	No immunizations within 48 h No recent antibiotics
Physical examination	Well appearing Unremarkable examination	Same	Same
Laboratory values			
Blood count	WBC ≥5000/mm³, ≤15,000/mm³ Absolute band count ≤1500/mm³	WBC ≤15,000/mm³ Band-to-neutrophil ratio ≤0.2	WBC ≤20,000/mm³
Urinalysis	WBC ≤10 per high-power field	WBC ≤10 per high-power field	WBC ≤10 per high-power field
Stool	WBC ≤5 per high-power field	—	—
Lumbar puncture and cerebrospinal fluid findings	None	WBC ≤8 per high-power field	WBC ≤10 per high-power field Negative Gram stain
Chest radiograph	None	Negative	Negative if obtained
Comments	Excluded lumbar puncture, so number of missed meningitis cases is unknown. UTIs missed in those with negative urinalysis. The least sensitive of the low-risk criteria.	Sensitivity of low-risk criteria for SBI 98%; specificity 44%; PPV 14%; NPV 99.7%	5% of low-risk neonates and infants had SBI (8 bacteremia, 8 UTI, 10 bacterial gastroenteritis); 96% sensitive to ceftriaxone

Abbreviations: NPV = negative predictive value; PPV = positive predictive value; SBI = serious bacterial illness; T = temperature; UTI = urinary tract infection.

[*]Any single deviation from the criteria is interpreted as failure of low-risk criteria.

Reproduced with permission from J.E. Tintinalli, J.S. Stapczynski, O.J. Ma, D. Yealy, G.D. Meckler, D.M. Cline: Tintinalli's Emergency Medicine: A Comprehensive Study Guide, 9th Edition. McGraw-Hill Education; 2020.

13. **The answer is B.** (Chapter 119) Clinical assessment of the severity of illness in infants ≤3 months of age can be difficult. Three commonly applied outpatient criteria for the management of fever in well appearing infants ≤3 months include the Rochester, Philadelphia, and Boston Criteria. For infants aged 29 to 56 days with a fever ≥38.2°C, the Philadelphia criteria are often suggested: complete blood cell count with differential, blood culture, urinalysis, urine culture, cerebrospinal fluid cell count/gram stain/culture, chest radiograph; risk stratify based on initial evaluation to high risk (intravenous antibiotics and hospitalization) or low risk (discharge home without antibiotics). In infants stratified to low risk based on Philadelphia Criteria, sensitivity is 98% and negative predictive value is 99.7% for serious bacterial infection (Table 10.3).

14. **The answer is D.** (Chapter 119) The most common serious bacterial infection in infants younger than 3 months is urinary tract infections, with an incidence between 2% and 8%. Urinary tract infections may not produce symptoms other than fever, so routinely obtain a urinalysis and urine culture in the evaluation of the febrile neonate or infant without a source. Diagnosis can be made with a microscopic urinalysis (white blood cell

[WBC] count of at least 5–10/high-power field [51%–91% sensitivity] or bacteria on gram stain [80%–87% sensitivity]) and urine culture (obtain a urine culture even if the initial urinalysis is negative in a patient at high risk for urinary tract infections, including infants ≤3 months).

15. **The answer is B.** (Chapter 120) The most common cause of bacterial meningitis in children in the United States, prior to advancements in immunizations, was *Haemophilus influenzae* type b followed by *Streptococcus pneumoniae*. Since the widespread implementation of standard vaccinations, *Neisseria meningitides* is now the primary cause of bacterial meningitis in the United States. However, the most common cause of meningitis in school aged children continues to be viral meningitis, with enterovirus being the most common etiology identified.

16. **The answer is A.** (Chapter 121) The child in the scenario meets criteria for initial observation for acute otitis media as he is older than 6 months, only has mild ear pain, symptoms have been present for less than 48 hours, and his fevers are less than 102.2°F, without any signs of perforation or history of myringotomy tubes. If he did not meet all of these criteria, the first-line antibiotic would be

TABLE 10.4	Indications for Consideration of Initial Observation for Acute Otitis Media (AOM)[7]

Children 6–23 mo old with *unilateral* AOM without severe signs or symptoms

- Mild ear pain for <48 h
- Temperature <39°C (102.2°F)

Children ≥24 mo old with *unilateral or bilateral* AOM without severe signs or symptoms

- Mild ear pain for <48 h
- Temperature <39°C (102.2°F)

Note: When observation is used, a mechanism must be in place to ensure follow-up and initiation of antibiotics if the child worsens or fails to improve within 48 to 72 hours of onset of symptoms.

Reproduced with permission from J.E. Tintinalli, J.S. Stapczynski, O.J. Ma, D. Yealy, G.D. Meckler, D.M. Cline: Tintinalli's Emergency Medicine: A Comprehensive Study Guide, 9th Edition. McGraw-Hill Education; 2020.

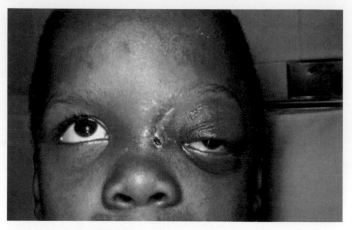

FIGURE 10.8   Photo contributor: Binita R. Shah, MD.

oral amoxicillin, 45 mg/kg, twice a day for 5 to 10 days, as the higher dose is needed to appropriately treat resistant forms of *Streptococcus pneumoniae*, the most common bacterial cause of acute otitis media. Ciprofloxacin drops would be the treatment of choice for acute otitis externa which based on the physical examination, this child does not have (Tables 10.4 and 10.5).

17. **The answer is C.** (Chapter 122) Periorbital cellulitis is characterized by swollen, erythematous, indurated, and tender eyelids without changes in visual acuity, conjunctival injection, proptosis, pain with eye movement, or impairment in extra ocular movements. Orbital cellulitis is characterized by swollen, erythematous, indurated, and tender eyelids, accompanied by proptosis, impaired extra ocular movements, pain with eye movement, changes in visual acuity, or conjunctival injection. If there is any ambiguity in the clinical examination or limitations due to the age of the patient, an orbital and sinus CT scan can be used to differentiate between the two (Figure 10.8).

TABLE 10.5	Indications for Initial Antibiotic Use for Acute Otitis Media (AOM): No Observation Period[7]

- All infants <6 mo old
- All children with severe signs or symptoms
  - Moderate or severe ear pain or
  - Ear pain for ≥48 h or
  - Temperature >39°C (102.2°F)
- Children <24 mo old with bilateral AOM
- Recurrent AOM (prior episode of AOM within 2–4 wk)
- AOM with perforation
- Patients with myringotomy (pressure-equalizing) tubes in place
- Patients with craniofacial abnormalities
- Immunocompromised patients
- Any child with AOM if the provider or caregiver is not comfortable with initial observation

Reproduced with permission from J.E. Tintinalli, J.S. Stapczynski, O.J. Ma, D. Yealy, G.D. Meckler, D.M. Cline: Tintinalli's Emergency Medicine: A Comprehensive Study Guide, 9th Edition. McGraw-Hill Education; 2020.

18. **The answer is C.** (Chapter 122) Age of presentation for newborn conjunctivitis can help determine etiology. Chemical conjunctivitis after exposure to the erythromycin ointment prophylaxis given in the newborn nursery usually presents within 24 hours of administration and requires no treatment except for reassurance. Infants who present between 2 and 7 days of life with conjunctivitis should be evaluated for Neisseria gonorrhoeae and treated with admission and intravenous antibiotics. The timing of presentation in this scenario, between 7 and 14 days of age, is most consistent with a chlamydial infection, which is treated with oral antibiotics, as long as there are no respiratory symptoms or evidence of pneumonia. If the child presented between 14 and 28 days of life, the most likely diagnosis would be viral conjunctivitis, such as herpes simplex virus, which requires treatment with intravenous and topical antivirals.

19. **The answer is A.** (Chapter 123) In an adolescent boy with profuse unilateral epistaxis requiring packing, juvenile nasal angiofibroma should be suspected and the patient should be evaluated with a CT scan. Rhinitis sicca is more common in winter months, with low humidity and dry air heating, causing nasal mucosa desiccation. Simple epistaxis should be considered when there is known trauma or the bleeding subsides within a few minutes with appropriate nasal pressure. Von Willebrand disease should be considered in patients with recurrent epistaxis, other sources of bleeding besides the nose, or a family history of a bleeding disorder.

20. **The answer is A.** (Chapter 124) Time is important in the survival of an avulsed tooth. If it is reimplanted within 5 minutes, there is an 85% to 97% chance of survival, but there is an almost 0% survival if it takes longer than 1 hour to reimplant the tooth. Scrubbing the debris off the tooth should be avoided as this can cause further damage to the

periodontal ligaments; only a gentle rinsing with water or saline should be used to remove debris. If the tooth cannot be immediately replanted it should be stored in ViaSpan, Hanks' Balanced Salt Solution, cold milk, saliva, saline, or water (in order of preference).

21. **The answer is C.** (Chapter 125) Thyroglossal duct cysts are midline and mostly infrahyoid in location. The pathognomonic feature of a thyroglossal duct cyst is a painless fluctuant mass that moves with swallowing and/or protrusion of the tongue, which can present in childhood and persist into adulthood. Brachial cleft cysts are often anterior to the sternocleidomastoid and near the angle of the mandible. Dermoid cysts usually occur in children younger than 3 years, are midline and often suprahyoid, and are mobile but do not move with tongue protrusion. The most common cause of thyroid cancer in children is papillary thyroid cancer and usually presents in an advanced stage with metastatic involvement.

22. **The answer is A.** (Chapter 126) Airway hemangioma should be considered in an infant with biphasic stridor that does not respond to nebulized racemic epinephrine, especially in an infant with cutaneous hemangiomas on the skin, particularly in the beard distribution. Laryngomalacia is very common in infants with stridor, but the stridor should improve with neck extension and prone positioning. Subglottic stenosis should be considered in an infant with a history of intubation post-delivery. An infant with viral croup is more likely to present with an acute onset of stridor associated with fever, nasal congestion, and "barky" cough, with the worst symptoms on illness day 3 to 4.

23. **The answer is B.** (Chapter 126) Irregular tracheal margins are associated with bacterial tracheitis, often found in unimmunized children aged 5 to 8 years, usually occurring after an upper respiratory infection, in a child with high fever, stridor, cough and toxic appearance. Retropharyngeal swelling is noted when the prevertebral soft tissue C2 is twice the diameter at C4, and associated with a retropharyngeal abscess, often found in children aged 1 to 4 years old, with preceding upper respiratory infection, severe inspiratory stridor, muffled hot potato voice, drooling and limitation to the range of motion of the neck. Steeple sign (subglottic narrowing) is seen on the AP neck radiographs of children with viral croup, often seen in children aged 6 months to 3 years, presenting with fever, nasal congestion, "barky" cough and hoarse voice. Thumbprint sign is seen on lateral neck radiographs in unimmunized children aged 1 to 7 years with epiglottitis, who often present in the "tripod position" with acute onset of fever, drooling, and inspiratory stridor.

24. **The answer is C.** (Chapter 127) The American Academy of Pediatrics suggest that the most important initial treatment for infants with bronchiolitis is instillation of saline into the nares followed by nasal suctioning and using supplemental oxygen to maintain SpO_2 >90%. There is no benefit documented in clinical course, admission rate, or length of hospital stay in response to albuterol or nebulized hypertonic saline use in bronchiolitis. Inhaled nebulized epinephrine may have a role in children who are acutely deteriorating from severe bronchiolitis, if used in conjunction with steroids. Heliox has not been proven to decrease length of stay in infants with bronchiolitis.

25. **The answer is C.** (Chapter 127) Inhaled corticosteroids have not been shown to have a role in the acute emergency department management of a child with status asthmaticus, but should be prescribed prior to discharge in a child with severe asthma. Inhaled ipratropium bromide is an anticholinergic that blocks the muscarinic receptors in the bronchiole leading to bronchodilation, and should be used in combination with short-acting B_2 agonists. Magnesium sulfate inhibits smooth muscle contraction leading to bronchodilation and can be used in the treatment of an acute asthma exacerbation, but should not be a first line treatment. Early administration of systemic corticosteroids has been shown to decrease emergency department length of stay, admission rate, and likelihood of relapse, and should be given as early in the emergency department visit as possible.

26. **The answer is C.** (Chapter 128) A chest radiograph should be obtained in all children younger than 3 months as part of a sepsis evaluation; however, it should not be routine in children >3 months of age. Fever and white blood cell count alone are not absolute indicators for a chest radiograph, regardless of the height. However, the combination of fevers greater than 39°C, white blood cell count >20,000, and no clear source of infection should prompt the provider to order a chest radiograph. Patients with a history of congenital anomalies, whether pulmonary or cardiac in origin, deserve a chest radiograph when presenting with features concerning for pneumonia.

27. **The answer is A.** (Chapter 129) The four components of tetralogy of Fallot are a large ventricular septal defect, right ventricular outflow tract obstruction, right ventricular hypertrophy, and an overriding aorta. ECG shows right-axis deviation and right ventricular hypertrophy. Chest radiograph shows the classic "boot-shaped heart." Tricuspid atresia presents with cyanosis, tachypnea, a single S_2, 3/6 regurgitant systolic murmur heard best at the left lower sternal border. ECG often shows a superior QRS axis, right and left atrial hypertrophy, and left ventricular

hypertrophy. Chest radiograph shows normal heart size with decreased pulmonary vascular markings. Total anomalous pulmonary venous return would reveal on physical examination cyanosis and tachypnea in addition to a right ventricular heave, fixed split S_2, 3/6 systolic ejection murmur at the left upper sternal border, and a mid-diastolic rumble. ECG shows right axis deviation and right ventricular hypertrophy. Chest radiograph shows significant cardiomegaly, increased pulmonary vascular markings, and is described as a "snowman" sign. A ventricular septal defect alone is an acyanotic cardiac lesion that would present with 2–5/6 holosystolic, harsh murmur at the left lower sternal border and a narrowly split S_2. ECG findings include left atrial and ventricular hypertrophy.

28. **The answer is A.** (Chapter 130) The child in this scenario most likely had a breath-holding spell, and with no other concerning features found on the history or physical examination, requires no specific evaluation or treatment. However, all children who present with syncope to the emergency department should receive an ECG to screen for cardiac etiology.

29. **The answer is C.** (Chapter 130) Class II antiarrhythmics are the mainstay of treatment for patients with long QT syndrome; however, they are ineffective for some long QT variants. Class Ib medications should be used with suspected long QT that is refractory to class II agents. Classes Ia and III agents should not be used if long QT syndrome is suspected as they prolong the QT interval.

30. **The answer is C.** (Chapter 131) Pyloric stenosis is a condition that is usually diagnosed by ultrasound and clinical history of progressive, nonbilious emesis in an infant younger than 10 weeks. The peak incidence is at 5 weeks of life. Emergency department stabilization includes correction of electrolytes and surgical consultation. The diagnosis is usually confirmed by ultrasound. Intussusception typically occurs in older infants (peaks at 12 months of age) and is characterized by colicky abdominal pain, which precedes emesis. Malrotation with (typically midgut) volvulus is characterized by bilious emesis, usually in an infant younger than 4 weeks. It requires immediate surgical intervention to prevent bowel necrosis. Acute gastroenteritis is the most common cause of vomiting and diarrhea in children. Though it can present as just vomiting in young infants, it is usually associated with loss of appetite.

31. **The answer is B.** (Chapter 133) Ondansetron can be used in children with persistent vomiting as an adjunct to oral rehydration therapy. Metoclopramide, prochlorperazine, and promethazine are dopamine receptor antagonists, and are not recommended as first line agents in children due to respiratory depression, extrapyramidal reactions, and lack of evidence of efficacy.

32. **The answer is C.** (Chapters 131 and 133) The ultrasound images show the typical findings of intussusception, with a classic target appearance on cross-section due to bowel inside of bowel. Intussusception is typically characterized by colicky abdominal pain, which precedes vomiting. It can also present as unexplained lethargy. "Currant jelly" stools, thought to be the "classic" presentation, occur in a minority of cases. Physical examination is often normal, though a mass in the right lower quadrant may be appreciated. Appendicitis is usually characterized by a noncompressible tubular structure on ultrasound. Classically, patients present with periumbilical pain that migrated to the right lower quadrant, with associated anorexia, nausea, and possibly fever. Constipation is a common cause of intermittent abdominal pain but is a diagnosis rarely made by ultrasound. A Meckel's diverticulum will often present as painless rectal bleeding, sometimes in significant quantities, not colicky abdominal pain. The study of choice for evaluation would be a nuclear medicine scan, not an ultrasound.

33. **The answer is D.** (Chapter 134) Hematemesis in a newborn is most likely swallowed maternal blood. As 5 months is much too far after delivery to be from blood ingested during the delivery itself, the most likely source is blood from mother's cracked nipples while breastfeeding. Asking the mother about breastfeeding and pain/bleeding, and examination of the mother, if allowed, will give you more information. An Apt test can be performed to distinguish maternal from infant blood but is not available at every hospital. Examination of the stool will not give you any further information in the setting of known hematemesis. Labs are often guided by the child's appearance and likely diagnosis. Since this child is well-appearing and the source is not likely the patient, laboratory studies will not help the management. Nasogastric lavage is unlikely to help in this situation and also does not rule out active bleeding in an infant that you are concerned about an upper gastrointestinal tract source.

34. **The answer is D.** (Chapter 135) In infants and children who are not toilet-trained, the preferred method for urine collection is bladder catheterization. Perineal bag collection of urine may yield inaccurate culture results. A blood culture is unlikely to yield more information with a known urinary source. As the definitive test for a urinary tract infection remains a urine culture, empiric antibiotics

should not be given prior to collection of urine for culture, unless the patient is in extremis and antibiotics need to be given immediately. A renal ultrasound would be unlikely to add any diagnostic information at this time, as renal abscesses are rare in children, and would be more likely to present as urinary tract infections and fever that do not resolve with oral antibiotics. A renal ultrasound may be ordered by the primary doctor after the urinary tract infection resolves, to evaluate for urinary tract anomalies. This testing is rarely done in the emergency department.

35. **The answer is A.** (Chapter 136) Recommended treatment of epididymitis is slightly controversial, but in this non sexually active boy without evidence of a urinary tract infection, analgesia and rest are acceptable treatment choices. Manual detorsion would only be recommended if there was concern for torsion, which is unlikely given the normal vascular flow seen on ultrasound. Urology consultation from the emergency department is not necessary for epididymitis, as it does not need surgical management. Delayed surgical management may be indicated in cases of fully reduced testicular torsion. Intravenous antibiotics would be appropriate for treatment of pyelonephritis in a child who cannot tolerate oral intake, but this patient has a negative urinalysis, and is unlikely to have pyelonephritis.

36. **The answer is C.** (Chapter 136) The description given is urethral prolapse, where venous congestion of the prolapsed distal urethra gives the tissue a purple color. The first treatment choice would be conservative management, with estrogen cream and sitz baths. If that fails or the tissue is necrotic, urology or gynecology should be consulted for surgical repair. Oral antibiotics and surgical referral or drainage would be appropriate for an abscess or Bartholin's gland cyst, which would be rare in this age group. Urethral prolapse is not a result of sexual abuse, and does not warrant a report to child protective services, unless there are other concerns. It can be exacerbated by constipation, which is common in young children, so treatment of that condition may be helpful.

37. **The answer is B.** (Chapter 137) This patient has new-onset nephrotic syndrome. In patients with nephrotic syndrome, diuretics for volume overload may not be useful in the setting of severe hypoalbuminemia, and an infusion of albumin should precede diuretics. Steroids should not be initiated until after consultation with nephrology in the setting of the initial episode of nephrotic syndrome. This patient may require intensive care, but not for renal biopsy. Biopsy is not indicated in all cases during the initial episode. This patient is not in renal failure with a normal creatinine and electrolytes and does not need renal replacement therapy at this time.

38. **The answer is A.** (Chapter 138) Second and third line treatment include fosphenytoin, levetiracetam, phenobarbital, and valproic acid, and should be initiated after two appropriate doses of benzodiazepines. Ketamine, though effective in aborting seizures in some studies, is not yet recommended, and would not be a second-line therapy. Intravenous lorazepam could be given at 0.1 mg/kg, but after two doses of benzodiazepines, treatment should move on to the next alternative, as increasing doses of benzodiazepines increase the chance of respiratory depression and are unlikely to be successful. Propofol is a fourth-line agent and should be reserved until second- and third-line therapies fail to result in cessation of the seizure.

39. **The answer is D.** (Chapter 138) By definition, a febrile seizure that recurs within 24 hours is considered a complex febrile seizure. However, routine labs are not recommended for children who return to baseline during or prior to their emergency department visit. The American Academy of Pediatrics recommends that evaluation focus on the source of the fever. In females in this age range, urinalysis and urine culture are recommended for workup of fever without other evidence of acute infection. MRI and EEG are usually recommended in children with first-time afebrile seizures, but those can be completed on an outpatient basis, and do not need to be facilitated in the emergency department.

40. **The answer is A.** (Chapter 139) Idiopathic intracranial hypertension (pseudotumor cerebri) is characterized by a chronic progressive headache and papilledema with a normal MRI (ruling out space-occupying lesions). The diagnostic gold standard is lumbar puncture, performed in lateral decubitus position, with opening pressure. There is no indication to repeat the MRI of this patient without acute changes in headache quality or severity. Ophthalmology will likely be consulted to monitor for progressive defects in visual acuity, but this does not need to be done urgently in the emergency department for papilledema caused by increased intracranial pressure. A drug screen and psychiatry consultation is not indicated in this patient, as papilledema is unlikely to be due to a psychiatric cause.

41. **The answer is C.** (Chapter 140) A point-of-care glucose is the quickest of the listed options, and in a child with altered mental status, especially with a history of vomiting and diarrhea, it will alert the clinician to hypoglycemia or severe hyperglycemia requiring treatment. This patient may require a CT head but currently has no focal neurologic findings on examination, and symptoms may resolve with treatment of hypoglycemia. Lumbar puncture may also be indicated during the emergency department course, depending on other findings, but in this afebrile patient, does not need to be done immediately. Intussusception

can cause lethargy, and an ultrasound of the abdomen may be ordered later if indicated upon further history, but is not the first test to order this acutely sick child.

42. **The answer is D.** (Chapter 111) This child has no concerning signs on her examination, and is acting appropriately, with only a frontal hematoma on examination. Intracranial injuries are more likely to be associated with non frontal hematomas. Anticipatory guidance and return precautions should be explained to parents prior to discharge home. Several diagnostic rules—PECARN, CHANCE, and CHALICE—indicate that this child is very low risk for serious intracranial injury and does not require observation overnight, neurosurgical consultation, or a CT of the head.

43. **The answer is B.** (Chapter 111) Concussions are becoming more recognized in student athletes and are characterized by short-lived neurologic impairment after a traumatic blow. Eighty percent of "same season" concussions occur within 10 days of each other, and are more common in athletes who return to play quickly. Immediate return to play puts a player at risk for second impact syndrome, a condition exclusive to pediatrics, with a high mortality rate due to cerebral edema. Amnesia of the event caused by a concussion may never resolve, and memories may not return. Adults with concussions tend to recover faster, with return to baseline on neurocognitive tests within 3 to 5 days, compared to high school students' 10 to 14 days.

44. **The answer is B.** (Chapter 112) Pseudo-subluxation is a relatively common finding in children younger than 8 years and may be mistaken for a cervical spine injury. The line of Swischuk distinguishes between subluxation and pseudo-subluxation. A line is drawn that connects the anterior aspect of the posterior arch of C1 to the anterior aspect of the posterior arch of C3. If the line falls more than 2 mm anterior to the spinous process of C2, there is more likely to be cervical spine pathology. In this patient, the spinous processes line up, and there is unlikely to be a cervical spine fracture, and the patient should be able to be clinically cleared. Emergent MRI of the spine and urgent neurosurgical consultation are not indicated in this patient, given that she has no focal neurologic findings, is moving all extremities, and does not have any pathology seen on x-ray. Even if ligamentous injury is suspected, flexion and extension view x-rays have little utility in evaluation for spinal injury in children in the emergency department (Figure 10.9).

45. **The answer is B.** (Chapter 141) The x-ray finding described is a toddler's fracture, a common fracture in children learning to walk, and can occur after insignificant

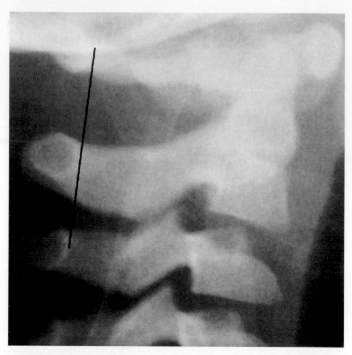

FIGURE 10.9 Reprinted with permission from Yamamoto L: Cervical spine malalignment—true or pseudosubluxation? In: Yamamoto LG, Inaba AS, DiMauro R (eds): Radiology Cases in Pediatric Emergency Medicine, Vol. 1, Case 5. Honolulu, HI: University of Hawaii John A. Burns School of Medicine, Department of Pediatrics, 1994. http://www.hawaii.edu/medicine/pediatrics/pemxray/v1c05.html.

trauma or an unwitnessed fall. Sometimes, the fracture is not evident on initial x-ray, but for radiologically evident fractures, the leg should be immobilized in a long leg cast or splint with adequate flexion to fit a car seat. Referral to child protective services is not indicated unless there are other concerns for abuse. A spica cast is used for femur fractures in young children, and is usually placed in the operating room. No immobilization would be acceptable if there was no visible fracture on radiographs, and the patient was able to follow up within a week for repeat x-rays, but referral to child protective services would still not be necessary.

46. **The answer is D.** (Chapter 141) The most common (Figures 10.10 and 10.11) elbow fracture in children is a supracondylar fracture, with 90% to 95% resulting from extension-type injuries, such as a fall onto an outstretched arm. Type 1 fractures are stable and can usually just be splinted in the emergency department. Types 2 and 3 often require surgical management and necessitate orthopedic consultation in the emergency department (Figures 10.10 and 10.11). If there are no other areas of tenderness or swelling in a cooperative patient, only imaging of the affected bones is indicated; no x-rays of the shoulder, hand, or wrist are needed. Medial epicondyle fractures are the third most common elbow fractures in children, following supracondylar and lateral condyle fractures.

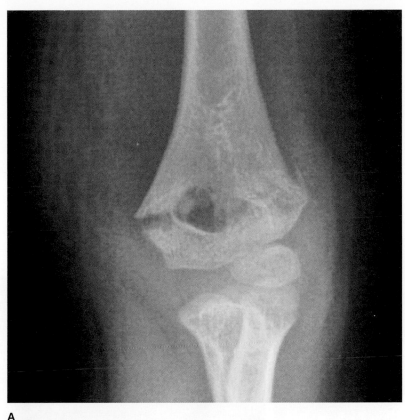

A

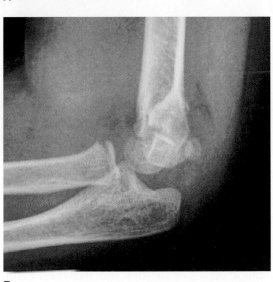

B

FIGURE 10.10 Image used with permission of Karen Black, BC Children's Hospital, Vancouver.

47. **The answer is A.** (Chapter 141) Transient synovitis may be difficult to distinguish from septic arthritis of the hip. However, in this patient with a normal white blood cell count, a low C-reactive protein, no fever, and ability to range the hip, though with pain, transient synovitis is the more likely diagnosis. The ultrasound of the hip without evidence of effusion confirms the diagnosis. It is an idiopathic inflammatory condition, though most believe it is a postviral condition, and resolves without intervention. Intravenous antibiotics and admission or orthopedic washout of the joint would be recommended if the patient had septic arthritis of the hip. Fever, leukocytosis, elevated inflammatory markers, refusal to move the joint, and an effusion on ultrasound would be classic findings of that condition. Bony changes do not occur with transient synovitis, and it is not related to Legg-Calvé-Perthes disease, which is characterized by avascular necrosis of the femoral head.

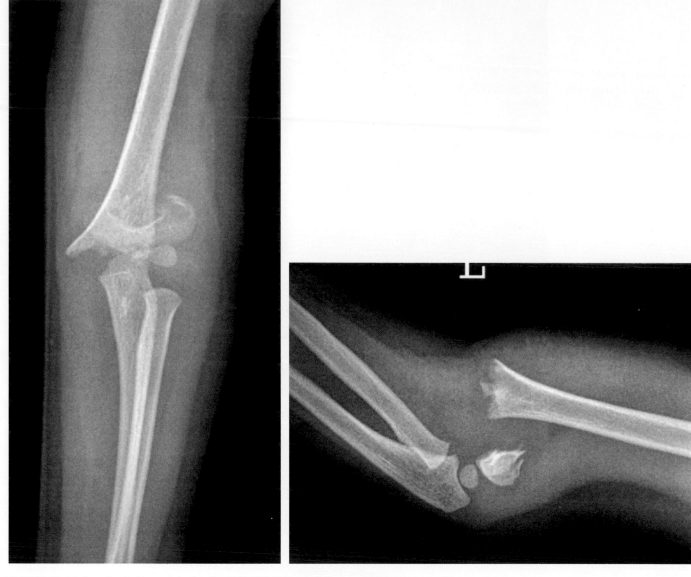

FIGURE 10.11   Reproduced with permission from Hospital for Sick Children 2018, Toronto, Canada.

48. **The answer is D.** (Chapter 142) The rash pictured is typical of Henoch-Schönlein purpura, the most common vasculitis of childhood. Renal disease occurs in about 50% of cases and is diagnosed by the presence of blood on urinalysis. Laboratory studies are not needed for straightforward cases, as it is a vasculitis and blood counts and coagulation factors are usually not affected. Ultrasound of the ankle(s) may be indicated if there was concern for septic arthritis, but the symmetrical joint involvement and lack of fever makes that diagnosis much less likely. Ultrasound of joints is not indicated in Henoch-Schönlein purpura, unless there is concern for bacterial infection.

49. **The answer is A.** (Chapter 142) The history and physical examination are consistent with a diagnosis of Kawasaki's disease. Classic criteria are a fever for 5 or more

days plus four of the following findings: bilateral nonexudative conjunctivitis, cervical lymphadenopathy (usually unilateral and bigger than 1.5 cm), erythema or cracking of the lips and strawberry tongue, peeling or other skin changes of the extremities, and nonvesicular rash. Treatment includes high-dose aspirin therapy and intravenous immunoglobulin infusion to reduce the risk of coronary aneurysms. Blood culture and intravenous antibiotics would be indicated if there was concern for bacteremia or sepsis, but Kawasaki's disease is an idiopathic vasculitis, not an infection. Intravenous steroids are not indicated, as they have not been shown to improve outcomes, and Kawasaki's disease is associated with various rashes, so dermatologic biopsy is not needed. Since the patient meets criteria for Kawasaki's disease at this time, supportive management is no longer appropriate.

50. **The answer is C.** (Chapter 142) Erythema toxicum neonatorum is a benign self-limited condition with an alarming name. It occurs in about 50% of neonates, usually before 7 days of life. The rash will resolve without intervention. Atopic dermatitis is a common skin condition in infants, but normally does not develop until 2 to 6 months of life. Transient neonatal pustular melanosis is less common, and more often seen in darker skinned infants. The diagnosis is normally made from the clinical appearance: small pustules that turn into macule with surrounding scale as the pustules rupture, and brown macule that fade over time. Microscopic evaluation of the skin scrapings or pustule contents are not needed. Seborrheic dermatitis is an inflammatory condition, not a fungal infection, though it may occur in infants that also have diaper dermatitis.

51. **The answer is A.** (Chapter 143) The incidence of acute chest syndrome is higher in children with sickle cell disease than adults, but has a better prognosis. Patients with sickle cell disease and asthma are four to six times as likely to develop acute chest syndrome, and more likely to have a complicated course. Infection is still the leading cause of death in children with sickle cell disease, and bacteremia rates remain higher than the general population even with prophylaxis. Invasive pneumococcal disease has decreased by over 90% since the development of the pneumococcal 7-valent conjugate vaccine, and is expected to fall further with the 13-valent conjugate vaccine. Parvovirus can cause a transient aplastic crisis, which may be more pronounced in children with sickle cell disease, due to the shortened life span of red blood cells in these patients. However, infection with parvovirus usually results in lifelong immunity and would be unlikely to cause recurrent aplastic crises. *Salmonella* and *Escherichia coli* infections are more likely causes of bacteremia and sepsis in this age group, while *Haemophilus influenzae* and *Streptococcus pneumoniae* remain more frequent in younger infants.

52. **The answer is C.** (Chapter 144) Even mild head trauma should be taken seriously in a patient with hemophilia, especially one that requires regular factor infusions, indicating severe disease. Patients may not have clinical manifestations of bleeding on initial presentation, as bleeding can occur at a slow rate. All reports of head injuries, especially one resulting in visible head trauma (an ecchymosis), should be immediately treated with 100% factor correction. In most patients, the dose will be 50 units/kg of factor VIII or 100 units/kg of factor IX. A head CT should be ordered immediately, but factor administration should not be delayed waiting for results. A hematologist should also be consulted for all hemophilic children with evidence of bleeding.

53. **The answer is D.** (Chapter 145) Chemotherapy or antileukemic agents are the definitive treatment for this condition, and an oncologist should be consulted as soon as possible for initiation of therapy. In symptomatic anemia, goals of transfusion would be to raise the hemoglobin level to 8 to 10 g/dL. However, in the setting of hyperleukocytosis (>100,000 white blood cells/mm^3), packed red blood cells can increase viscosity and increase complications, and transfusions should be to much lower levels. Platelets do not increase blood viscosity but are normally reserved in asymptomatic patients for platelet counts less than 10,000 to 20,000 cells/mm^3. Leukapheresis is a temporizing measure until chemotherapy can be started and may be difficult to initiate in the emergency department. The insertion of the catheter may also increase bleeding rash in the setting of thrombocytopenia. Emergent leukapheresis should be reserved for symptomatic patients: headache, mental status changes, visual changes, seizures, stroke, dyspnea, hypoxemia, or respiratory failure. A specialist should be involved with the decision to start leukapheresis. Aggressive intravenous hydration may decrease blood viscosity and decrease risks of leukostasis complications.

54. **The answer is B.** (Chapter 146) Blood glucose level is the most important immediate diagnostic test for any critically ill child, as it can be done rapidly and results can be immediately treated. Hypoglycemia is a common feature of inborn errors of metabolism, and correction of glucose levels can quickly improve the patient's clinical picture. Blood ammonia level may be important for continuing treatment by a metabolic disease specialist, but is not needed for the initial resuscitation. Lactic acidosis is a common finding in many critically ill children, and a lactate level may be trended over time, but the initial resuscitation of this infant does not depend on lactate level. Urinary ketones may help in the initial diagnosis of an inborn error of metabolism, but this child has a known diagnosis, and the presence of ketones will not affect the initial management.

55. **The answer is D.** (Chapter 146) Cerebral edema is a rare complication of diabetic ketoacidosis and typically presents hours after the start of therapy. Standard treatment for cerebral edema is mannitol, though more recent studies show 3% normal saline may be as efficacious. A head CT should be emergently ordered, but treatment of the suspected cerebral edema should not be delayed. Intubation may be needed in some patients who the first sign of cerebral edema was respiratory depression or arrest. However, this patient is still talking, and therefore protecting her airway. Sodium bicarbonate is not a treatment for

cerebral edema, and in studies has been shown to increase the risk for cerebral edema when used in the treatment of diabetic ketoacidosis.

56. **The answer is C.** (Chapter 148) Though increased ventricle size increases the likelihood of a shunt malfunction, unchanged ventricle size does not rule out a malfunction. The brain tissue surrounding abnormal ventricles often demonstrates loss of compliance, which can conceal shunt malfunction. Shunt infections are most prevalent within 6 months from the last revision, and without fever or documentation of infection, immediate intravenous antibiotics are not recommended. Unless there is concern for cerebral or cerebellar herniation or other signs of significantly increased intracranial pressure, such as Cushing's triad, shunt aspiration should be done by the Neurosurgeon. Observation in the emergency department without neurosurgical consultation is not recommended in a patient who is high-risk for having increased intracranial pressure.

57. **The answer is D.** (Chapter 149) Oppositional defiant disorder is characterized by non compliant behavior in a patient who is easily angered and hostile toward others. Attention-deficit/hyperactivity disorder is characterized by difficulty in school, and difficulty concentrating, without specific anger or non compliance concerns. Bipolar disorder is characterized by episodes of manic behavior (excessive spending, risk taking, insomnia) interspersed with episodes of depression. Conduct disorder is characterized by serious rule-breaking, destruction of property, and aggressive behavior toward people and animals.

58. **The answer is A.** (Chapter 150) Bruises to the ear, especially in a non ambulatory infant, are concerning for physical abuse and warrant further investigation and referral to child protective services. Femur fractures can be concerning for abuse, especially in young infants, but the story of falling off the jungle gym is an appropriate mechanism for the fracture. A 3-year-old may be verbal and could tell their own story of the injury. Linear skull fractures can be accidental or non accidental injuries, and could occur in an infant falling from their parent's arms. A spiral tibia fracture in a 2-year-old is most likely a toddler's fracture, and is not indicative of abuse. All injuries should be viewed in light of the clinical picture, and if there are other concerning bruises or injuries, further workup and referral to child protective services may still be needed.

59. **The answer is B.** (Chapter 150) All suspected or alleged abuse (physical, sexual, medical, or neglect) should be reported to child protective services, regardless of physical examination findings. A normal physical examination does not rule out sexual abuse, as often sexually abusive activities in children do not leave physical marks, and remote injuries may have healed without obvious scarring. Speculum examinations are not needed in young children, as visual inspection can be performed in the frog-leg or knee-chest positions. As the reported incident occurred a week ago or longer, immediate forensic collection is unnecessary, as findings are unlikely after 24 hours.

Systemic Infectious Disorders

11

QUESTIONS

1. A 22-year-old woman presents for a second visit to the emergency department 3 days after being evaluated for dysuria. She has persistent dysuria despite being prescribed nitrofurantoin. Review of her urinalysis from 3 days ago reveals multiple WBCs, a negative pregnancy test, and a negative culture. Which of the following may be a complication if this infection is not treated appropriately?
   (A) Meningitis
   (B) Pelvic inflammatory disease
   (C) Pustular skin lesions
   (D) Septic arthritis

2. A 19-year-old woman presents to the emergency department with the rash on her right arm, as shown in Figure 11.1. She is sexually active with a new partner for 2 months and not using protection. Treatment for which of the following disease processes should be considered?

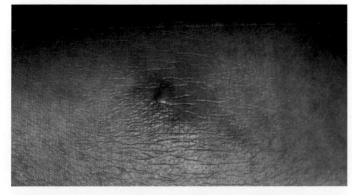

FIGURE 11.1 J.E. Tintinalli, J.S. Stapczynski, O.J. Ma, D. Yearly, G.D. Meckler, D.M. Cline: Tintinalli's Emergency Medicine: A Comprehensive Study Guide, 9th Edition: Copyright © McGraw-Hill Education. All rights reserved.

(A) *Chlamydia trachomatis*
(B) Herpes simplex virus
(C) *Neisseria gonorrhoeae*
(D) *Trichomonas vaginalis*

3. Which of the following sexually transmitted infections is commonly associated with genital ulcers?
   (A) *Chlamydia trachomatis*
   (B) *Neisseria gonorrhoeae*
   (C) Syphilis
   (D) *Trichomonas vaginalis*

4. A 20-year-old man presents with a painless lesion on his penis (Figure 11.2). He states that he has had six sexual partners in the last 4 months, including both men and women, and he rarely uses protection. Which of the following is the MOST APPROPRIATE treatment?
   (A) Acyclovir
   (B) Benzathine penicillin G
   (C) Clindamycin
   (D) Metronidazole

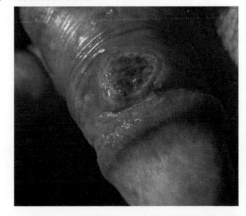

FIGURE 11.2 Reproduced with permission from Wolff KL, Johnson R, Suurmond R: Fitzpatrick's Color Atlas & Synopsis of Clinical Dermatology, 5th ed. 2005, McGraw-Hill, Inc., New York.

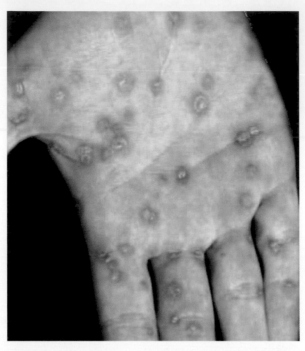

FIGURE 11.3 Reproduced with permission from Goldsmith LA, Katz SI, Gilchrest BA, et al: Fitzpatrick's Dermatology in General Medicine, 8th ed. 2012 by McGraw-Hill, Inc., New York.

5. A 20-year-old man presents with a sore throat, headache, malaise, and a rash as seen in Figure 11.3. He states that he has had unprotected sex with multiple partners. Which of the following is the MOST APPROPRIATE treatment?
   (A) Acyclovir
   (B) Benzathine penicillin G
   (C) Clindamycin
   (D) Metronidazole

6. A 28-year-old woman presents for urinary retention. She describes 1 day of dysuria and vaginal burning but no hematuria or vaginal discharge. She denies abdominal or flank pain. On external vaginal examination, you note the picture finding (Figure 11.4). Which of the following is the MOST APPROPRIATE treatment?
   (A) Acyclovir
   (B) Benzathine penicillin G
   (C) Clindamycin
   (D) Metronidazole

7. Which of the following sexually transmitted infections presents with a painful genital ulcer?
   (A) Chancroid
   (B) Granuloma inguinale (donovanosis)
   (C) Lymphogranuloma venereum
   (D) Syphilis

8. Which of the following medications used to treat sexually transmitted infections is considered safe for use during pregnancy?
   (A) Acyclovir
   (B) Doxycycline
   (C) Ofloxacin
   (D) Tinidazole

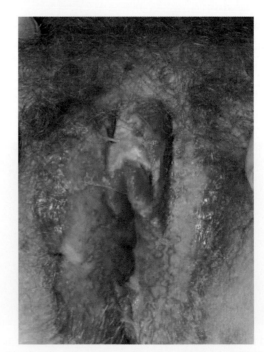

FIGURE 11.4 Reproduced with permission from Goldsmith LA, Katz SI, Gilchrest BA, et al: Fitzpatrick's Dermatology in General Medicine, 8th ed. 2012 by McGraw-Hill, Inc., New York.

9. Which of the following risk factors is more commonly associated with staphylococcal toxic shock syndrome, as opposed to streptococcal toxic shock syndrome?
   (A) Influenza
   (B) Retained foreign body (tampon, nasal packing)
   (C) Surgery
   (D) Varicella

10. Which of the following is a characteristic feature of staphylococcal toxic shock syndrome (TSS) erythroderma?
    (A) Involves the palms
    (B) Painful
    (C) Petechial
    (D) Spares the mucosa

11. A 76-year-old man presents to the emergency department 3 days after having a right-sided nasal packing placed for epistaxis with fever, headache, sore throat, myalgias, and abdominal pain. He is ill appearing and tachycardic. On examination, you notice a red, macular rash that involves his palms and soles as well as conjunctival injection. He states that it is not painful. What is the MOST LIKELY diagnosis?
    (A) Kawasaki's disease
    (B) Meningococcemia
    (C) Staphylococcal toxic shock syndrome
    (D) Toxic epidermal necrolysis

12. An 88-year-old woman with a history of coronary artery disease, chronic renal insufficiency, and diabetes mellitus presents to the emergency department with family for 3 days of fever and now altered mentation. On examination, the patient is febrile, there is a wound on the right leg with purulent drainage and crepitus, and you notice a red, macular rash that involves her palms and soles. The rash does not seem painful to palpation. What is the MOST LIKELY diagnosis?
    (A) Kawasaki's disease
    (B) Meningococcemia
    (C) Streptococcal toxic shock syndrome
    (D) Toxic epidermal necrolysis

13. Outside of the surgical setting, what is the predominant pathogen of sepsis?

    (A) Fungi
    (B) Gram-negative bacteria
    (C) Gram-positive bacteria
    (D) Viruses

14. A 90-year-old woman presents to the emergency department from a nursing home with fever and altered mentation. Vitals reveal a sinus tachycardia of 128, respiratory rate of 28, and blood pressure 85/55. Laboratory abnormalities include a white blood cell count of 19.8×10^9/L and lactic acid of 5.5. Which of the following etiologies MOST LIKELY accounts for her presentation?
    (A) Cellulitis
    (B) Meningitis
    (C) Pneumonia
    (D) Pyelonephritis

15. A 55-year-old man with chronic kidney disease on hemodialysis presents to the emergency department for fever and increased weakness today. His wife has noticed that he seems confused about the events of the last 2 days. Vital signs reveal fever, tachycardia, and hypotension. Which of the following organisms is the MOST LIKELY cause of bacteremia in this patient?
    (A) *Escherichia coli*
    (B) *Pseudomonas aeruginosa*
    (C) *Staphylococcus aureus*
    (D) *Streptococcus pyogenes*

16. An 87-year-old woman presents to the emergency department from a nursing home with fever and altered mentation. Vitals reveal a sinus tachycardia of 129 and blood pressure 79/55. She has an indwelling urinary catheter with purulent drainage. Laboratory abnormalities include a white blood cell count of 21.3×10^9/L, lactic acid level of 5.5, and glucose of 391. Which of the following is the BEST first step in management of this patient?
    (A) Acetaminophen per rectum
    (B) Intramuscular hydrocortisone
    (C) Intravenous access
    (D) Subcutaneous insulin

17. A 52-year-old diabetic man presents to the emergency department for 2 days of increasing pain, swelling, and erythema to the right lower extremity. He reports subjective fevers and chills with generalized malaise today. On examination, you note warmth, erythema, and mild edema, but no fluctuance or crepitus (Figure 11.5). Which of the following is the MOST APPROPRIATE management?

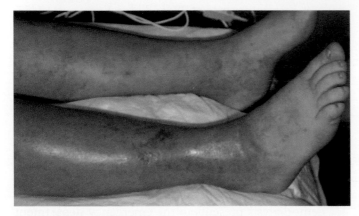

FIGURE 11.5 Photo contributed by Lawrence B. Stack, MD. Reproduced with permission from Knoop K, Stack L, Storrow A, Thurman RJ: Atlas of Emergency Medicine, 3rd ed. 2010, McGraw-Hill, Inc., New York.

(A) Incision and drainage to obtain wound culture
(B) Intravenous antibiotics and admission
(C) Oral antibiotics and discharge with 24-hour reevaluation
(D) Surgery consultation and admission

18. A 22-year-old healthy man presents to the emergency department for "pimples" that are spreading on his body. He states that he otherwise feels well and has no medical history. He is afebrile and well appearing on examination. Examining the skin, you see a patch of carbuncles on the anterior chest wall and a well-circumscribed 1-cm abscess on the inner left thigh without cellulitis. Bedside glucose is 88. Which of the following is the MOST APPROPRIATE management?
(A) Incision and drainage and discharge with oral antibiotics
(B) Incision and drainage and discharge with wound care
(C) Warm compresses and discharge with oral antibiotics
(D) Warm compresses and discharge with wound care

19. A 44-year-old diabetic man presents to the emergency department for 2 days of increasing pain, swelling, and erythema to the left lower extremity despite oral antibiotics and wound care at home. He reports subjective fevers and chills with generalized malaise today and the development of a blister. On examination, you note swelling, warmth, and erythema to the left leg surrounding the blister with crepitus (Figure 11.6). Which of the following is the MOST APPROPRIATE management?

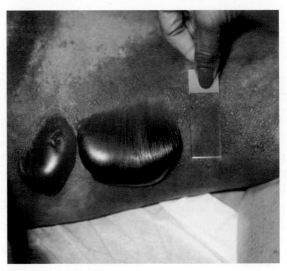

FIGURE 11.6 Photo contributed by Lawrence B. Stack, MD. Reproduced with permission from Knoop K, Stack L, Storrow A, Thurman RJ: Atlas of Emergency Medicine, 3rd ed. 2010, McGraw-Hill, Inc., New York.

(A) Add a second oral antibiotic and discharge with 24-hour reevaluation
(B) Incision and drainage to obtain wound culture
(C) Intravenous antibiotics and admission
(D) Surgical consultation and admission

20. A 35-year-old healthy female florist presents to the emergency department for a nonhealing nodule on her right arm despite daily warm soaks and topical antibiotic ointment (Figure 11.7). Which of the following organisms should be considered when choosing an appropriate antibiotic?
(A) *Aeromonas hydrophila*
(B) *Mycobacterium marinum*
(C) *Sporothrix schenckii*
(D) *Vibrio parahaemolyticus*

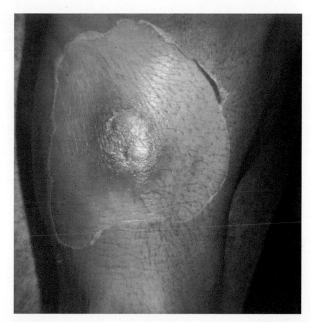

FIGURE 11.7 Reproduced with permission from Knoop K, Stack L, Storrow A: Atlas of Emergency Medicine, 2nd ed. 2002, McGraw-Hill, Inc., New York.

21. A 33-year-old woman with no significant medical history presents to the emergency department in January for fevers, chills, myalgias, malaise, headache, nasal congestion, and dry cough. She is 22 weeks pregnant with her first child. She states that she is a second-grade teacher and multiple children in her classroom have been ill with similar symptoms. Which of the following therapies should be offered to this patient?
    (A) Amantadine
    (B) Azithromycin
    (C) Oseltamivir
    (D) Supportive measures

22. Which of the following statements regarding herpes simplex virus (HSV) infections is TRUE?
    (A) HSV-1 infection is most often implicated in genital herpes.
    (B) Most HSV infections are subclinical.
    (C) Primary infections most commonly occur in the winter.
    (D) Secondary infections typically produce more extensive lesions.

23. A 79-year-old male kidney transplant recipient presents to the emergency department with family for fever and altered mentation. He was started on oral antibiotics 2 days ago by his primary care physician for an ulcer with surrounding cellulitis that was developing on his lower lip. The rash has progressed and is now generalized on his body (Figure 11.8). Which of the following is the MOST LIKELY diagnosis?

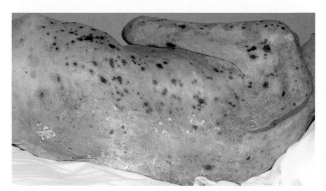

FIGURE 11.8 Reproduced with permission from Wolff K, Johnson RA: Fitzpatrick's Color Atlas and Synopsis of Clinical Dermatology, 5th ed., 2005 by McGraw-Hill, Inc., New York.

    (A) Erythema multiforme
    (B) Herpes simplex virus
    (C) Meningococcemia
    (D) Staphylococcal toxic shock syndrome

24. A healthy 22-year-old man presents to the emergency department with 2 days of aching left shoulder pain after working out. On examination, you observe a rash (Figure 11.9). Which of the following statements regarding this condition is TRUE?

    (A) The patient also likely has oral lesions on examination.
    (B) The patient should be tested for human immunodeficiency virus infection.
    (C) The rash commonly crosses the midline.
    (D) The rash is easily treated with topical antifungals.

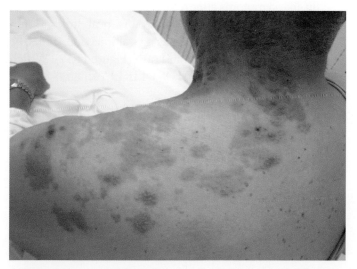

FIGURE 11.9 J.E. Tintinalli, J.S. Stapczynski, O.J. Ma, D. Yearly, G.D. Meckler, D.M. Cline: Tintinalli's Emergency Medicine: A Comprehensive Study Guide, 9th Edition: Copyright © McGraw-Hill Education. All rights reserved.

25. A 16-year-old boy presents for fever, headache, sore throat, and odynophagia, upper abdominal pain and fatigue. He is tolerating his secretions without difficulty and speaking clearly. On oropharyngeal examination, you note the following. Laboratory testing reveals lymphocytosis (Figure 11.10). Which of the following is TRUE regarding this condition?

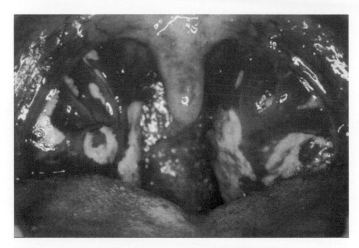

FIGURE 11.10 Reproduced with permission from Shah BR, Lucchesi M: Atlas of Pediatric Emergency Medicine, © 2006 by McGraw-Hill, Inc., New York.

(A) Antibiotics are the mainstay of treatment.
(B) College students experience the lowest morbidity.
(C) It is associated with cancers such as B-cell lymphoma.
(D) Peak incidence occurs in middle aged adults.

26. A 35-year-old otherwise healthy man presents to the emergency department with 3 days of fever, rash, and flu-like symptoms after returning from a business trip to South America. He was evaluated in a local clinic in South America and told that he has a viral infection. Today he has worsening headache and rash (Figure 11.11). Which of the following is the MOST LIKELY diagnosis?
(A) Dengue
(B) Ehrlichiosis
(C) Malaria
(D) Syphilis

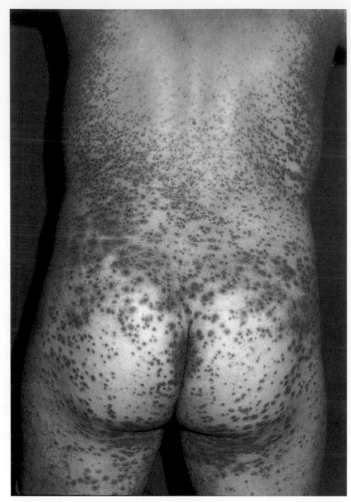

FIGURE 11.11 Reproduced with permission from Wolff K, Johnson RA: Fitzpatrick's Color Atlas and Synopsis of Clinical Dermatology, 6th ed., © 2009 by McGraw-Hill, Inc., New York.

27. Which patient characteristic is associated with the highest pretest risk of acquiring human immunodeficiency virus infection?
(A) African American
(B) Heterosexual
(C) Marijuana user
(D) White female

28. In a human immunodeficiency virus infection-positive patient, thrush is likely to occur when the CD4+ T-cell count drops below what level?
(A) 200 cells/mm^3
(B) 500 cells/mm^3
(C) 700 cells/mm^3
(D) 900 cells/mm^3

29. A 37-year-old man with human immunodeficiency virus presents to the emergency department with two days of fever and a new-onset seizure tonight. After completing a thorough physical and neurologic examination, what is the NEXT BEST step in management?
    (A) Head CT
    (B) Intravenous lorazepam
    (C) Lumbar puncture
    (D) Measure CD4+ T-cell counts

30. A 47-year-old woman with human immunodeficiency virus infection presents to the emergency department with 2 days of headache, increasing left-sided weakness, and new-onset seizure tonight. Contrast-enhanced CT scan shows multiple ring-enhancing lesions with surrounding areas of edema. Which of the following statements regarding this condition is TRUE?
    (A) Serologic tests are useful in making or excluding the diagnosis.
    (B) Symptoms may also include fever and altered mental status.
    (C) This condition commonly occurs in patients with normal CD4+ cell counts.
    (D) This patient can be discharged with oral sulfamethoxazole-trimethoprim and dexamethasone.

31. A 55-year-old man with human immunodeficiency virus infection presents to the emergency department with 2 weeks of hemoptysis, night sweats, prolonged fevers, weight loss, and anorexia. Which of the following statements regarding this condition is TRUE?
    (A) Approximately 50% of new cases in the United States occur in HIV-infected persons.
    (B) Definitive diagnosis is commonly made through positive blood cultures.
    (C) Frequently occurs in patients with CD4+ T-cell counts less than 100 cells/mm^3.
    (D) Negative purified protein derivative skin test results are common among HIV patients.

32. A 65-year-old woman with a history of a prosthetic mitral valve secondary to rheumatic fever presents for a procedure. For which of the following procedures is endocarditis prophylaxis indicated?
    (A) Incision and drainage of a periapical abscess
    (B) Laceration repair

(C) Urethral catheterization
(D) Uterine dilation and curettage

33. A 28-year-old male migrant worker from California presents with painful muscular contraction and spasm of his neck after working 10 hours. On examination, he has spasm and contraction of his neck muscles with palpation. He also has difficulty opening his mouth for examination of the oropharynx. You notice a healing puncture wound on his right hand. Which of the following is the appropriate first-line treatment for this condition?
    (A) Benzodiazepines
    (B) Clindamycin
    (C) Intravenous calcium
    (D) Tetanus immunoglobulin

34. Which of the following antibiotics can potentiate the effects of tetanospasmin when administered?
    (A) Azithromycin
    (B) Clindamycin
    (C) Metronidazole
    (D) Penicillin

35. Which of the following exposures mandates rabies postexposure prophylaxis?
    (A) Awakening in a room with a bat present
    (B) Cleaning a stray dog with unknown origins
    (C) Contact with rabid dog blood on intact skin
    (D) Petting a cat with raccoon saliva on its coat

36. A 42-year-old female veterinarian presents to the emergency department with complaints of paresthesias in her right arm, headache, nausea, vomiting, and hypersalivation. On examination, she has a scratch on her right forearm from a stray dog that she was caring for 5 days earlier. Which of the following treatments is contraindicated for this condition?
    (A) Amantadine
    (B) Corticosteroids
    (C) Ketamine
    (D) Ribavirin

37. A 37-year-old man presents with fever, malaise, myalgias and arthralgias, headache, and intermittent abdominal pain. On further discussion, the patient returned 3 weeks ago from Haiti and states that he did suffer from mosquito bites. Which species of this protozoan causes the MOST deaths worldwide?
    (A) *Plasmodium falciparum*
    (B) *Plasmodium malariae*
    (C) *Plasmodium ovale*
    (D) *Plasmodium vivax*

38. An 8-year-old girl who was recently adopted from Africa presents with seizure. Her parents state that for the last 2 days she has been complaining of intermittent abdominal pain with fever, chills, myalgias, and headache. On eye examination, you notice the following (Figure 11.12). Which of the following is the appropriate definitive treatment for this condition?
    (A) Benzodiazepines
    (B) Quinidine + clindamycin
    (C) Ribavirin
    (D) Supportive measures

39. A husband and wife present together to the emergency department with flushing, headache, abdominal cramping, and vomiting 60 minutes after eating tuna that they prepared at home. In addition to supportive measures, which of the following is the APPROPRIATE treatment?
    (A) Azithromycin
    (B) Ciprofloxacin
    (C) Diphenhydramine
    (D) Mannitol

40. A 52-year-old man presents for generalized weakness, intermittent vomiting, double vision, and difficulty swallowing. There has been no recent travel. He and his wife own a farm with poultry and cattle and can their own vegetables. Which of the following is the MOST LIKELY causative organism?
    (A) *Brucella*
    (B) *Clostridium botulinum*
    (C) *Clostridium perfringens*
    (D) *Listeria monocytogenes*

41. A 52-year-old man presents to the emergency department for 2 weeks of a painful indurated lesion on his thumb. Symptoms began shortly after returning home from a trip to the gulf coast of Florida. He states that he initially had scratched his hand on a shell in the ocean (Figure 11.13). Which of the following is the MOST LIKELY causative organism?
    (A) *Aeromonas hydrophila*
    (B) *Legionella pneumophila*
    (C) *Mycobacterium marinum*
    (D) *Pseudomonas aeruginosa*

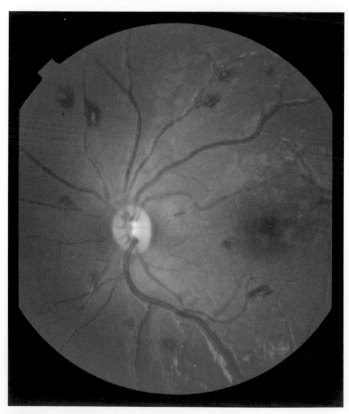

FIGURE 11.12 Photo contributed by Ian MacCormick, MD.

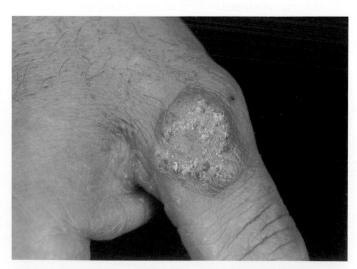

FIGURE 11.13 Reproduced with permission from Wolff K, Johnson RA: Color Atlas and Synopsis of Clinical Dermatology, 5th ed, © 2005, McGraw-Hill, Inc., New York.

42. A 42-year-old man presents to the emergency department for 7 days of a painful red rash that has now developed blisters. Symptoms began shortly after returning home from a trip to the gulf coast of Florida. He states that he initially had scratched his feet while walking through shells in the ocean (Figure 11.14). Which of the following is the MOST LIKELY causative organism?

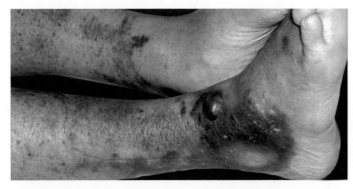

FIGURE 11.14 Reproduced with permission from Wolff K, Johnson R: Fitzpatrick's Color Atlas and Synopsis of Clinical Dermatology, 6th ed, © 2009 McGraw-Hill, Inc., New York.

(A) *Aeromonas hydrophila*
(B) *Mycobacterium marinum*
(C) *Pseudomonas aeruginosa*
(D) *Vibrio vulnificus*

43. An 8-year-old girl presents to the emergency department in early January for fever, myalgias, headache, nausea, vomiting, and diarrhea. Her family recently returned from a trip to North Carolina during her school holiday break. On examination, she appears ill and you notice small, blanching pink macules on her palms and wrists. Which of the following is the MOST APPROPRIATE treatment for this condition?

(A) Azithromycin
(B) Doxycycline
(C) Supportive measures
(D) Vancomycin

44. A 22-year-old woman presents to the emergency department with complaints of fever, headache, arthralgias, and right-sided facial weakness. Three weeks ago, after returning from a trip to the eastern coast of the United States, she was ill with 3 days of fever and myalgias, which resolved spontaneously. On examination, she is ill-appearing with a right facial droop that involves the forehead. There are no other neurological deficits on examination. What is the MOST APPROPRIATE treatment for this condition?
(A) Azithromycin
(B) Ceftriaxone
(C) Doxycycline
(D) Streptomycin

45. A 42-year-old man with his wife presents to the emergency department for fever and confusion. He returned early from a fishing trip to North Carolina 5 days ago secondary to flu-like illness. He has been experiencing intermittent fever, headache, malaise, nausea, diarrhea, abdominal pain, and arthralgias. His wife states that he was confused about his whereabouts and acting very bizarre. On examination, he is ill-appearing, febrile, and difficult to arouse. No rash is noted. Which of the following should be considered in the differential diagnosis?
(A) Babesiosis
(B) Ehrlichiosis
(C) Rocky Mountain spotted fever
(D) Tularemia

ANSWERS

1. The answer is B. (Chapter 153) Urethral chlamydial infection should be considered in the differential diagnosis of sterile pyuria for men and women. Complication of untreated infection may include pelvic inflammatory disease. Other complications may include ectopic pregnancy and infertility. Pustular skin lesions, meningitis, and septic arthritis are more commonly associated with gonococcal infections.

2. The answer is C. (Chapter 153) Petechial or pustular acral skin lesions on an erythematous base are one of the symptoms of disseminated gonococcemia. Herpes simplex virus involves vesicles on an erythematous base and the tense center umbilicates to form a depressed center. Chlamydia and Trichomonas are not commonly associated with skin lesions.

3. The answer is C. (Chapter 153) Genital ulcers are associated with infections caused by syphilis, herpes virus infection, chancroid, lymphogranuloma venereum, and granuloma inguinale (donovanosis). Skin lesions associated with gonococcemia are petechial or pustular acral lesions on an erythematous base. Chlamydia and Trichomonas are not commonly associated with genital ulcers or skin lesions.

4. The answer is B. (Chapter 153) Primary syphilis is characterized by a painless chancre with indurated borders on the penis, as in this case. Painless ulcers may be found on the vulva in women or other areas of sexual contact. *Treponema pallidum*, the spirochete that causes syphilis, remains very sensitive to penicillin and this is considered first-line treatment. Acyclovir is used to treat herpes simplex virus, which presents with painful genital ulcers. Metronidazole and clindamycin are used to treat bacterial vaginosis, which is not commonly associated with genital ulcers.

5. The answer is B. (Chapter 153) Secondary syphilis develops 3 to 6 weeks after the end of the primary stage and is characterized by rash and lymphadenopathy. Nonspecific symptoms of sore throat, malaise, fever, and headaches are common. The rash often starts on the trunk and flexor surfaces of the extremities, spreading to the palms and soles. The rash is often dull red-pink and papular. Primary syphilis is characterized by a painless chancre with indurated borders on the penis. *Treponema pallidum*, the spirochete that causes syphilis, remains very sensitive to penicillin and this is considered first-line treatment. Acyclovir is used to treat herpes simplex virus, which presents

with painful genital ulcers. Metronidazole and clindamycin are used to treat bacterial vaginosis, which is not commonly associated with genital ulcers.

6. The answer is A. (Chapter 153) In women, the painful ulcers of herpes simplex virus (HSV) can occur on the introitus, urethral meatus, labia, and perineum. In men, HSV ulcers often appear on the shaft or glans of the penis. Lesions are exquisitely painful and sometimes are associated with serous discharge. In both sexes, lesions may be found on the perianal area, thighs, or buttocks. Dysuria is common in women and may progress to urinary retention secondary to severe pain. Primary syphilis is characterized by painless ulcers that may be found on the vulva in women or other areas of sexual contact and first-line treatment remains penicillin. Metronidazole and clindamycin are used to treat bacterial vaginosis, which is not commonly associated with genital ulcers.

7. The answer is A. (Chapter 153, Table 11.1) *Haemophilus ducreyi* is the pleomorphic gram-negative bacillus that causes chancroid, which presents as painful genital ulcers and lymphadenitis. The ulcers are 1 to 2 cm in diameter with sharp, undermined margins. Painful inguinal lymphadenopathy develops 1 to 2 weeks after primary infection and a bubo will develop if left untreated. Lymphogranuloma venereum, Granuloma inguinale (donovanosis), and syphilis all present with painless genital ulcers.

8. The answer is A. (Chapter 153, Table 11.2) Penicillin, ceftriaxone, azithromycin, cefixime, metronidazole, erythromycin, and acyclovir are thought to be safe for use during pregnancy. Tetracyclines and fluoroquinolones should be avoided during pregnancy. Tinidazole should be avoided in the first 3 months of pregnancy.

9. The answer is B. (Chapter 249) The vagina and nares are known sites of *Staphylococcus aureus* colonization. Retained foreign bodies such as tampons, female barrier contraceptives, and nasal packing material are risk factors for developing staphylococcal toxic shock syndrome (TSS). Influenza, surgery, and varicella are associated with both staphylococcal and streptococcal TSS.

10. The answer is A. (Chapter 249) Toxic shock syndrome erythroderma is characterized as a painless, diffuse, red, macular rash resembling "sunburn" and involves the palms and soles. Mucosal involvement can include conjunctival and scleral hemorrhage as well as vaginal, cervical, or oropharyngeal hyperemia ("strawberry tongue").

TABLE 11.1	Clinical Features of Genital Ulcerative Infections				
Disease	Clinical Diagnosis	Presence of Pain	Inguinal Adenopathy	Comment	
Syphilis	Indurated, relatively clean base; heals spontaneously	No	Firm, rubbery, discrete nodes; not tender	Primary: chancre Secondary: rash, mucocutaneous lesions, lymphadenopathy Tertiary: cardiac, ophthalmic, auditory, CNS lesions	
Herpes simplex virus infection	Multiple small, grouped vesicles coalescing and forming shallow ulcers; vulvovaginitis	Yes	Tender bilateral adenopathy	Cytologic detection insensitive; false-negative culture results common; type-specific serologic test	
Chancroid (*Haemophilus ducreyi*)	Multiple painful, irregular, purulent ulcers with potential exudative base	Yes	50% painful, suppurative, inguinal lymph nodes potentially requiring drainage	Cofactor for human immunodeficiency virus transmission; 10% have coinfections with herpes simplex virus infection or syphilis	
Lymphogranuloma venereum	Small and shallow ulcer, associated proctocolitis with fistulas and strictures	No	Tender lymph nodes	Caused by *Chlamydia trachomatis* L1, L2, L3	
Granuloma inguinale (donovanosis)	Painless, beefy red, bleeding ulcers	No	No	Endemic in Africa, Australia, India, New Guinea; rare in United States	

Reproduced with permission from J.E. Tintinalli, J.S. Stapczynski, O.J. Ma, D. Yealy, G.D. Meckler, D.M. Cline: Tintinalli's Emergency Medicine: A Comprehensive Study Guide, 9th Edition. McGraw-Hill Education; 2020.

11. The answer is C. (Chapter 249) Staphylococcal toxic shock syndrome (TSS) erythroderma is characterized as a painless, diffuse, red, macular rash resembling "sunburn" and involves the palms and soles. Mucosal involvement can include conjunctival and scleral hemorrhage as well as vaginal, cervical, or oropharyngeal hyperemia ("strawberry tongue"). The vagina and nares are known sites of *Staphylococcus aureus* colonization. Retained foreign bodies such as tampons, female barrier contraceptives, and nasal packing material are risk factors for developing staphylococcal TSS.

12. The answer is C. (Chapters 152 and 249) Streptococcal toxic shock syndrome (STSS) is a complication of infections involving group A *Streptococcus* (GAS, *S. pyogenes*), especially skin and soft tissue infections associated with necrotizing fasciitis and myositis. It is also a complication of GAS pneumonia and bloodstream infections. Incidence rates for GAS are highest in those age 65 years and older or under the age of 1. GAS infections are also more common in those with underlying medical conditions. Associated comorbidities include heart, liver, and kidney disease; diabetes mellitus; alcoholism; and drug abuse. STSS may be preceded by a nonspecific prodrome of fever, chills, sweats, malaise, arthralgias, cough, sore throat, rhinorrhea, anorexia, nausea, vomiting, abdominal pain, and diarrhea. This may be followed by confusion, somnolence, and agitation. A diffusely erythematous and macular rash may also be seen in STSS and progress to desquamation but is not required to make the diagnosis.

13. The answer is C. (Chapter 151) Outside of the surgical setting, since 1987, gram-positive bacteria are the predominant pathogens of sepsis. With increased antimicrobial resistance, methicillin-resistant *Staphylococcus aureus*, vancomycin-resistant *Enterococcus*, and other multidrug-resistant organisms have become more common.

14. The answer is C. (Chapter 151) Sepsis is a clinical diagnosis in the emergency department when the practitioner has suspicion or confirmation of infection, systemic inflammation, and new organ dysfunction or tissue hypoperfusion. The most common etiology of sepsis is acute bacterial pneumonia and the most common causative organisms are *Streptococcus pneumoniae*, *Staphylococcus aureus*, gram-negative bacilli, and *Legionella pneumophila*. Cellulitis and pyelonephritis are also common causes of sepsis but less common than pneumonia. Meningitis is a rare but devastating cause of sepsis.

15. The answer is C. (Chapter 151) Bacteremia from indwelling medical devices such as intraperitoneal or intravascular dialysis catheters may be a source of septic shock. The most prevalent causes of bacteremia are *Staphylococcus aureus*, *Streptococcus pneumoniae*, and *Neisseria meningitidis*. *Pseudomonas aeruginosa* and other gram-negative bacteria are occasional causes of bacteremia in injection drug users. *Streptococcus pyogenes* is more commonly associated with necrotizing soft tissue infection leading to sepsis.

16. The answer is C. (Chapter 151) The initial treatment of sepsis is early recognition, reversal of hemodynamic compromise, and infection control. Intravenous access should be obtained as the initial resuscitation includes administering fluids and appropriate antimicrobials

TABLE 11.2 Treatment of Sexually Transmitted Infections

Sexually Transmitted Infection	First-Line Treatment	Alternative(s)	Pregnancy/Lactation
Bacterial vaginosis	Metronidazole, 500 mg PO two times daily × 7 d or Metronidazole vaginal gel 0.75%, 5 grams intravaginally daily × 5 d or Clindamycin vaginal cream 2%, 5 grams intravaginally at bedtime × 7 d	Tinidazole, 2 grams PO daily × 2 d or Tinidazole, 1 gram PO daily × 5 d or Clindamycin, 300 mg PO twice daily × 7 d or Clindamycin ovules, 100 mg intravaginally at bedtime × 3 d	Metronidazole, 500 mg PO two times daily × 7 d or Metronidazole vaginal gel 0.75%, 5 grams intravaginally daily × 5 d
Chancroid	Azithromycin, 1 gram PO single dose or Ceftriaxone, 250 mg IM single dose∗ or Ciprofloxacin, 500 mg PO, two times daily × 3 d or Erythromycin base, 500 mg PO three times daily × 7 d		Azithromycin, 1 gram PO single dose or Ceftriaxone, 250 mg IM single dose∗
Chlamydia (treat for *Neisseria gonorrhoeae* concurrently)	Azithromycin, 1 g PO single dose or Doxycycline, 100 mg PO two times daily × 7 d	Erythromycin base, 500 mg PO four times daily × 7 d or Erythromycin ethylsuccinate, 800 mg PO four times daily × 7 d or Levofloxacin, 500 mg PO once daily × 7 d or Ofloxacin, 300 mg PO twice daily × 7 d	Azithromycin, 1 g PO single dose PLUS test of cure in 3–4 wk or Amoxicillin, 500 mg PO three times daily × 7 d PLUS test of cure in 3–4 wk or Erythromycin base, 500 mg PO four times a day for 7 d PLUS test of cure in 3–4 wk or Erythromycin base, 250 mg PO four times a day for 14 d PLUS test of cure in 3–4 wk or Erythromycin ethylsuccinate, 800 mg orally four times a day for 7 d PLUS test of cure in 3–4 wk or Erythromycin ethylsuccinate, 400 mg orally four times a day for 14 d PLUS test of cure in 3–4 wk
Gonorrhea (treat for *Chlamydia trachomatis* concurrently)	Ceftriaxone∗, 250 mg IM single dose, AND azithromycin, 1 g PO single dose or Ceftriaxone∗, 250 mg IM single dose, AND doxycycline, 100 mg PO twice a day for 7 d	Cefixime, 400 mg PO single dose, AND azithromycin, 1 gram PO single dose or Cefixime, 400 mg PO single dose, AND doxycycline, 100 mg PO twice a day for 7 d or Azithromycin, 2 g PO single dose, PLUS gemifloxacin, 320 mg PO single dose	Ceftriaxone∗, 250 mg IM single dose, AND azithromycin, 1 gram PO single dose or Spectinomycin 2 g IM single dose
Granuloma inguinale (donovanosis)	Azithromycin, 1 g PO *weekly* for at least 3 wk and until lesions completely healed or Azithromycin, 500 mg PO *daily* for at least 3 wk and until lesions completely healed	Doxycycline, 100 mg PO two times daily for at least 3 wk and until lesions completely healed or Ciprofloxacin, 750 mg PO two times daily for at least 3 wk and until lesions completely healed or Erythromycin base, 500 mg PO four times daily for at least 3 wk until lesions completely healed or Trimethoprim-sulfamethoxazole, 1 double-strength (160/800 mg) tablet PO two times daily for at least 3 wk and until lesions completely healed	Erythromycin base, 500 mg PO four times daily for at least 3 wk and until lesions completely healed or Azithromycin, 1 g PO weekly for at least 3 wk and until lesions completely healed or Gentamicin 1 mg/kg IV every 8 h (if the above therapy is ineffective)

(Continued)

TABLE 11.2	Treatment of Sexually Transmitted Infections (*Continued*)		
Sexually Transmitted Infection	First-Line Treatment	Alternative(s)	Pregnancy/Lactation
Herpes simplex *First episode*	Acyclovir, 400 mg PO three times daily × 7–10 d *or* Acyclovir, 200 mg PO five times daily × 7–10 d *or* Valacyclovir, 1 g PO two times daily × 7–10 d *or* Famciclovir, 250 mg PO three times daily × 7–10 d		Acyclovir, 400 mg PO three times daily × 7–10 d *or* Acyclovir, 200 mg PO five times daily × 7–10 d *or* Valacyclovir, 1 g PO two times daily × 7–10 d
Suppressive therapy for recurrent genital herpes in patients without human immunodeficiency virus	Acyclovir, 400 milligrams orally twice a day *or* Valacyclovir 500-1000 mg orally once a day (500 mg may not be as effective as 1000) *or* Famciclovir 250 mg orally twice a day		Acyclovir, 400 mg PO three times daily *or* Valacyclovir, 500 mg PO daily
Severe	Acyclovir, 5–10 mg/kg IV every 8 h × 2–7 d then oral medications for total treatment time of 10 d		Acyclovir, 5–10 mg/kg IV every 8 h × 2–7 d then oral medications for total treatment time of 10 d
Lymphogranuloma venereum	Doxycycline, 100 mg PO two times daily × 21 d	Erythromycin base, 500 mg PO four times daily × 21 d	Erythromycin base, 500 mg PO four times daily × 21 d
Syphilis *Primary, secondary, and early latent*	Benzathine penicillin G, 2.4 million units IM single dose	Doxycycline, 100 mg PO two times daily × 14 d *or* Tetracycline, 500 mg PO four times daily × 14 d *or* Ceftriaxone, 1–2 g IM or IV daily × 10–14 d *or* Azithromycin, 1 g PO single dose. Use only if treatment with penicillin or doxycycline is not feasible.	Benzathine penicillin G, 2.4 million units IM single dose
Latent	Benzathine penicillin G, 2.4 million units IM one time a week × 3 wk	Doxycycline, 100 mg PO two times daily × 28 d *or* Tetracycline, 500 mg PO four times daily × 28 d	Benzathine penicillin G, 2.4 million units IM one time a week × 3 wk
Trichomoniasis	Metronidazole, 2 g PO single dose *or* Tinidazole, 2 g PO single dose	Metronidazole, 500 mg PO two times daily × 7 d	Metronidazole, 2 g PO single dose (weigh risks and benefits of treatment)

*Ceftriaxone is painful IM and may be mixed with lidocaine 1% to decrease patient discomfort with administration.

Reproduced with permission from J.E. Tintinalli, J.S. Stapczynski, O.J. Ma, D. Yealy, G.D. Meckler, D.M. Cline: Tintinalli's Emergency Medicine: A Comprehensive Study Guide, 9th Edition. McGraw-Hill Education; 2020.

to patients with suspected sepsis as soon as possible. Adjunct therapies may include vasopressors and removing the nidus of infection based on the presenting conditions. Once the patient is stabilized, other interventions may include management of oxygenation and ventilation, fever control to reduce metabolic demand, and control of hyperglycemia. Acetaminophen may be administered as an antipyretic but is not a management priority until appropriate resuscitation with intravenous fluids and antibiotics has been addressed. Intramuscular hydrocortisone is not a standard treatment for sepsis.

17. **The answer is B.** (Chapter 152) Patients with cellulitis and evidence of systemic toxicity and those with underlying comorbidities such as diabetes mellitus, alcoholism, or immunosuppression should be admitted. Healthy patients without systemic toxicity can be discharged with close reevaluation and a list of warning signs to prompt return to the emergency department. Incision and drainage should be reserved for abscesses. Consider necrotizing fasciitis in patients with severe infection or systemic toxicity; early surgical evaluation should be obtained when necrotizing fasciitis is suspected, but this patient's examination is not suggestive of this diagnosis.

18. **The answer is A.** (Chapter 152) Incision and drainage is the recommended treatment for large furuncles, carbuncles, and skin abscesses. Antibiotics are recommended for patients with multiple lesions, extensive surrounding cellulitis, immunosuppression, or signs of systemic infection.

19. **The answer is D.** (Chapter 152) Necrotizing soft tissue infection or gas gangrene is characterized by fulminant, extensive soft tissue necrosis, systemic toxicity, and high mortality. These infections can appear benign early in their course but rapidly progress. Risk factors include advanced age, diabetes mellitus, alcoholism, peripheral vascular disease, heart disease, renal failure, human immunodeficiency virus, cancer, nonsteroidal anti-inflammatory drug use, decubitus ulcers, chronic skin infections, intravenous drug abuse, and immune system impairment. Antibiotics alone are rarely effective and immediate surgical consultation should be obtained for management, which may include fasciotomy, debridement, and/or amputation.

20. **The answer is C.** (Chapter 152) Sporotrichosis is a mycotic infection caused by the fungus *Sporothrix schenckii* and is commonly found in soil, sphagnum moss, and decaying vegetable matter. It is most common in tropical and subtropical zones but can be found among florists, gardeners, and agricultural workers. Inoculation is often secondary to penetrating trauma from plant thorns, wood splinters, or contaminated organic materials. After the fungus enters the body through a break in the skin, lesions restricted to the site of inoculation may appear as a crusted ulcer or verrucous plaque. The surrounding skin may then become erythematous and ulcerate, resulting in a chancre with local lymphadenitis. If left untreated, the initial painless nodule or papule at the site of inoculation can go on to develop subcutaneous nodules with skip areas along local lymphatic channels. Aeromonas hydrophilia is associated with freshwater laceration exposures. *Mycobacterium marinum* is associated with fish tanks. *Vibrio parahaemolyticus* is associated with saltwater exposure, lacerations from fish or fishbones, and underlying hepatic cirrhosis.

21. **The answer is C.** (Chapter 154) Patients with influenza typically present with fevers, aches and respiratory symptoms. Most cases are self-limited and in otherwise healthy individuals require only supportive measures. However, current guidelines from the Centers for Disease Control recommend treating patients with risk factors for severe influenza. Treatment with a neuraminidase inhibitor such as oseltamivir should be offered. Risk factors for severe influenza include children younger than 2 years, adults older than 65 years, patients with comorbid conditions, immunocompromised patients, pregnant patients, patients younger than 19 years receiving long-term aspirin, American Indians/Alaskan natives, morbidly obese patients, and residents of nursing homes and long-term care facilities. Amantadine and azithromycin would not be recommended for empiric influenza treatment.

22. **The answer is B.** (Chapter 154) Herpes simplex virus (HSV) infections occur year-round without a predilection for season. Symptoms of HSV vary widely and depend on multiple factors: the anatomic site involved, the immune status of the host, virus type, and primary versus recurrent infection. Most HSV infections are subclinical without the host realizing that they were infected. Symptomatic HSV-1 infection most commonly results in orolabial lesions, whereas HSV-2 is most often associated with genital herpes. Primary HSV infection typically produces more extensive lesions involving both mucosal and extramucosal sites and can be accompanied by systemic signs and symptoms.

23. **The answer is B.** (Chapter 154) Herpes simplex virus (HSV) infection in immunocompromised hosts can lead to widespread dissemination with multiorgan involvement. HSV encephalitis is acute onset of fever and neurologic symptoms. Organ transplant patients may also develop esophagitis, hepatitis, colitis, and pneumonia. The rash in an immunocompromised host who develops disseminated herpes simplex begins as vesicular lesions on an erythematous base, which may umbilicate, blister, and crust over. The rash pictured is not consistent with the target lesions of erythema multiforme or the erythrodermic appearance associated with staphylococcal toxic shock syndrome. Meningococcemia can present with fever and altered mental status but results from the underlying central nervous infection rather than starting as an ulcerating lesion and generalizing.

24. **The answer is B.** (Chapter 154) The presence of herpes zoster in a young, otherwise healthy person may be a sign of human immunodeficiency virus infection or immune suppressed condition. Herpes zoster involving more than three dermatomes should also prompt consideration to an immunodeficient condition. Herpes zoster often begins with a prodrome of pain, itching, and paresthesias in one or more dermatomes. These symptoms are followed by the development of a maculopapular rash that becomes vesicular with lesions in different stages of development. The eruption of herpes zoster does not cross the midline and is not treated with topical antifungal treatments. Herpes simplex infections can present with oral lesions, but herpes zoster is not associated with oral lesions.

25. The answer is C. (Chapter 154) Epstein-Barr virus (EBV) is the causative agent of heterophile-positive infectious mononucleosis. EBV infection is also associated with cancers such as B-cell lymphoma, Hodgkin's disease, Burkitt's lymphoma, and nasopharyngeal carcinoma. There are two age-related peaks of infection: early childhood and young adulthood with college students and military recruits experiencing the highest morbidity. EBV requires close contact for transmission via salivary secretions. Rest and analgesia are the mainstays of treatment with supportive management and symptom control.

26. The answer is A. (Chapter 154) Dengue virus is a common cause of fever and rash in tropical areas with large mosquito populations, and dengue hemorrhagic fever can develop in people who are exposed to a second infection with a different serotype. Dengue, yellow fever, Rift Valley fever, and chikungunya viruses are among the viruses causing hemorrhagic fever syndromes. These diseases typically cause mild nonspecific illness in a healthy infected individual. They less commonly progress to fever and myalgia, arthritis and rash, encephalitis, or hemorrhagic fever. Ehrlichiosis, malaria, and syphilis are not associated with hemorrhagic fever.

27. The answer is A. (Chapter 155) African Americans represent only 14% of the total U.S. population, but this group accounted for almost half (44%) of new human immunodeficiency virus (HIV) infections in the year 2010. The rate of new infections among black men was the highest of any group by race and sex, notably in men having sex with men. Risk factors associated with acquiring HIV infection include homosexuality or bisexuality, injection drug use, receipt of a blood transfusion prior to 1985, and maternal HIV infection.

28. The answer is B. (Chapter 155) Thrush, persistent vulvovaginal candidiasis, peripheral neuropathy, cervical dysplasia, recurrent herpes zoster, and idiopathic thrombocytopenic purpura are more likely to occur as the CD4+ T-cell count drops below 500 cells/mm³. If the CD4+ T-cell count drops below 200 cells/mm³, the frequency of serious opportunistic infections increases.

29. The answer is A. (Chapter 155) Initial emergency department evaluation of human immunodeficiency virus (HIV) patients presenting with new neurologic symptoms or deficits should include non–contrast-enhanced CT is the first neuroimaging study to be obtained. Contrast-enhanced CT or MRI may be obtained next if the non–contrast-enhanced CT is equivocal or there is concern for malignancy or abscess. The patient should undergo lumbar puncture for further infectious

evaluation if head imaging is unremarkable, but a space-occupying lesion should be ruled out with CT before this is attempted. This patient may require intravenous lorazepam if he has another seizure but does not currently need it. Determining his CD4+ T cell count may assist in guiding treatment if an infectious cause is found but should not delay head CT.

30. The answer is B. (Chapter 155) Toxoplasmosis most commonly occurs in patients with CD4+ cell counts <100 cells/mm³. Symptoms may include headache, fever, focal neurologic deficits, altered mental status, and seizures. Serologic tests are not useful in making or excluding the diagnosis because antibodies to *Toxoplasma gondii* are prevalent in the general population. The presence of antibodies to *T. gondii* in the CSF is helpful, although there is a high rate of false-negative results. On unenhanced CT scan, toxoplasmosis typically appears as multiple subcortical lesions with a predilection for the basal ganglia. Contrast-enhanced CT scan typically shows multiple ring-enhancing lesions with surrounding areas of edema. Patients with suspected toxoplasmosis are admitted and treated with a combination of IV pyrimethamine plus sulfadiazine plus leucovorin (folinic acid) and steroids (dexamethasone 4 mg IV every 6 hours) when edema or a mass effect exists.

31. The answer is D. (Chapter 155) Classic manifestations of tuberculosis include cough with hemoptysis, night sweats, prolonged fevers, weight loss, and anorexia. Approximately 10% of new cases of tuberculosis in the United States occur in human immunodeficiency virus (HIV) infected persons. Tuberculosis frequently occurs in patients with CD4+ T-cell counts of 200 to 500 cells/mm³. Negative purified protein derivative skin tuberculosis test results are frequent among AIDS patients due to immunosuppression. Definitive diagnosis of tuberculosis is made by stain and culture of expectorated sputum, although some cases require bronchoscopy.

32. The answer is A. (Chapter 156) High-risk conditions for endocarditis include prosthetic heart valves, prosthetic material used for valve repair, history of previous infective endocarditis, unrepaired cyanotic congenital heart disease, repaired congenital heart defect with prosthetic material or device, repaired congenital heart disease with residual defects, and cardiac transplant recipients with valve regurgitation due to a structurally abnormal valve. For high-risk patients, provide antibiotic prophylaxis before dental procedures that involve manipulation of gingival tissue, the periapical region of teeth, or perforation of the oral mucosa. Prophylaxis is not needed for nondental procedures, such as local injections, laceration suturing, intravenous line placement, blood drawing, endotracheal intubation, endoscopy, vaginal delivery, oral trauma and bleeding, urethral catheterization, or uterine dilation and curettage.

33. **The answer is D.** (Chapter 157) For the treatment of tetanus, the usual recommended dose of tetanus immunoglobulin is 3000 to 6000 units IM, administered in a separate syringe and opposite the site of tetanus toxoid administration. At least a portion of the tetanus immunoglobulin dose should be administered around the wound itself. Tetanus immunoglobulin should be given before wound debridement, because exotoxin may be released during wound manipulation. Tetanus is defined as a syndrome of acute onset of hypertonia and/or painful muscular contractions (usually of the muscles of the jaw and neck) and generalized muscle spasms without other apparent medical cause as reported by a health professional. The majority of tetanus cases are reported from five states: California, Florida, Texas, New York, and Pennsylvania. Most patients who develop tetanus have inadequate immunity to the disease secondary to waning immunity and failure to receive routine boosters.

34. **The answer is D.** (Chapter 157) Antibiotics are of limited value for the treatment of tetanus but are traditionally administered. Parenteral metronidazole is the antibiotic of choice. Penicillin should not be administered as it may potentiate the effects of tetanospasmin.

35. **The answer is A.** (Chapter 158, Table 11.3) Any direct contact between a human and a bat should be evaluated for a rabies exposure. Seeing a bat does not constitute an exposure. Postexposure prophylaxis is recommended for persons who were in the same room as a bat and who were unaware if a bite or direct contact had occurred (e.g., a sleeping person awakens to find a bat in the room, or an adult witnesses a bat in a room with an unattended child, mentally disabled person, or intoxicated person). A nonbite exposure is contamination of scratches, abrasions, open wounds, or mucous membranes with saliva or brain tissue from a rabid animal. For example, animal licks to nonintact skin have transmitted rabies. Nonbite exposures from animals very rarely cause rabies. If the material containing the virus is dry, the virus can be considered noninfectious. Petting a rabid animal or contact with blood, urine, or feces of a rabid animal does not constitute an exposure and is not an indication for prophylaxis.

36. **The answer is B.** (Chapter 158) In animal models tested for response to treatment of rabies, the use of corticosteroids shortens the incubation time of the virus and increases mortality. For this reason, steroids are

TABLE 11.3	Summary of Risk of Acquiring Rabies in the United States
Risk	**Exposures**
Moderate to high	Bite by skunk, raccoon, fox, and other wild carnivores (unless animal tested negative for rabies)
	Bite or direct contact with bat (unless animal tested negative for rabies)
	Exposure by percutaneous injury, mucous membrane exposure, or inhalation to live rabies virus in a laboratory
	Dog bite in a country with endemic rabies and inadequate immunization of dogs (or bite by feral dog)
Very low to low	Bite by inadequately vaccinated cat or dog that has access to the outdoors (or feral cat or dog)
	Contamination of open wound or abrasion (including scratches) with, or mucous membrane exposure to, saliva or other potentially infectious material (e.g., neural tissue) from a possibly rabid animal (skunk, raccoon, fox, and other wild carnivores, bat)
	Awakening in a room with a bat present
No risk identified	Contact of animal fluids (e.g., saliva, blood, neural tissue) with intact skin
	Indirect contact with saliva from a wild animal (e.g., by cleaning a dog or cat that has had contact with a wild animal)

Reproduced with permission from J.E. Tintinalli, J.S. Stapczynski, O.J. Ma, D. Yealy, G.D. Meckler, D.M. Cline: Tintinalli's Emergency Medicine: A Comprehensive Study Guide, 9th Edition. McGraw-Hill Education; 2020.

contraindicated in the treatment of rabies. Unfortunately, no specific therapies have demonstrated benefit in clinical rabies. Treatment with rabies vaccine, rabies immunoglobulin, IV ribavirin, or interferon is often tried but has not proven to be effective. Survival with normal neurologic function was reported for a 15-year-old girl in whom coma was induced and treatment with ketamine, midazolam, ribavirin, and amantadine was provided. However, similar regimens have been used for other patients without success. Specific therapies should be directed at the clinical complications of the disease.

37. **The answer is A.** (Chapter 159) Five species of the genus *Plasmodium* infect humans: *P. vivax*, *P. ovale*, *P. malariae*, *P. falciparum*, and *P. knowlesi*. Most malaria deaths are due to *P. falciparum* infections. *P. falciparum* is most prevalent in Africa, Haiti, and New Guinea. The *Plasmodium* is transmitted primarily by the bite of an infected female Anopheles mosquito but can also be transmitted by transfusion of infected blood, by needlestick accident, or across the placenta from mother to fetus.

38. **The answer is B.** (Chapter 159, Table 11.4) Quinidine gluconate plus doxycycline in adults or clindamycin in children is an appropriate antimalarial drug option for severe malaria. The figure is a retinal examination in a child with cerebral malaria demonstrating patches of whitening around the fovea and scattered white-centered hemorrhages. Malaria is described as severe when it includes one or more of the following: coma with or without seizures ("cerebral

TABLE 11.4	Antimalarial Drug Options for Severe (Complicated) Malaria	
Drug	Adult Dose	Pediatric Dose
Artesunate* (available from the CDC if quinidine fails to provide improvement; call 770-488-7788)	2.4 mg/kg IV at 0, 8, and 24 h, then daily. Artesunate can be given IM if necessary.	2.4 mg/kg IV at 0, 8, and 24 h, then daily. Artesunate can be given IM if necessary.
Quinidine gluconate (plus doxycycline or clindamycin)†	6.25 mg base (= 10 mg salt)/kg IV load over 2 h (maximum, 600 mg), follow with 0.0125 mg base (= 0.02 mg salt)/kg/min continuous infusion.	6.25 mg base (= 10 mg salt)/kg IV load over 2 h (maximum, 600 mg), follow with 0.0125 mg base (= 0.02 mg salt)/kg/min continuous infusion.
Plus		
Doxycycline	2.2 mg/kg IV (up to adult dose of 100 mg) every 12 h for 7 d.	2.2 mg/kg IV (up to adult dose of 100 mg) every 12 h for 7 d.
Or in children under age 8 y		
Clindamycin		10 mg base/kg loading dose IV followed by 5 mg base/kg IV every 8 h for 7 d.

Abbreviation: CDC = Centers for Disease Control and Prevention.

*Artesunate is considered the drug of choice by World Health Organization guidelines.

†Quinine dihydrochloride is an alternative to quinidine gluconate (20 mg [salt]/kg infused IV over 2–4 hours, then 10 mg/kg every 8 hours, can be given IM if necessary, as 50 mg/mL solution).

Reproduced with permission from J.E. Tintinalli, J.S. Stapczynski, O.J. Ma, D. Yealy, G.D. Meckler, D.M. Cline: Tintinalli's Emergency Medicine: A Comprehensive Study Guide, 9th Edition. McGraw-Hill Education; 2020.

malaria"), prostration, severe anemia, acidosis, hypoglycemia, acute renal failure, acute respiratory distress syndrome, pulmonary edema, jaundice, intravascular hemolysis, shock, and disseminated intravascular coagulation.

39. **The answer is C.** (Chapter 160) Scombroid fish poisoning may occur after ingestion of tuna, mackerel, bonito, mahi-mahi, bluefish, herring, and sardines. Scombroid fish poisoning occurs when histidine is metabolized by bacteria into histamine and other bioactive amines inside of improperly prepared fish, allowing these substances to accumulate. Symptoms usually begin 30 minutes to 24 hours after ingestion and include flushing, headache, abdominal cramping, vomiting, and diarrhea. Treatment is with antihistamines such as diphenhydramine and cimetidine. Antibiotic treatment is not indicated. Intravenous mannitol has been reported as a potential treatment for severe neurologic symptoms from ciguatera poisoning, although the evidence is not strong.

40. **The answer is B.** (Chapter 160) Ingestion of the preformed toxin of *Clostridium botulinum* results in an illness characterized by vomiting, diarrhea, blurred vision, diplopia, dysphagia, descending muscle weakness, and paralysis. Symptoms can be seen days to months after the ingestion. Food implicated in this illness include canned foods, canned fish, foods kept warm in dishes, herbed oils, and cheese sauce. Treatment may require intubation as well as botulism antitoxin. Brucella may occur after ingestion of raw milk, unpasteurized goat's milk or cheese, or contaminated meat and is characterized by fever, chills, myalgias, arthralgias, weakness, and bloody diarrhea but would not explain this patient's double vision. *Clostridium perfringens* may be found in meat, poultry, dried or precooked foods and meals with poor temperature control and infection is characterized by watery diarrhea, nausea, and cramping. *Listeria monocytogenes* may be found in fresh soft cheeses, poorly pasteurized dairy products, deli meats, and hot dogs. Infection is characterized by fever, myalgias, nausea, diarrhea, meningitis, and premature delivery if pregnant.

41. **The answer is C.** (Chapter 160) Nontuberculous *Mycobacterium* such as *Mycobacterium marinum* or *avium* is found in salt and fresh water and can cause illness. *M. marinum* is associated with granulomatous skin infections similar to the painful indurated plaque pictured in the question stem. Aeromonas species are found in fresh and marine water and can cause gastroenteritis and wound infections that can range from simple cellulitis to necrotizing infections and septic arthritis. *Legionella* is a common inhabitant of fresh water. Infection occurs from inhalation of contaminated aerosols, resulting in one of two syndromes: Legionnaires disease or Pontiac fever. *Pseudomonas aeruginosa* is found in fresh water and can cause otitis externa, keratitis in contact lens wearers, and folliculitis.

42. **The answer is D.** (Chapter 160) *Vibrio vulnificus* infection may present after recent exposure to salt water with skin infections that can range from simple cellulitis to hemorrhagic bullae (as seen in the figure) and necrotizing infection. *Mycobacterium marinum* is associated with granulomatous skin infections. *Aeromonas* species are found in fresh and marine water and can cause gastroenteritis and wound infections that can range from simple cellulitis to necrotizing infections and septic arthritis. *Pseudomonas aeruginosa* is found in fresh water and can cause otitis externa, keratitis in contact lens wearers, and folliculitis.

43. **The answer is B.** (Chapter 161) Rocky Mountain spotted fever (RMSF) is one of the most severe of the tickborne illnesses in the United States, with more than 60% of reported cases originating from five states: North Carolina, Tennessee, Oklahoma, Missouri, and Arkansas. The causative organism is *Rickettsia rickettsii*. Vectors in the United States are the *Dermacentor* (*D. variabilis* and

D. andersoni, the American dog tick) and *Rhipicephalus sanguineus* ticks (the brown dog tick, found in the American southwest). Typical hosts include deer, rodents, horses, cattle, cats, and dogs. Early signs and symptoms of RMSF are fever, headache, myalgia, and malaise with other nonspecific findings of lymphadenopathy, abdominal pain, nausea, vomiting, diarrhea, and headache. If left untreated, it may progress to confusion, meningismus, renal failure, respiratory failure, and myocarditis. The classic triad of fever, rash, and tick bite may not be seen as 20% of patients do not develop rash and only about half of patients recall a tick bite. Doxycycline therapy is the recommended treatment for all rickettsial diseases, including RMSF, in adults and children of all ages by the American Academy of Pediatrics and by the Centers for Disease Control and Prevention. Vancomycin and azithromycin are not recommended first-line treatments for RMSF, and supportive care alone would be inappropriate as this disease can progress to severe illness or death without appropriate antimicrobial treatment.

44. **The answer is B.** (Chapter 161) Lyme disease is the most common vector-borne zoonotic infection in the United States, with majority of cases reported in the northeast and upper midwestern states. The infecting organism is *Borrelia. burgdorferi*, a spirochete, transmitted by the *Ixodes* deer tick, also known as the black-legged tick. Lyme disease has three clinical stages. The first stage is local and classically characterized by a rash, erythema migrans, with other nonspecific symptoms of fever, chills, fatigue, myalgias, arthralgias, and lymphadenopathy. The second stage, early disseminated disease, is characterized by fever, adenopathy, neuropathies, cardiac abnormalities, arthritic complaints, and skin lesions. One of the most common neurologic symptoms in the secondary stage of illness is unilateral or bilateral facial nerve palsy. The third stage, late disseminated stage, occurs months to years after the initial infection and is characterized by chronic arthritis, myocarditis, subacute encephalopathy, axonal polyneuropathy, and leukoencephalopathy. The preferred treatment of Lyme disease is with doxycycline. However, severe disease or neurologic symptoms require ceftriaxone therapy.

45. **The answer is B.** (Chapter 161) Ehrlichiosis is a group of zoonotic diseases caused by the *Ehrlichia* genus, gram-negative pleomorphic coccobacilli, and is transmitted by the lone star tick, *Amblyomma americanum*. The white-tailed deer in the southeastern United States is the major animal reservoir. Within 1 to 2 weeks of a tick bite, infected individuals may develop headache, malaise, nausea, vomiting, diarrhea, abdominal pain, and arthralgias. A minority of patients may go on to develop renal failure, respiratory failure, and encephalitis. Treatment is with doxycycline. Babesiosis is a malaria-like disease transmitted by ticks with clinical features of generalized malaise, anorexia, fever, and chills that can progress to intermittent sweats, myalgia, headache, and hemolytic anemia. Rocky Mountain spotted fever is one of the most severe of the tickborne illnesses in the United States with typical clinical features of rash that is petechial or purpuric, pulmonary infiltrates, jaundice, myocarditis, hepatosplenomegaly, meningitis, encephalitis, and lymphadenopathy. Tularemia is contracted through tick/fly bites, by inhalation, or through open wounds with clinical presentation depending on the method of inoculation: the clinical forms are called ulceroglandular, glandular, typhoidal, pneumonic, oculoglandular, and oropharyngeal.

Nervous System Disorders

12

QUESTIONS

1. A patient presenting with vertigo and admits to some confusion understanding the different components of the HINTs (head impulse, nystagmus type, test of skew) examination. Which of the following statements is CORRECT?
   (A) A peripheral lesion is suggested if a vertical skew gaze is provoked by alternately covering each eye.
   (B) A rapid corrective saccade back to the target during the head impulse component suggests a central lesion.
   (C) Fatiguing lateral nystagmus assessed during movement of the eyes suggests a central lesion.
   (D) The HINTs examination should be reserved for those patients who are symptomatic with acute vertigo.

2. A 66-year-old man presents to the emergency department with severe acute onset headache. The pain is diffuse and stabbing. He has no prior history of headaches. What is the MOST LIKELY diagnosis?
   (A) Cluster headache
   (B) Migraine headache
   (C) Subarachnoid hemorrhage
   (D) Tension headache

3. A 34-year-old man presents to the emergency department with severe headache. His headaches started abruptly approximately 1 month ago. They are a sharp stabbing pain located in the right side of his face lasting for approximately 15 minutes. They resolve spontaneously but abruptly return. He has had approximately seven episodes in the last week, prompting his visit. On examination, he is tearing from his right eye with mild conjunctival injection and miosis. What is the MOST LIKELY diagnosis?

   (A) Cluster headache
   (B) Migraine headache
   (C) Subarachnoid hemorrhage
   (D) Tension headache

4. In which of the following patients is it safe to perform a lumbar puncture prior to CT scan imaging?
   (A) A 23-year-old woman with a history of renal transplant who presents with headache and nuchal rigidity
   (B) A 23-year-old woman with a history of VP shunt placement for obstructive hydrocephalus who presents with headache and nuchal rigidity
   (C) A 23-year-old woman with active intravenous drug use who presents with altered mental status and fever
   (D) A 23-year-old woman with no past medical history who presents with altered mental status and fever

5. You suspect bacterial meningitis in a patient who presents with fever and a Glasgow coma score of 10. Which of the following is the MOST APPROPRIATE sequence of actions?
   (A) First administer antibiotics, next obtain a CT scan of the brain, and then perform a lumbar puncture
   (B) First administer antibiotics, next perform a lumbar puncture, and then obtain a CT scan of the brain
   (C) First perform a lumbar puncture, next administer antibiotics, and then obtain a CT scan of the brain
   (D) First perform a lumbar puncture, next obtain a CT scan of the brain, and then administer antibiotics

6. A 38-year-old G1P1 6-week postpartum woman presents due to new onset seizure at 2:00 AM. According to her husband, she has been complaining of a headache in the last month. She had no prior history of headache. She has had two prior visits to the emergency department for headache in the last month. Each time she was diagnosed with a headache secondary to sleep deprivation due to her newborn, was treated for migraine, and was discharged. This evening her husband was awakened to the patient having a seizure in bed and he called 911. Upon arrival to the emergency department, the patient is confused and actively vomiting. Which of the following conditions is the MOST LIKELY cause of her headache?
   (A) Migraine headache
   (B) Subdural hematoma
   (C) Temporal arteritis
   (D) Venous thrombosis

7. A 25-year-old obese woman presents to the emergency department with headache and double vision. Her headaches started approximately 2 weeks ago and have progressively worsened. She was started on oral contraception approximately 1 month ago. On funduscopic examination, you see Figure 12.1. What is the MOST serious sequelae of her condition if left untreated?

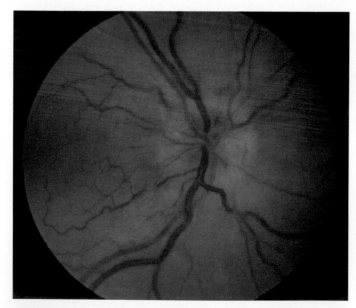

FIGURE 12.1 Reproduced with permission from Knoop K, Stack L, Storrow A: Atlas of Emergency Medicine, 2nd ed. 2002, McGraw-Hill, New York.

   (A) Chronic hearing loss
   (B) Midbrain stroke
   (C) Permanent vision loss
   (D) Severe migraine

8. What is the treatment for posterior reversible encephalopathy syndrome?
   (A) Antihypertensive medications
   (B) Chemotherapeutic agents
   (C) Intravenous antivirals
   (D) Intravenous gamma-globulins

9. What type of hemorrhage is demonstrated in Figure 12.2?

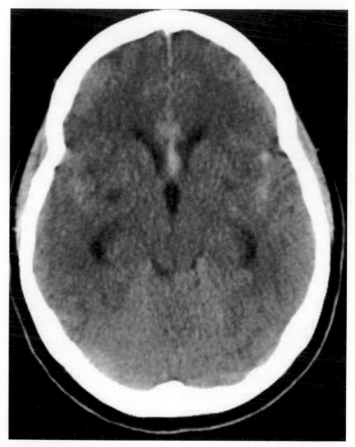

FIGURE 12.2 Image used with permission of James Anderson, MD, Department of Radiology, Oregon Health & Science University.

   (A) Epidural hemorrhage
   (B) Intracerebral hemorrhage
   (C) Subarachnoid hemorrhage
   (D) Subdural hemorrhage

10. What is the MOST LIKELY cause of this intracranial hemorrhage (Figure 12.3)?

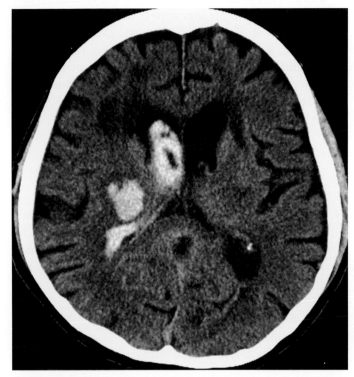

(A) Hypertension
(B) Infection
(C) Trauma
(D) Vomiting

11. Which of the following is a risk factor for thrombotic stroke?
(A) Atrial fibrillation
(B) Diabetes mellitus
(C) Myocardial infarction
(D) Valve replacement

12. A 55-year-old man with a past medical history of diabetes mellitus and 40 pack-year smoking history presents with left lower extremity weakness and paresthesias as well as confusion. His neuro examination reveals normal cranial nerves, 5/5 muscle strength of his bilateral upper extremities and right lower extremity, and 4/5 muscle strength of his left lower extremity. He has decreased sensation of his left lower extremity. Which artery is MOST LIKELY infarcted?

(A) Left anterior cerebellar artery
(B) Left anterior cerebral artery
(C) Right anterior cerebellar artery
(D) Right anterior cerebral artery

13. Which clinical presentation is MOST LIKELY for a patient with this nonenhanced CT scan (Figure 12.4)?

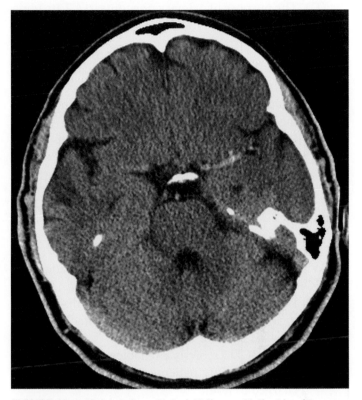

(A) Left lower extremity sensory loss, left lower extremity weakness, confusion and motor hemineglect
(B) Left lower facial droop, left upper extremity weakness, left lower extremity weakness, and neologism
(C) Right lower extremity sensory loss, right lower extremity weakness, confusion, and motor hemineglect
(D) Right lower facial droop, right upper extremity weakness, right lower extremity weakness, and neologism

14. Which of the following statements regarding imaging of stroke patients is CORRECT?
    (A) Brain imaging and interpretation should be completed within 60 minutes of patient arrival.
    (B) Current thrombolytic inclusion/exclusion criteria require CT imaging.
    (C) MRI is the initial imaging modality of choice in acute stroke presentations.
    (D) The purpose of primary noncontrast CT imaging is to identify location of the occlusion.

15. Which of the following is an absolute contraindication to thrombolytic therapy?
    (A) Major surgery or serious trauma within preceding 14 days
    (B) Pretreatment systolic blood pressure >185 despite therapy
    (C) Previous myocardial infarction within the preceding 3 months
    (D) Seizure at onset with postictal residual neurologic impairments

16. Which statement about transient ischemic attacks is CORRECT?
    (A) Duration of symptoms is a reliable discriminator between a transient ischemic attack versus a cerebral vascular accident.
    (B) The ABCD2 score is a reliable score that can be used to identify patients who can be safely discharged to home.
    (C) The combinations of aspirin and dipyridamole or aspirin and clopidogrel are less effective in stroke prevention than aspirin alone.
    (D) Use of direct oral anticoagulants in patients with atrial fibrillation has demonstrated equal efficacy compared to warfarin in stroke prevention.

17. A 75-year-old woman presents with her family secondary to confusion and difficulty walking. She initially developed urinary incontinence approximately 2 weeks ago and this has gradually worsened. CT scan imaging of the brain reveals excessively large ventricles. What is the MOST LIKELY diagnosis?
    (A) Dementia of the elderly
    (B) Normal pressure hydrocephalus
    (C) Spinal epidural abscess
    (D) Urinary tract infection

18. A mother brings her 2-year-old son to the emergency department for repeated falls. She states that since he has learned how to walk he has not had any difficulties and has been steady. In the last week, he has fallen three times and his legs appear unsteady. He has no other recent illnesses. Upon initial evaluation of the patient, he is awake, alert, and appropriate for his age but had two instances of rapid uncontrolled eye movement. Which of the following conditions does this patient MOST LIKELY have?
    (A) A mass in his chest or abdomen
    (B) A post viral metabolic syndrome
    (C) A toxic alcohol ingestion
    (D) A tumor in the central cerebellum

19. A 27-year-old woman presents to the emergency department with acute vertigo. She reports that the symptoms began after she recently had her neck adjusted at a chiropractor's office. What is the MOST LIKELY diagnosis?
    (A) Bacterial labyrinthitis
    (B) Benign positional vertigo
    (C) Transient ischemic attack
    (D) Vertebral artery dissection

20. What is status epilepticus?
    (A) Seizure activity for ≥5 minutes or two or more seizures without regaining consciousness between seizures
    (B) Seizure activity for ≥5 minutes or two or more seizures within a 24-hour period
    (C) Seizure activity for ≥10 minutes or two or more seizures without regaining consciousness between seizures
    (D) Seizure activity for ≥10 minutes or two or more seizures within a 24-hour period

21. A 26-year-old man presents to the emergency department after a first-time seizure. The patient returned to baseline mental status shortly after arrival. After unremarkable imaging and an unremarkable metabolic evaluation, your next action should include which of the following?
    (A) Obtaining an emergent electroencephalogram prior to discharge
    (B) Obtaining emergent magnetic resonance imaging of the brain
    (C) Reporting the seizure to the government agency in charge of driving privileges as determined by state law
    (D) Starting the patient on an antiepileptic medication

22. What is the initial agent of choice in the treatment of status epilepticus?
    (A) Lorazepam
    (B) Phenobarbital
    (C) Phenytoin
    (D) Valproate

23. A 65-year-old woman is brought to the emergency department via ambulance for new-onset seizures. She received 5 mg of intramuscular midazolam en route and continues to have seizure activity. Upon arrival she was given intravenous lorazepam and intravenous levetiracetam, which resolved her tonic-clonic movements. Upon reevaluation, the patient remains altered and demonstrates a very faint rhythmic movement of her mouth and slight continued rhythmic eye saccades. Which condition should this patient be treated for?
    (A) Dystonic reaction with akathisia
    (B) Generalized partial seizure
    (C) Nonconvulsive status epilepticus
    (D) Tuberous sclerosis syndrome

24. A 46-year-old woman presents to the emergency department with a complaint of weakness in both of her legs. Initially she felt unbalanced, but now she cannot walk because her knees repeated give out bilaterally. She admits to having a cough and cold approximately 1 month ago. On examination, she demonstrates 4/5 muscle weakness at her ankles and knees with both flexion and extension, but 5/5 muscle strength at the hips bilaterally. She has one out of four reflexes at her Achilles and her patellar tendons bilaterally. What is the MOST LIKELY diagnosis?
    (A) Clostridium botulinum toxicity
    (B) Guillain-Barré syndrome
    (C) Lumbosacral plexopathy
    (D) Ramsey Hunt syndrome

25. A 52-year-old man presents to the emergency department secondary to weakness. He states that he feels fine each morning upon awakening but gradually gets weaker throughout the day. He denies fatigue. His vital signs are normal. On examination, he has a mild ptosis of his left eye, but otherwise his cranial nerve examination is normal. He has 5/5 muscle strength at his bilateral wrists, elbows, ankles, and knees. He has 4/5 muscle strength at his bilateral shoulders and hips. He has a normal gait and his cerebellar evaluation is normal. On laboratory evaluation, his metabolic workup is normal. What is the NEXT MOST APPROPRIATE test?

    (A) CT scan of the brain
    (B) Edrophonium challenge
    (C) Electroencephalogram
    (D) X-ray of the chest

26. A 25-year-old woman presents to the emergency department with the complaint of paresthesias in her left arm. Upon review of her medical records, she has presented three other times in the past year. She initially complained of right hand numbness, then vision changes in her right eye, followed by the complaint of a weak grip in her left hand. All of those symptoms have since resolved. She now reports a vibration sensation in her left arm. On examination, she has increased tone in left arm with 3/4 reflexes at the elbow and brachioradialis muscle. Additionally, she has decreased vibratory and temperature sensation in her left arm. What is the MOST LIKELY diagnosis?
    (A) Guillain-Barré syndrome
    (B) Intracranial mass
    (C) Multiple sclerosis
    (D) Myasthenia gravis

27. What is the MOST significant emergency department complication of myasthenia gravis?
    (A) Labile hypotension
    (B) Respiratory failure
    (C) Seizure disorder
    (D) Urinary tract infection

28. In the United States, what is the MOST COMMON cause of bacterial meningitis in immunocompetent adults?
    (A) Group B *Streptococcus*
    (B) *Neisseria meningitides*
    (C) *Staphylococcus aureus*
    (D) *Streptococcus pneumoniae*

29. Which of the following is the MOST COMMON presenting symptom of meningitis?
    (A) Confusion
    (B) Fever
    (C) Headache
    (D) Stiff neck

30. Older alcoholic patients presenting with bacterial meningitis are at highest risk for which causative organism?
    (A) *Listeria monocytogenes*
    (B) *Neisseria meningitides*
    (C) *Staphylococcus aureus*
    (D) *Streptococcus pneumoniae*

31. With regard to meningitis, a cerebrospinal fluid analysis with a white blood count <300/mm³, lymphocytic predominance, normal glucose and protein <200 mg/dL is MOST suggestive of which etiology?
    (A) Bacterial
    (B) Fungal
    (C) Neoplastic
    (D) Viral

32. A 55-year-old otherwise healthy woman arrives to the emergency department via ambulance secondary to altered mental status and new onset seizures. Upon arrival, the patient is altered and cannot provide a history. She spontaneously moves all her extremities but does not follow commands. She has a vesicular rash in her left ear. The following is her magnetic resonance imaging. What is the MOST LIKELY diagnosis (Figure 12.5)?

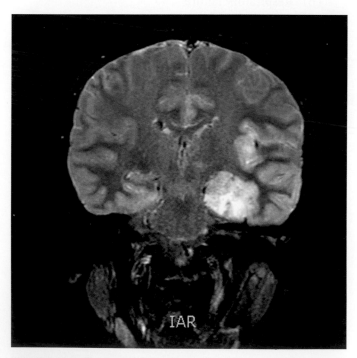

FIGURE 12.5 Photo contributed by Elizabeth Yutan, Department of Radiology, Oregon Health & Science University.

(A) Herpes simplex encephalitis
(B) Rabies encephalitis
(C) West Nile encephalitis
(D) Western equine encephalitis

33. A 33-year-old man presents with the complaint of a severe headache 2 weeks after he sustained a skull fracture in a motorcycle accident. A CT scan of the brain reveals an intracranial abscess. What is the MOST LIKELY causative organism?
    (A) Group B *Streptococcus*
    (B) *Neisseria meningitides*
    (C) *Staphylococcus aureus*
    (D) *Streptococcus pneumoniae*

34. A 33-year-old man presents with a complaint of back pain. He denies trauma, urinary, or bowel incontinence, leg weakness, or saddle anesthesia. On physical examination, the patient has normal vital signs, evidence of intravenous drug use on both arms, and severe diffuse pain of his lumbar spine. Which statement about this patient is MOST LIKELY to be CORRECT?
    (A) He has a paraspinal lumbar muscle strain.
    (B) He is at high risk for a spinal epidural abscess.
    (C) He is malingering with the goal of drug seeking.
    (D) He should have an x-ray of the spine to evaluate for a compression fracture.

35. What is the MOST COMMON type of ventriculoperitoneal (VP) shunt malfunction?
    (A) Abdominal complication
    (B) Mechanical failure
    (C) Obstruction
    (D) Overdrainage

ANSWERS

1. **The answer is D.** (Chapter 164) Vertigo is often a symptom of vestibular system dysfunction but may also result from a central nervous system disorder such as posterior circulation stroke. The horizontal head impulse test is a bedside maneuver to detect peripheral vestibular disease. This test should be reserved for patients who are currently experiencing vertigo. A normal (negative) finding of the horizontal head impulse test reliably identifies patients with a central cause of acute vertigo, but an abnormal test (positive) may occur with both peripheral and central causes of vertigo. A rapid corrective saccade back to the target during head rotation suggests a peripheral vestibular etiology. Two additional maneuvers are employed in conjunction with the horizontal head impulse test to reliably exclude central causes of vertigo: examination for nystagmus and assessment for skew gaze. Nystagmus that changes direction with gaze to either side is predictive of a central lesion, as is spontaneous vertical or multidirectional nystagmus. Skew deviation refers to misalignment of the eyes. Though subtle at times, it may be unmasked by alternately covering each eye while the patient fixes gaze on the examiner. Vertical skew gaze suggests a central lesion.

2. **The answer is C.** (Chapter 165) Patients >50 years of age, with a new or worsening headache, represent a high-risk group. The incidence of migraine, cluster, and tension headaches decreases with age, raising the likelihood of ominous pathology for older patients. Causes of thunder clap headache include intracranial hemorrhage, "sentinel" aneurysmal hemorrhage, spontaneous intracerebral hemorrhage, carotid or vertebrobasilar dissection, reversible cerebral vasoconstriction syndrome, cerebral venous thrombosis, posterior reversible encephalopathy syndrome, coital headache, valsalva-associated headache, spontaneous intracranial hypotension, acute hydrocephalus, and pituitary apoplexy.

3. **The answer is A.** (Chapter 165) Patients presenting with cluster headaches have at least five attacks that are severe, unilateral, lasting 15 to 180 minutes if untreated, with a circadian/circannual pattern. Associated ipsilateral symptoms include at least one of the following: lacrimation, conjunctival injection, nasal congestion or rhinorrhea, ptosis and/or miosis, edema of the eyelid and/or face, and sweating of the forehead and/or face. Although migraine headache symptoms can vary, they typically last hours and are less likely to feature unilateral tearing. Subarachnoid hemorrhage presents with sudden severe headache that would be unlikely to resolve in 15 minutes.

Tension headaches would likewise not be expected to cause unilateral lacrimation or resolve so quickly.

4. **The answer is D.** (Chapter 165) The possibility of herniation in association with lumbar puncture (LP) is a frequent concern of emergency providers. There is no randomized controlled trial assessing the question of when it is safe to perform an LP. The cumulative evidence suggests that in patients without a history of immunosuppression, who have a normal sensorium, and who have no focal neurologic deficits, it is safe to proceed with LP without imaging prior to LP. Risk of an abnormal CT scan is elevated in patients with any of the following clinical features: a deteriorating or altered level of consciousness (particularly a Glasgow coma scale score of ≤11), brainstem signs (including pupillary changes, posturing, or irregular respirations), focal neurologic deficit, history of recent seizure, history of a preexisting neurologic disorder, or history of immunocompromised state. In patients with these clinical features, imaging prior to LP is appropriate.

5. **The answer is A.** (Chapter 165) A lumbar puncture (LP) is indicated for suspected meningitis. If the LP is delayed (e.g., CT, coagulopathy, thrombocytopenia, agitation) and meningitis is strongly suspected, administer antibiotics without delay. For many patients who are awake, are alert with no evidence of papilledema or focal neurologic deficit, and have no history to suggest immunocompromised state or new-onset seizure, the head CT can be delayed until after the LP. However, this patient is altered with a Glasgow coma scale score of 10, so CT imaging should proceed LP to rule out edema or space-occupying lesions, which might increase the risk of herniation with CSF removal.

6. **The answer is D.** (Chapter 165) Cerebral venous thrombosis is a rare, but dangerous, cause of headache. Consider this diagnosis in patients presenting with new headache symptoms, especially in the presence of certain known risk factors. Cerebral venous thrombosis is more common in women, especially in the peripartum period, and in patients with a recent surgical history. It is associated with hypercoagulable states such as use of oral contraceptives, hematologic disorders, factor V Leiden homozygous mutation, protein S or protein C deficiency, and anti–thrombin III deficiency. The presentation can vary widely, from a progressive headache developing over days to weeks to, in some instances, a "thunderclap" headache. Similarly, the patient's clinical appearance can

be quite benign, especially early on in the course of the illness, or in more severe cases, patients may present with seizures, stroke symptoms, and even coma. Migraine headaches will not progress to seizure activity. A spontaneous subdural in this patient is unlikely given her lack of risk factors. Patients with temporal arteritis are >50 years old.

7. **The answer is C.** (Chapter 165) The fundoscopic examination demonstrates papilledema. This patient has idiopathic intracranial hypertension. Idiopathic intracranial hypertension, also known as pseudotumor cerebri, is most common in obese women. The incidence is 19.3 per 100,000 obese women between the ages of 20 and 44 years and has increased along with the obesity epidemic. The most prominent symptoms include headache (84%), transient visual obscurations (68%), back pain (53%), and pulsatile tinnitus (52%). The diagnostic criteria include papilledema with an otherwise normal neurologic examination and elevated opening pressure on lumbar puncture. Lumbar puncture is necessary to make the diagnosis of idiopathic intracranial hypertension, and concomitant removal of a volume of cerebrospinal fluid can provide temporary relief of symptoms. If left untreated, idiopathic intracranial hypertension can lead to permanent visual impairment.

8. **The answer is A.** (Chapter 165) Patients with posterior reversible encephalopathy syndrome can present with severe headache, visual changes, seizures, and encephalopathy in the setting of marked blood pressure elevation (usually rapidly developing). It is most common in patients undergoing active treatment with immune-suppressing or modulating medications or chemotherapeutic agents, as well as in patients with end-stage renal disease. MRI typically shows evidence of symmetrical vasogenic edema in the occipital area of the brain, although other areas of the brain can be involved. Treatment involves blood pressure control and supportive care.

9. **The answer is C.** (Chapter 166) This image demonstrates a subarachnoid hemorrhage. Newer-generation CT scanners provide increased sensitivity for detecting subarachnoid hemorrhage, especially in the setting of (1) patients presenting within 6 hours of symptom onset and (2) greater availability of a timely interpretation by a neuroradiologist. The probability of excluding a subarachnoid hemorrhage following CT/CTA is about 99.4%. The usefulness of MRI, particularly fluid-attenuated inversion recovery MRI sequences, is limited. A negative MRI result would still need to be followed by a lumbar puncture (LP). In general, normal findings on head CT, the absence of xanthochromia, and zero or few RBCs ($<5 \times 10^6$ RBCs/L) in the cerebrospinal fluid (CSF) help reliably exclude subarachnoid hemorrhage.

10. **The answer is A.** (Chapter 166) Risk factors for intracerebral hemorrhage include long-standing hypertension, arteriovenous malformations, arterial aneurysm, anticoagulant therapy, use of sympathomimetic drugs (particularly cocaine and phenylpropanolamine), intracranial tumors, and amyloid angiopathy in the elderly. In hypertensive intracerebral hemorrhage, bleeding is usually localized to the putamen, thalamus, pons, or cerebellum (in decreasing order of frequency), and clinical examination findings may be relatable to those areas. Cerebellar hemorrhage is commonly associated with dizziness, vomiting, marked truncal ataxia, gaze palsies, and depressed level of consciousness. Patients with cerebellar hemorrhage are more likely to have rapidly progressive symptoms and may require more aggressive intervention than patients with other forms of intracerebral hemorrhage. Patients who develop a subarachnoid hemorrhage from aneurysm rupture may experience their symptoms during an activity that raises blood pressure, such as vomiting. Trauma is a common cause of intracranial bleeding, but it would be more likely to cause an epidural or subdural hematoma or traumatic subarachnoid hemorrhage. Infection is unlikely to cause this type of hemorrhage.

11. **The answer is B.** (Chapter 167) Risk factors for vessel thrombus include hypertension, diabetes mellitus, and coronary atherosclerotic disease. In contrast, atrial fibrillation, valvular replacement, or recent myocardial infarction suggest an embolic stroke etiology.

12. **The answer is D.** (Chapter 167) Occlusion of the anterior cerebral artery is uncommon (0.5%–3% of all strokes), but when unilateral occlusion occurs, it can cause contralateral sensory and motor symptoms in the lower extremity, with sparing of the hands and face. In addition, a left-sided lesion is typically associated with akinetic mutism and transcortical motor aphasia (repetition ability retained), whereas right-sided infarction can result in confusion and motor hemineglect. Bilateral occlusion can cause a combination of the above symptoms but was particularly associated with mutism, incontinence, and poor outcome in one small series. Cerebellar artery infarctions can present nonspecifically with dizziness but would be suggested by vertigo, gait disturbances, limb ataxia, nystagmus, or nausea and vomiting. A cerebellar artery infarct would be less likely to cause focal left lower extremity weakness and sensory loss.

13. **The answer is D.** (Chapter 167) The middle cerebral artery is the vessel most commonly involved in stroke, and clinical findings can be quite variable, depending on exactly where the lesion is located and which brain hemisphere is dominant. (In right-handed patients and in up to 80% of left-handed patients, the left hemisphere is dominant.) A middle cerebral artery stroke typically presents with hemiparesis, facial plegia, and sensory loss contralateral to the affected cortex. These deficits variably affect the face and upper extremity more than the lower extremity. If the dominant hemisphere is involved, aphasia (receptive, expressive, or both) is often present. If the nondominant hemisphere is involved, inattention, neglect, extinction on double-simultaneous stimulation, dysarthria without aphasia, and constructional apraxia (difficulty in drawing complex two-dimensional or three-dimensional figures) may occur. A homonymous hemianopsia and gaze preference toward the side of the infarct may also be seen, regardless of the side of the infarction. Lesions affecting lower extremities without facial or upper extremity involvement are suggestive of anterior cerebral artery etiologies.

14. **The answer is B.** (Chapter 167) According to the American Heart Association/American Stroke Association (AHA/ASA), time recommendations for acute ischemic stroke, head CT interpretation should be completed within 45 minutes of patient arrival. Diffusion-weighted MRI is superior to non–contrast-enhanced CT or other types of MRI (T1/T2 weighted, fluid-attenuated inversion recovery) in the detection of acute infarction. However, at this time, the role of MRI for acute stroke in the emergency department is limited because of MRI's uncertain accuracy in detecting acute hemorrhage, lack of rapid availability, patient-specific contraindications (lack of cooperation, claustrophobia, metallic implants or pacemakers, and diminished access to the patient), relative inexperience in some practitioners in interpreting MRI scans in acute stroke, and cost-effectiveness. Despite these caveats, the current AHA/ASA acute ischemic stroke guidelines recommend either non–contrast-enhanced CT or MRI as the initial imaging in the acute stroke patient. Most acute ischemic strokes are not visualized by a non–contrast brain CT in the early hours of a stroke. Therefore, the utility of the first brain CT is primarily to exclude intracranial bleeding, abscess, tumor, and other stroke mimics, as well as to detect current contraindications to thrombolytics.

15. **The answer is B.** (Chapter 167) All other options are relative exclusion criteria. The only absolute contraindication listed is a pretreatment systolic blood pressure >185.

Blood pressures higher than this were found to have increased hemorrhagic conversion following thrombolytic therapy.

16. **The answer is D.** (Chapter 167) Direct oral anticoagulants demonstrate equal efficacy in stroke prevention with a reduce incidence of intracerebral hemorrhage when compared to warfarin. Duration of symptoms is not a reliable discriminator between transient ischemic attacks and cerebral vascular accidents. The ABCD2 score should NOT be used to identify patients with transient ischemic attack who can be safely discharged home. The combination of aspirin with either dipyridamole or clopidogrel is more effective in stroke prevention than aspirin alone.

17. **The answer is B.** (Chapter 168) Normal-pressure hydrocephalus is suggested by the presence of excessively large ventricles on head CT and can prompt consideration of a trial of lumbar puncture with cerebrospinal fluid drainage or ventricular shunting. Consider normal-pressure hydrocephalus if urinary incontinence and gait disturbance develop early in the disease process. The onset of symptoms in this patient is more rapid than would be seen with progressive dementia and that should not cause excessively enlarged ventricles. Spinal epidural abscess usually presents with back pain, infectious symptoms, or neurologic deficits secondary to spinal cord compression and should not cause changes on head CT. Urinary tract is less likely given the time course of her symptoms and the head CT findings.

18. **The answer is A.** (Chapter 169) This child is presenting with opsoclonus-myoclonus. Acute ataxia associated with rapid chaotic eye movements (opsoclonus) and myoclonic extremity jerks of the head and extremities are the striking syndrome of opsoclonus-myoclonus. This may be a postviral syndrome, but that is unlikely in this patient given his lack of recent illness. Opsoclonus-myoclonus is often a paraneoplastic syndrome associated with a neuroblastoma located in the abdomen or chest. The patient would not be awake, alert, and appropriate for his age if he was symptomatic from a toxic alcohol ingestion. A central cerebellar lesion would result in truncal ataxia rather than limb ataxia.

19. **The answer is D.** (Chapter 170) Recent head or neck trauma is a risk factor for dissection of the vertebral artery. In patients with acute vertigo, a recent history of trauma should spark concern for dissection even if pain is absent. The other answer options would be uncommon in this age group and less likely to begin immediately following neck manipulation.

20. The answer is A. (Chapter 171) Status epilepticus is seizure activity for ≥5 minutes or two or more seizures without regaining consciousness between seizures. Refractory status epilepticus is persistent seizure activity despite the intravenous administration of adequate doses of two antiepileptic agents.

21. The answer is C. (Chapter 171) Driving is prohibited until cleared by the neurologist or primary care physician. Reporting of conditions that may affect driving privileges should conform to state law, and it may be up to the emergency physician to document seizure activity for the Department of Motor Vehicles. Although EEG is very helpful, it is often not readily available in most emergency departments. Emergent EEG can be considered in the evaluation of a patient with persistent, unexplained altered mental status to evaluate for nonconvulsive status epilepticus, subtle status epilepticus, paroxysmal attack when a seizure is suspected, or ongoing status epilepticus after chemical paralysis for intubation. Almost one-quarter of adults with new-onset seizure will have visualized pathology on follow-up MRI, but this imaging is not required in the emergency department. Guidelines do not recommend hospital admission or initiation of anticonvulsant therapy in the patient with a first unprovoked seizure, as long as the patient has returned to neurologic baseline.

22. The answer is A. (Chapter 171) Intravenous lorazepam is considered the initial agent of choice. Lorazepam is more effective than phenytoin or phenobarbital as the initial drug. Valproic acid is effective but has serious side effects compared to other agents.

23. The answer is C. (Chapter 171) In nonconvulsive status epilepticus, the patient is comatose or has fluctuating abnormal mental status or confusion, but no overt seizure activity is present. The diagnosis is challenging and is typically made by EEG. Findings suggestive of nonconvulsive status epilepticus include a prolonged postictal period after a generalized seizure; subtle motor signs such as twitching, blinking, and eye deviation; fluctuating alterations in mental status; or unexplained stupor and confusion in the elderly. This patient is having seizures rather than a dystonic reaction based on the description of her clinical course, and a dystonic reaction would not be expected to cause altered mental status. She does not have a history of tuberous sclerosis, which is genetic condition that is typically diagnosed well before age 65.

24. The answer is B. (Chapter 172) Guillain-Barré syndrome is an acute polyneuropathy characterized by immune-mediated peripheral nerve myelin sheath or axon destruction. The prevailing theory is that antibodies directed against myelin sheath and axons of peripheral nerves are formed in response to a preceding viral or bacterial illness. Symptoms are at their worst in 2 to 4 weeks, and recovery can vary from weeks to a year. Classically, Guillain-Barré syndrome is preceded by a viral illness, followed by ascending symmetric weakness or paralysis and areflexia or hyporeflexia. Paralysis may ascend to the diaphragm, compromising respiratory function and requiring mechanical ventilation in one-third of patients. Botulism presents as a descending symmetric paralysis, not ascending like this patient. Lumbosacral plexopathies result in proximal weakness. Ramsey Hunt syndrome does not involve the extremities.

25. The answer is B. (Chapter 173) Myasthenia gravis is an autoimmune disease characterized by muscle weakness and fatigue, which is seen especially with repetitive use of voluntary muscles. In the normal neuromuscular junction, acetylcholine release by the nerve fiber causes a localized end-plate potential that leads to muscle fiber contraction. In myasthenia gravis, there is a marked decrease in the number and function of the muscle fiber acetylcholine receptors, despite normal nerve anatomy and function. Most myasthenia gravis patients have general weakness, especially of the proximal extremity muscle groups, neck extensors, and facial or bulbar muscles. Consider the diagnosis of myasthenia gravis in any patient who complains specifically of ocular disturbances or proximal limb muscle weakness not associated with systemic causes of generalized fatigue. The diagnosis is established through the administration of edrophonium chloride (an acetylcholinesterase inhibitor); electromyography, which demonstrates a postsynaptic neuromuscular junctional dysfunction with repetitive nerve stimulation; and serologic testing for acetylcholine receptor antibodies. It can be associated with a thymoma, which may be visible on chest x-ray, but this is not the next most appropriate test. A CT scan of the brain or electroencephalogram would not be diagnostic for myasthenia gravis.

26. The answer is C. (Chapter 173) Multiple sclerosis (MS) is a neurologic disorder that causes variable motor, sensory, visual, and cerebellar dysfunction as a result of multifocal areas of CNS myelin destruction. Multiple sclerosis causes a dysfunction in oligodendrocytes such that the axonal myelin sheaths are damaged, slowing nerve impulse conduction. Scattered cerebral and spinal plaques cause gliosis primarily in the white matter, with relative axon sparing. Plaques occur in multiple areas, including the cerebrum, brainstem, spinal cord, and cranial nerves. MS is suggested when a young person presents multiple times with neurologic symptoms that suggest different areas of pathology, often with resolution of the earlier symptoms. The physical examination may reveal decreased strength, increased tone, hyperreflexia, clonus, a positive Babinski reflex, a decrease in both vibration sense and joint proprioception, and a reduction in pain and temperature sensation. Although sensory and motor deficits are present initially in only one-third of patients, all patients will experience these findings at some point during the disease course. Patients describe these deficits as a heaviness, weakness, stiffness, or extremity numbness. Guillain-Barré syndrome is an acute polyneuropathy that causes ascending symmetric weakness and paralysis. Neurologic symptoms from an intracranial mass would be likely to come and go without intervention like this patient's symptoms have. Myasthenia gravis is an autoimmune disease characterized by muscle weakness and fatigue, which is seen especially with repetitive use of voluntary muscles.

27. **The answer is B.** (Chapter 173) The most significant emergency department complication of myasthenia gravis is respiratory failure, which is usually precipitated by infection, surgery, or the rapid tapering of immunosuppressive drugs. Although intubation should be considered in patients with a low forced vital capacity or in the presence of abnormal blood gas analysis, this decision is made primarily on clinical grounds. Because of the increased sensitivity of myasthenia gravis patients to neuromuscular junction inhibitors and an unpredictable reaction to succinylcholine in particular avoid the administration of depolarizing or nondepolarizing paralytic agents in preparation for intubation.

28. **The answer is D.** (Chapter 174) In the United States, the most common causes of bacterial meningitis are *Streptococcus pneumoniae* (58.0%), group B *Streptococcus* (18.1%), *Neisseria meningitidis* (13.9%), *Haemophilus*

influenzae (6.7%), and *Listeria monocytogenes* (3.4%). *Escherichia coli* in the neonatal population and *Mycobacterium tuberculosis* in immunocompromised hosts are also important considerations.

29. **The answer is C.** (Chapter 174) The presentation of fever, headache, stiff neck, and altered mental status is commonly seen in patients with bacterial meningitis. Although most patients have at least two of four of these symptoms, their absence does not exclude meningitis. Headache is the most common symptom and is seen in more than 85% of patients. Fever is the second most common symptom. Seizures and focal neurologic deficits are seen in 25% to 30% of patients.

30. **The answer is A.** (Chapter 174) Assess historical data in order to elicit risk factors suggestive of certain pathogens. *N. meningitidis* is associated with close living quarters, such as in military barracks and college dormitories. Unvaccinated patients are at risk for *H. influenzae*. Consider *L. monocytogenes* in older adults and alcoholics. Penetrating head trauma makes *S. pneumoniae* more likely. *Staphylococcus aureus*, coagulase-negative staphylococci, and streptococci are the most commonly implicated organisms after craniotomy, whereas coagulase-negative staphylococci are commonly seen after ventriculoperitoneal shunt and spinal surgery. Immunocompromised patients, such as those with human immunodeficiency virus, on chronic steroids, or with a history of splenectomy, are susceptible to meningitis with encapsulated organisms.

31. **The answer is D.** (Chapter 174) Viral meningitis is associated with a normal opening pressure and clear to bloody fluid with a negative gram stain. WBCs are generally <300/mm^3 with lymphocytic predominance. Glucose is normal and protein <200 mg/dL (Table 12.1).

TABLE 12.1	Cerebrospinal Fluid (CSF) Diagnostic Evaluation of Meningitis and Encephalitis						
	Opening Pressure (<170 mm H$_2$0)*	Color (clear)	Gram Stain (negative)	Cell Count (<5 WBC, 0 PMN)	Glucose (>40 milligrams/dL)	Protein (<50 milligrams/dL)	Cytology (negative)
Bacterial	Elevated	Cloudy, turbid	Positive (60%–80% before antibiotic, 7%–41% after antibiotic)	>1000–2000/mm^3 WBC, neutrophilic predominance, >80% PMN	<40 milligrams/dL, CSF/blood glucose ratio <0.3–0.4	>200 milligrams/dL	Negative
Viral	Normal	Clear or cloudy	Negative	<300/mm^3 WBC, lymphocytic predominance, <20% PMN	Normal	<200 milligrams/dL	Negative
Fungal	Normal to elevated	Clear or cloudy	Negative	<500/mm^3	Normal to slightly low	>200 milligrams/dL	Negative
Neoplastic	Normal	Clear or cloudy	Negative	<300/mm^3	Normal to slightly low	>200 milligrams/dL	Negative

*Normal values and findings are in parentheses.

Abbreviation: PMN = polymorphonuclear lymphocyte.

Reproduced with permission from J.E. Tintinalli, J.S. Stapczynski, O.J. Ma, D. Yealy, G.D. Meckler, D.M. Cline: Tintinalli's Emergency Medicine: A Comprehensive Study Guide, 9th Edition. McGraw-Hill Education; 2020.

32. **The answer is A.** (Chapter 174) Viral encephalitis is clinically distinguished from viral meningitis with the presence of neurologic findings such as altered level of consciousness, focal weakness, or seizures, although the two often coexist. Herpes simplex virus (HSV) accounts for 40% to 50% of cases where a cause is determined. HSV involves limbic structures of the temporal and frontal lobes with prominent psychiatric features, memory disturbance, and aphasia.

33. **The answer is C.** (Chapter 174) It is important to investigate for the source of a brain abscess in order to determine the likely bacterial etiology and to treat the source itself. Otogenic brain abscesses are often caused by gram-negative rods and are located adjacent to the temporal lobe or cerebellum. Sinogenic or odontogenic abscesses are often caused by anaerobic and microaerophilic streptococci and are commonly located in the frontal lobes. Abscesses formed from hematogenous spread are usually polymicrobial, with anaerobic and microaerophilic streptococci commonly represented. Direct implantation or traumatic injuries yield staphylococci, with gram-negative rods also seen in cases related to neurologic surgery.

34. **The answer is B.** (Chapter 174) Although the patient may have a muscle strain, he is at high risk for a spinal epidural abscess, an emergent diagnosis that should be ruled out in this patient before attributing his symptoms to a benign muscle strain. Back pain is the most common presenting complaint in spinal epidural abscess and is seen in 70% to 90% of cases. Fever is another common symptom, followed by the presence of a neurologic deficit. However, the classic triad of back pain, fever, and neurologic symptoms is seen in a minority of patients (8%–37%) on initial presentation. This patient is in the early stages of initial presentation. Intravenous drug use puts him at high risk for a spinal epidural abscess. It is not appropriate to assume a high-risk patient is just malingering instead of evaluating for a spinal emergency. An x-ray would provide little diagnostic value as there is more concern for a spinal epidural abscess, which would not appear on plain films, than for an atraumatic compression fracture as a 33-year-old patient.

35. **The answer is C.** (Chapter 175) Obstruction is the most common type of shunt malfunction. The most frequent location of obstruction is the proximal tubing, followed by the distal tubing, and then the valve chamber. Proximal obstructions usually occur within the first years after shunt insertion.

Toxicologic Disorders

13

QUESTIONS

1. A 44-year-old man ingests lye in a suicide attempt and presents to the emergency department immediately thereafter. You evaluate him upon arrival and note that he is mildly tachypneic. The remainder of his vital signs are normal. His examination is remarkable for audible stridor and difficulty with phonation. No oral burns are present, and the remainder of his examination is nondiagnostic. After you secure his airway, what is the NEXT BEST course of action?
   (A) Administer activated charcoal to adsorb any remaining alkali
   (B) Administer broad-spectrum antibiotics in case perforation is present
   (C) Arrange for emergent endoscopic evaluation of the upper gastrointestinal tract
   (D) Neutralize the alkali with instillation of sterile water via an orogastric tube

2. A 62-year-old man is brought to the emergency department in status epilepticus. His family found him convulsing in his bed; no evidence of trauma was noted at the scene. They report that he has "struggled with depression for a long time," and was recently diagnosed with pulmonary tuberculosis after a trip to India. The family found an empty bottle of isoniazid on his nightstand.

   Which of the following would represent definitive antidotal care for this patient?

   (A) Diazepam
   (B) Hydroxocobalamin
   (C) Pyridoxine
   (D) Sodium bicarbonate

3. You are evaluating a 16-year-old man who intentionally overdosed on his father's "heart pills" approximately 6 hours prior to his emergency department arrival. He is unwilling to provide any additional history other than stating that he is "seeing haloes around things" and feels like his heart is "fluttering." Vital signs are normal, and examination is unremarkable. His electrocardiogram shows frequent multifocal premature ventricular complexes, with a QRS duration of 92 ms and a QTc interval of 392 ms. The patient's renal function is normal, and urine output is brisk. Serum potassium concentration is 6.6 mEq/L, and other electrolytes are normal. Acetaminophen and salicylate concentrations are undetectable. Which of the following statements is TRUE?
   (A) Immediate sodium bicarbonate administration is necessary
   (B) Intravenous crystalloid hydration is the only indicated therapy.
   (C) Overdrive pacing is the best choice in managing this patient's ectopy.
   (D) This patient requires digoxin-specific antibody fragment administration.

4. You call the regional poison center regarding a 50-year-old woman with a well-documented history of ethanol abuse who presents with confusion. Family members who accompany her to the emergency department state that "she hasn't really been eating much over the past few days." She takes no medications and has no other known medical issues. Vital signs are remarkable for a HR 102, BP 149/82, and RR 24. She appears disheveled and is moderately confused. Her examination shows no hyperreflexia and/or clonus. Laboratory studies include a serum glucose concentration of 263 mg/dL and an anion gap of 22. Serum ketones are reported by the laboratory. The poison center recommends which of the following therapies?
(A) Benzodiazepines
(B) Dextrose-containing crystalloid
(C) Insulin infusion
(D) Psychiatric evaluation

5. A 26-year-old woman presents to the emergency department from her university, where she works as a graduate assistant in the chemistry laboratory. She complains of moderate skin and eye irritation after being exposed to "chemical reagents." You take a detailed history and learn that she is researching novel wastewater treatments and uses chlorine in her experiments. She was not wearing proper personal protective equipment when she spilled a small amount of dilute liquid chlorine on her shirt and hands. She states that she coughed "once or twice" at the time of the exposure, but has had no respiratory complaints since. The patient's vital signs are unremarkable. She exudes a pungent odor on examination. Her conjunctivae are injected but visual acuity is normal. No foreign bodies are seen on fluorescein staining. She is not coughing, and her pulmonary examination is remarkable only for very minimal wheezing. The remainder of her examination is nondiagnostic. What is the BEST course of emergency department treatment?
(A) Cutaneous decontamination and supportive care
(B) Immediate intubation and mechanical ventilation
(C) Methylene blue administration
(D) Prophylactic antibiotic administration

6. A patient presents to the emergency department 45 minutes after "drinking pesticide." He is immediately brought to the resuscitation area, where he is noted to have a respiratory rate of 36. His other vital signs are normal. He smells of hydrocarbon, his pupils are miotic, and he is coughing on your evaluation. He speaks in full sentences and phonates normally. After 3 minutes of your examination, you note muscle fasciculations, lacrimation, and rhinorrhea. The patient then proceeds to vomit nonbloody, nonbilious material. Which of the following is the NEXT BEST immediate action?
(A) Administration of atropine and pralidoxime
(B) Gastrointestinal decontamination with activated charcoal
(C) Initiation of high-flux hemodialysis
(D) Vitamin K_1 administration

7. You are evaluating a 10-month-old boy who was brought to the emergency department by his parents after "turning blue and getting short of breath." The mother states that the patient has been increasingly fussy recently, which she attributes to teething. She has been treating him with an over-the-counter teething gel with an active ingredient of 10% benzocaine. Vital signs are remarkable for a respiratory rate of 32 and a pulse oximetry reading of 88% on room air. The child appears somewhat bluish-grayish and dyspneic, but the remainder of his examination is nondiagnostic. His condition does not improve with supplemental oxygen administration. Which of the following is the MOST APPROPRIATE treatment at this time?
(A) Botulinum antitoxin
(B) Deferoxamine
(C) Methylene blue
(D) Prostaglandin E1

8. A 27-year-old man is found unresponsive at a party. Bystanders who brought him to the emergency department provide no history and leave immediately for fear of arrest. No additional history is available. Vital signs include T 36°C, HR 55, BP 100/62, and RR 14. Examination reveals complete unresponsiveness, absent gag reflex, and briskly-reactive, and normally-sized pupils. The patient's electrocardiogram is normal, and his rapid bedside fingerstick blood glucose is 127 mg/dL. He does not respond to appropriately dosed naloxone. You intubate the patient without sedation. Subsequent electrolyte panel, complete blood cell (CBC) count, and noncontrast CT head are normal. Acetaminophen, salicylate, and ethanol concentrations are undetectable. The patient remains intubated and unresponsive without additional chemical sedation for 1 hour while awaiting an intensive care unit bed, after which he rapidly awakens, self-extubates, and elopes. Which of the following agents is MOST LIKELY responsible for the patient's presentation?

(A) Carisoprodol
(B) Gamma-hydroxybutyrate (GHB)
(C) Methadone
(D) Methylenedioxymethamphetamine (MDMA)

9. A 60-year-old woman presents to the emergency department for evaluation of slurred speech and inability to ambulate. Her family states that she is a "serious alcoholic" and has recently become unable to recall even basic recent events. However, her long-term memory appears to be preserved, per the family's report. Examination is remarkable for ataxia, slurred speech, and paralysis of extraocular movements with lateral gaze. She is considerably confused but not delirious. Vital signs are normal and there is no hyperreflexia or clonus. This patient is suffering from which of the following?
   (A) Alcoholic hallucinosis
   (B) Korsakoff psychosis
   (C) Osmotic demyelination syndrome
   (D) Wernicke encephalopathy

10. A 37-year-old man with bipolar disorder and hypertension presents to the emergency department from his group home with "neurologic problems." The home also reports that he has had a "stomach bug" with vomiting and diarrhea over the past several days. Vital signs are normal, but the patient is significantly ataxic and tremulous. He is mildly confused and diffusely hyperreflexic, but he is not delirious. There is no cogwheeling or lead-pipe rigidity. His mucous membrane examination is normal. His medication list includes alprazolam, gabapentin, lithium, and metoprolol. Which of the following statements is TRUE regarding the drug responsible for this patient's symptom complex?
   (A) Activated charcoal is effective at reducing the offending drug's serum half-life.
   (B) Chronic toxicity is typically the result of volume depletion and/or renal insufficiency.
   (C) Diabetes mellitus is a complication of long-term therapy.
   (D) This medication is associated with neuroleptic malignant syndrome.

11. Which of the following medications is associated with hyperammonemia, both in therapeutic use and overdose?
   (A) Carbamazepine
   (B) Lithium
   (C) Topirimate
   (D) Valproic acid

12. A 13-year-old boy is brought to the emergency department completely naked and hallucinating. He is alert but delirious, exhibits mumbling speech, and is picking at his monitor leads and intravenous lines. His core temperature is 39.1°C and his pulse rate is 126; the remainder of his vital signs are normal. His examination is notable for impressive mydriasis, a flushed appearance to his skin, and dry axillae. His electrocardiogram reveals a QRS complex of normal morphology and duration; however, his QTc is prolonged. What is the MOST APPROPRIATE NEXT course of action?
   (A) Benzodiazepine administration
   (B) Gastrointestinal decontamination with gastric lavage
   (C) Psychiatric consultation for psychosis
   (D) Sodium bicarbonate administration

13. A 19-year-old man is brought in by friends from a "rave." The patient's acquaintances state that he suffered a generalized tonic-clonic seizure at the party after "doing a lot of Ecstasy and dancing really hard." The patient's vital signs are remarkable only for a respiratory rate of 22, and he is clearly postictal. There are no signs of trauma, and the only remarkable physical examination findings are those of urinary incontinence and a small abrasion overlying the anterior tongue. Which of the following laboratory studies is MOST LIKELY to be significantly abnormal?
   (A) Ammonia
   (B) Creatinine
   (C) Potassium
   (D) Sodium

14. A patient presents to the emergency department with severe finger pain after "accidentally touching a fish in his home salt-water fishtank" while cleaning the glass. He shows you a photograph of the offending organism on his smartphone (Figure 13.1). His vital signs are normal and his examination is notable for mild erythroderma at the site of his pain. You perform a bedside ultrasound and a radiograph, neither of which reveals evidence of a retained foreign body.

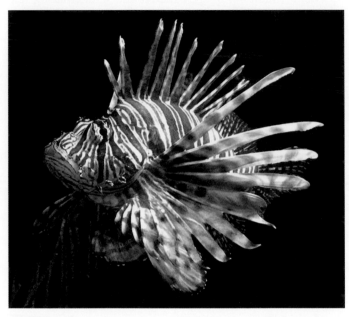

FIGURE 13.1

Which of the following therapies is MOST APPRO-PRIATE to treat the patient's pain?
(A) Acetic acid application to the envenomation site
(B) Cold water immersion
(C) Hot water immersion
(D) Immersion of the affected area in salt water

15. You are evaluating a 2-year-old boy who was brought to the emergency department by his parents after they witnessed ingestion of a single pellet of "rat poison." They pulled the pellet from his mouth, but fear that "some of it may have dissolved on his tongue." They brought the product to the emergency department, and the only active ingredient is 0.005% brodifacoum. The remainder of the product is constituted of inert/nontoxic substances. Which of the following is the NEXT BEST course of action?

(A) Gastric lavage and consideration of immediate chelation with succimer
(B) Immediate vitamin K_1 administration and admission for serial laboratory studies
(C) Immediate vitamin K_1 administration and intensive care unit admission for hemodialysis
(D) Obtain a prothrombin time/international normalized ratio (PT/INR) in the emergency department and discharge the patient with instructions for repeat PT/INR in 24 to 48 hours

16. A 15-year-old woman with a history of major depression and anemia presents to the emergency department after ingesting several handfuls of her prescription medication. Her vital signs are normal, but she complains of nausea and vomiting. An abdominal radiograph is obtained, which displays many radio-opaque tablets within the stomach. After placing two large-bore intravenous catheters and starting a crystalloid infusion, what is the NEXT BEST step in management?
(A) Administer a single dose of activated charcoal
(B) Administer an empiric dose of deferoxamine
(C) Consult gastroenterology for emergent endoscopic removal of tablet fragments
(D) Place a nasogastric tube and start whole-bowel irrigation

17. A 29-year-old man was brought to the emergency department by his significant other after he ingested several of her medications. He was initially noted to be hypertensive and bradycardic, with obtundation and miosis. He was given 0.4 mg of intravenous naloxone without change in his mental status. He underwent emergent head CT for fear of intracranial hemorrhage, which was normal. As he returned from radiology, he was noted to be hypotensive. Crystalloid resuscitation was undertaken, and his blood pressure slightly improved. Which of the following medications is the MOST LIKELY etiology of the patient's presentation?
(A) Clonidine
(B) Metoprolol
(C) Nifedipine
(D) Oxycodone

18. A 59-year-old woman was recently started on a new medication for her chronic migraines. She was involved in a verbal altercation with her spouse and subsequently overdosed on the entire bottle of her new medication. She quickly became somnolent and her spouse activated EMS. En route to the hospital, she was noted to be tachycardic and hypotensive. She also suffered a generalized tonic-clonic seizure in the ambulance. EMS was concerned about her electrocardiogram (Figure 13.2) and called the emergency department for recommendations. What is the BEST initial treatment for this overdose?
    (A) Hemodialysis
    (B) Normal saline
    (C) Sodium bicarbonate
    (D) Synchronized cardioversion

19. A 20-year-old man from a local university presents to the emergency department with altered mental status and agitation. Housemates who accompany him state he has a history of depression but no other medical problems. His only medication is citalopram, which he reportedly takes daily. While at a party tonight, he drank a large bottle of cough medication to "get high." Soon thereafter, he became confused and agitated. In the emergency department, he is noted to be hyperthermic, tachycardic, and hypertensive. His examination is remarkable for impressive bilateral lower extremity hyperreflexia and clonus. Reflexes in the upper limbs are normal. He was given multiple doses of benzodiazepines and several liters of crystalloid without improvement. He was admitted to the intensive care unit (ICU) overnight for continued therapy. What is the MOST LIKELY admitting diagnosis?
    (A) Antimuscarinic (anticholinergic) toxicity
    (B) Ethanol intoxication
    (C) Neuroleptic malignant syndrome
    (D) Serotonin syndrome

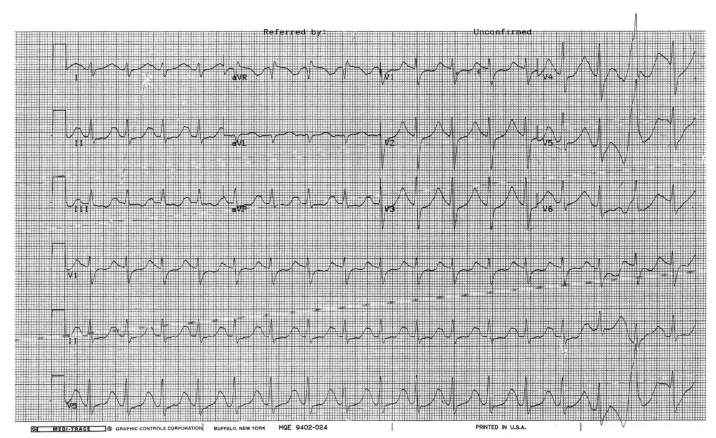

FIGURE 13.2 Reproduced with permission from J.E. Tintinalli, J.S. Stapczynski, O.J. Ma, D. Yealy, G.D. Meckler, D.M. Cline: Tintinalli's Emergency Medicine: A Comprehensive Study Guide, 9th Edition. McGraw-Hill Education; 2020.

20. A 47-year-old former alcoholic presents from a rehabilitation facility with altered mental status, slurred speech, and ataxia. He exhibits no signs of trauma. Staff at the referring institution state that they do not keep any type of liquor at the facility. An ethanol concentration returned as undetectable; additionally, his serum pH and bicarbonate are normal. Serum osmolality, however, was elevated and ketones were noted in the urine. What is the NEXT BEST step in management?
    (A) Administer fomepizole
    (B) Head CT
    (C) Insert a hemodialysis catheter
    (D) Supportive care and await sobriety

21. A 12-kg 18-month-old boy was playing at his grandparents' home where he "got into the medicine cabinet." His grandparents bring him to the emergency department several hours later. In the examination room, the patient is noted to be tachycardic, tachypneic, and somnolent. An intravenous line is placed, and a weight-based crystalloid bolus is given. His laboratory studies display a mixed metabolic acidosis with respiratory alkalosis. The grandparents show you a bottle of minty-smelling liquid, from which they suspect the patient drank. You have a high suspicion for what ingestion?
    (A) Acetaminophen
    (B) Isopropanol
    (C) Salicylate
    (D) Sodium hydroxide

22. A 3-year-old girl discovers a bottle of liquid in her parents' bedroom. She takes a sip of the solution and begins to vomit. Her parents activate EMS, who note agitation followed by lethargy. She arrives in the emergency department bradycardic and hypotensive, with evidence of bronchorrhea and respiratory distress. She suffers a generalized tonic-clonic seizure shortly after arrival. The patient's parents identified the bottle as containing liquid nicotine, from which they fill their electronic cigarettes. Administration of atropine will help reverse which of the patient's symptoms?
    (A) Bradycardia
    (B) Diaphragm paralysis
    (C) Hypotension
    (D) Wheezing

23. A 16-year-old man was huffing gas from a bag in his family's garage. He was startled by his father, who witnessed him collapse. The father noted no pulse immediately after the event and quickly called EMS. He then initiated cardiopulmonary resuscitation (CPR). The patient was taken to the local emergency department where his initial cardiac rhythm was polymorphic ventricular tachycardia. He was defibrillated once, and his rhythm degraded to ventricular fibrillation. Which is the MOST APPROPRIATE pharmacologic treatment for the patient's condition?
    (A) Amiodarone
    (B) Epinephrine
    (C) Esmolol
    (D) Procainamide

24. A 20-year-old foreign exchange student is in central Africa when he is diagnosed with malaria. He is prescribed quinine as monotherapy and discharged from clinic. He soon learns about a tragedy at home and overdoses on his newly prescribed medication. He quickly regrets his decision and returns to clinic. He is found to be nauseated, vomiting, and complains of tinnitus. He is noted to be hypotensive and an electrocardiogram displays significant QRS widening and QTc prolongation with intermittent runs of polymorphic ventricular tachycardia. Which is the MOST useful therapy in this scenario?
    (A) Amiodarone
    (B) Hemodialysis
    (C) High-dose diazepam
    (D) Multidose activated charcoal

25. A 33-year-old woman is flying alone from Bogota to Washington, DC. Flight attendants observe her to be anxious and diaphoretic. Vital signs obtained in flight display tachycardia and hypertension. She subsequently complains of chest pain, which results in an emergency landing so she can seek care. She is taken to the local emergency department, where she complains of severe abdominal pain. Her vital signs are remarkable for HR 136 and BP 262/157. An abdominal radiograph displays no fewer than 40 radiopaque foreign bodies in the patient's gastrointestinal tract. What is the MOST definitive therapy for this situation?
    (A) Benzodiazepine administration
    (B) Emergent laparotomy
    (C) Initiation of whole bowel irrigation
    (D) Symptomatic and supportive care

26. A 37-year-old woman without significant medical history presents to the emergency department for the second time in the past 2 weeks. Her chief complaint at the initial visit was nausea and vomiting; history-taking at that time revealed that her symptoms began after having a meal with her ex-husband. She was treated with crystalloid infusion and reported symptomatic improvement at that time. She was discharged with a diagnosis of foodborne illness without further evaluation at that visit. Since that visit, her feet have become "extremely painful," so much so that she can barely tolerate the bedsheets touching her feet at night. She also noted that her hair "started to fall out," and she has experienced sharp chest pain with deep inspiration over the past 48 hours. At the time of her second emergency department visit, she is noted to be persistently tachycardic despite crystalloid administration. You have a suspicion that she may have been poisoned at the encounter with her former spouse. What is the BEST treatment for this patient's condition?
    (A) Calcium disodium ethylenediamine tetraacetic acid (EDTA)
    (B) Dimercaprol (British anti-Lewisite [BAL])
    (C) Prussian blue
    (D) Succimer

27. A 54-year-old law enforcement officer is rushed to the emergency department where he is noted to be unconscious, tachycardic, and hypotensive. His police unit was dispatched to a parking lot where a person was noticed to be unconscious within a vehicle with the engine off. His squad partner waited in the car while the patient investigated the scene; the partner witnessed the patient collapse as he opened the car's door. The partner rushed to the patient's aid, but immediately noted a strong smell of rotten eggs. The partner managed to move the patient away from the vehicle. EMS was activated, who placed on a nonrebreather and transported him to the local emergency department. He was decontaminated outside; interestingly, all the coins in his pocket were noted to be oxidized a deep blue-black color. Which of the following is the BEST treatment for this patient's exposure?
    (A) Hydroxocobalamin
    (B) Hyperbaric oxygen
    (C) Sodium nitrate
    (D) Sodium thiosulfate

28. Extracorporeal elimination of a toxin is an important tool that toxicologists may employ with certain overdoses. Hemodialysis is the most commonly used enhanced elimination technique. Which of the following describes a property of a toxin that can be removed by hemodialysis?
    (A) High protein binding
    (B) High water solubility
    (C) Large molecular weight
    (D) Large volume of distribution

29. A 19-year-old man living in Texas read online about the mystical properties of toad venom. He locates one of these toads and "milks" the venom, which he then smokes. He begins to hallucinate but becomes extremely nauseated. He vomits and experiences severe abdominal pain. He presents to an emergency department, where he describes this misadventure. He is noted to be hyperkalemic, hypotensive, and bradycardic. In addition to psychedelic tryptamines, what other substances can be found in the venom of certain toads?
    (A) Alpha-2 agonists
    (B) Cardioactive steroids
    (C) Lithium-like substances
    (D) Opioid-like substances

30. An 18-month-old boy is brought to the emergency department unresponsive after he was found with one of his mother's "pain pills." The patient is noted to be bradypneic, hypopneic, and bradycardic. His respirations are quickly assisted, and intravenous access is obtained. You note pinpoint pupils and administer 0.1 mg/kg of naloxone. The patient's heart and respiratory rates quickly improve. An electrocardiogram shows sinus bradycardia with a prolonged QTc. Forty-five minutes after naloxone administration, he is noted to be increasingly somnolent and therefore given a second dose of naloxone. What is the BEST course of action for this patient?
    (A) Administer a dose of activated charcoal
    (B) Await sobriety in the emergency department
    (C) Initiate a naloxone drip and admit
    (D) Obtain an abdominal radiograph

ANSWERS

1. **The answer is C.** (Chapter 200) Caustic ingestion is a relatively common chief complaint in emergency departments, primarily as an accidental exposure in the pediatric population or intentional ingestion with self-harm intent. Caustics can be broadly divided into acidic substances that cause coagulation necrosis and alkali that cause liquefactive necrosis. Coagulation necrosis forms a surface eschar after injuring the superficial tissues, while liquefactive necrosis (typically thought to be more severe) does not form an eschar; the alkali instead penetrates through epithelial tight junctions and continue to burn the deeper tissues. Management of these cases centers upon supportive care and endoscopic evaluation of the gastrointestinal (GI) tract. Activated charcoal does not effectively bind caustics. Broad-spectrum antibiotic administration is indicated in cases involving perforation; however, perforation should be strongly suspected or confirmed before antibiotics are administered. Neutralization of the caustic substance via instillation of sterile water is not indicated; this would cause an exothermic reaction and liberate heat, thereby causing a thermal burn in addition to chemical injury.

2. **The answer is C.** (Chapters 205 and 207) This patient has overdosed on the hydrazine isoniazid, and is suffering from seizures secondary to pharmacologic pyridoxine depletion. Pyridoxine administration would be rapidly curative. While benzodiazepines such as diazepam are not contraindicated in this scenario, they are unlikely to terminate this patient's convulsions. Hydroxocobalamin is an antidote used to treat cyanide toxicity. Sodium bicarbonate is used to treat wide-complex dysrhythmias secondary to toxins and would not be helpful in this scenario.

3. **The answer is D.** (Chapter 193) This case describes an acute cardiac glycoside overdose. Digoxin-specific antibody fragment administration is indicated, given the patient's potassium concentration of >6.0 mEq/L. Given that his QRS duration is normal, sodium bicarbonate is unlikely to be beneficial. Crystalloid administration alone is incorrect because the patient's hyperkalemia is an indication for digoxin-specific antibody fragment. While it has been successfully described, overdrive pacing is not as preferable as digoxin-specific antibody fragment administration in managing this patient.

4. **The answer is B.** (Chapter 226) This patient is suffering from alcoholic ketoacidosis. The treatment of choice is dextrose-containing crystalloid, which provides volume repletion along with glucose, which stimulates insulin production and halts further ketone production. Glucose administration also increases oxidation of nicotinamide adenine dinucleotide + hydrogen (NADH) to NAD+, thereby further stopping ketone production. Benzodiazepines are not expected to be helpful here, considering this patient is not experiencing gamma-aminobutyric acid (GABA) withdrawal. Insulin is not beneficial and may actually be harmful, as patients often have depleted glycogen stores and normal or low glucose levels. Psychiatric evaluation may be required once the patient recovers, but is unlikely to be of assistance prior to resuscitation.

5. **The answer is A.** (Chapter 204) This patient is suffering from mild chlorine toxicity. This agent is widely available in industry and laboratories. Chlorine is water-soluble, and patients will typically exhibit mucous membrane and upper airway irritation. Removal of contaminated clothing/cutaneous decontamination to prevent further exposure and supportive care are the hallmarks of therapy; humidified oxygen and bronchodilators will treat the vast majority of mild exposures. Neutralizing therapy with nebulized sodium bicarbonate is sometimes helpful. While chlorine may cause severe airway damage and pulmonary edema, the patient does not exhibit any signs or symptoms of severe toxicity; therefore, intubation is not advisable at this time. Methylene blue is the antidote for methemoglobinemia and will not be helpful in this scenario. Prophylactic antibiotics are not recommended.

6. **The answer is A.** (Chapter 201) The stem presents a relatively classic case of organophosphate toxicity. These agents are cholinergic poisons. The preferred mnemonic for cholinergic toxicity is "DUMMBBBELS": "Defecation," "Urination," "Miosis," "Muscle weakness," "Bronchorrhea," "Bronchospasm," "Bradycardia," "Emesis," "Lacrimation," and "Salivation." Most medical toxicologists prefer "DUMMBBBELS" over "SLUDGE," since the later does not include the "killer B's"; that is, most patients die from the cardiopulmonary effects left out by "SLUDGE." Immediate administration of atropine and pralidoxime is indicated in this situation since antidotal therapy must be undertaken prior to organophosphate aging in order to be effective. Activated charcoal administration has not been shown to improve clinical outcomes, and may delay administration of helpful therapy. Hemodialysis is not indicated at this time. Vitamin K_1 delivery is not expected to be helpful in this case.

7. **The answer is C.** (Chapter 207) Benzocaine is a common etiology of methemoglobinemia, which is described in the question stem. The cutaneous discoloration associated with methemoglobinemia typically correlates with a

methemoglobin concentration of 10% to 15%, while the classic "chocolate brown" discoloration of blood occurs at concentrations above 20%. Methylene blue administration is the antidote for pharmaceutical-associated methemoglobinemia. Botulinum antitoxin would not be helpful in this situation. Deferoxamine is the antidote for iron toxicity. Prostaglandin E1 would be indicated in a child with a ductal-dependent lesion.

8. **The answer is B.** (Chapter 184) The question stem describes a relatively classic case of gamma-hydroxybutyrate (GHB) intoxication. This agent has been used historically as an anesthetic; the sodium salt (sodium oxybate) is currently Food and Drug Administration (FDA) approved as a treatment for narcolepsy. GHB is most commonly encountered as an illicit drug used as a sedative-hypnotic, to facilitate sexual assault, and to help bodybuilders reduce fat and increase muscle mass. GHB is typically ingested and peak effects are seen in approximately 60 minutes. This agent has a very short half-life and is therefore difficult to detect once effects have dissipated. Carisoprodol is marketed as a centrally-acting "muscle relaxant"; toxicity typically involves sedation and prominent myoclonic jerking. Methylenedioxymethamphetamine (MDMA) or "ecstasy" is an amphetamine derivative and would not be expected to cause the symptoms described. Methadone is an opioid with a long half-life; therefore, rapid improvement of symptoms would not be expected.

9. **The answer is D.** (Chapters 185 and 205) The patient in the question stem displays confusion, ataxia, and oculomotor abnormalities. These are classic findings in Wernicke encephalopathy. The exact cause of this syndrome is unknown, but thiamine deficiency has been implicated. Many chronic alcoholics are thiamine-deficient, and this population is where Wernicke encephalopathy is most frequently observed. Along with alcoholic tremulousness, gamma-aminobutyric acid (GABA) withdrawal seizures, and delirium tremens, alcoholic hallucinosis (A) is one of the cardinal ethanol withdrawal syndromes; the fact that the patient's vital signs are normal and she has no hyperreflexia/clonus make withdrawal less likely here. Osmotic demyelination syndrome results from myelin destruction, most commonly secondary to rapid correction of hyponatremia. Often occurring in conjunction with Wernicke encephalopathy, Korsakoff psychosis is an irreversible clinical syndrome hallmarked by short-term memory defects and confabulation.

10. **The answer is B.** (Chapter 181) This is a classic case of chronic lithium toxicity, including tremulousness and ataxia. The other agents taken by this patient would not be expected to produce the clinical effects described. Chronic toxicity from this drug is typically a result of decreased

renal clearance from volume depletion or impaired glomerular filtration. Lithium is a metal and therefore not bound by activated charcoal. This drug causes decreased renal tubule response to arginine vasopressin and is thereby associated with diabetes insipidus, not diabetes mellitus, in long-term usage. Lithium is serotonergic and therefore associated with serotonin syndrome, not neuroleptic malignant syndrome.

11. **The answer is D.** (Chapter 197) Valproic acid (also called valproate) is commonly prescribed to treat seizures, migraine headaches, neuropathic pain, and various psychiatric conditions. This drug affects neurotransmitters and the function of electrically-excitable cells; it increases gamma-aminobutyric acid (GABA) concentrations and blocks N-methyl-d-aspartate (NMDA) receptors. It also prolongs recovery of activated sodium channels, enhances potassium conductance, and reduces T-type calcium current firing. This agent is metabolized by glucuronidation and mitochondrial beta-oxidation; it enters the mitochondria using levocarnitine as a cofactor. Valproate increases renal ammonia production and blocks hepatic ammonia metabolism by a complex mechanism. Carbamazepine, lithium, and topiramate would not be expected to cause hyperammonemia.

12. **The answer is A.** (Chapter 202) This is a classic presentation of anticholinergic syndrome, which may result from use/abuse of a myriad of such substances. Diphenhydramine, cyclic antidepressants, and various plants (Datura stramonium, commonly termed "jimsonweed") are common etiologies. Benzodiazepine administration is a hallmark of good supportive care in these cases; physostigmine may also be used to control symptoms. Considering that these patients are at risk of seizure, gastric lavage is rather controversial and frequently advised against by medical toxicologists. While the patient may eventually require psychiatric consultation if an underlying psychiatric disorder or pattern of substance abuse is diagnosed during admission, it is unlikely to be helpful in the acute setting. While these patients may indeed develop QRS prolongation from sodium channel blockade in the setting of severe poisoning, this patient does not require sodium bicarbonate administration to treat such a finding at this time.

13. **The answer is D.** (Chapter 188) Methylenedioxymethamphetamine (MDMA or "ecstasy") is the best-known designer hallucinogenic amphetamine. This agent is used for both its psychedelic properties and unique effects on mood, commonly at dance clubs and "raves." MDMA has complex effects due to its interaction with a multitude of receptors and neurotransmitters; use and

abuse can result in serious complications and death. The most common electrolyte disturbance seen in MDMA is hyponatremia, which is thought to be multifactorial. Excessive water consumption, both due to perspiration while dancing and syndrome of inappropriate antidiuretic hormone secretion (SIADH), are thought to play roles. Ammonia concentrations would not be expected to be elevated in this scenario. While volume depletion and subsequent elevation in creatinine and potassium can be seen in these cases, the stem does not suggest these processes.

14. **The answer is C.** (Chapter 213) This patient was envenomated by touching the dorsal spines of a lionfish (Pterosis spp.). Clinical effects are typically limited to immediate-onset pain and erythema at the envenomation site, which may radiate proximally. Untreated, the symptoms typically peak at 30 to 90 minutes post-envenomation and persist for 4 to 6 hours; however, this is highly variable. Nonspecific systemic effects such as diaphoresis and, nausea/vomiting may occur, but vital sign abnormalities are rather uncommon. Management centers upon excluding a retained foreign body and pain control. Hot water immersion is indicated in lion fish envenomations, since the toxin is heat-labile. Acetic acid application to the envenomation site may be helpful in patients stung by jellyfish. Cold water immersion is unlikely to be helpful in this scenario. Immersion of the affected area in saltwater would be indicated in a situation involving fire coral or various jellyfish species.

15. **The answer is D.** (Chapter 201) Most modern rodenticides are based upon an ultra-long-acting warfarin ("superwarfarin") moiety and cause clinical effects in both rodents and humans via delayed anticoagulant effects. Intentional ingestions may be serious; however, unintentional exploratory ingestions in the pediatric population are unlikely to be dangerous. The best course of action is this case would be to obtain a PT/INR in the emergency department with outpatient follow-up along with parental reassurance. Exploratory exposures are typically benign and do not require vitamin K1 administration.

16. **The answer is D.** (Chapter 198) Iron can be found in many homes. There are numerous formulations, each with a varying amount of elemental iron. Common formulations include ferrous sulfate (20% elemental iron), fumarate (33%), and chloride (28%). It is a significant gastroesophageal irritant and many patients present with nausea, vomiting, diarrhea, and abdominal pain from mucosal injury. Iron enters the mitochondria where it interferes with oxidative phosphorylation and disrupts the electron transport chain, producing metabolic acidosis with lactate formation. Toxic effects have been demonstrated at doses as low as 10 to 20 mg/kg of elemental iron. Moderate toxicity tends to occur at dosages of 20 to 60 mg/kg and severe toxicity is seen at greater than 60 mg/kg. Use of activated charcoal is not advised, as it does not adsorb iron well and can make emergent endoscopy difficult. Emergent endoscopy is typically not needed unless the patient fails gastrointestinal decontamination with whole-bowel irrigation. Whole bowel irrigation is performed with polyethylene glycol given through a nasogastric or orogastric tube at a rate of 1 to 2 L/h in adults and 250 to 500 mL/h in children. Deferoxamine should be given for systemic toxicity with metabolic acidosis, repeated vomiting, signs of shock, and/or in patients with an iron concentration above 500 mcg/dL. Most iron formulations are quite adherent to the gastric mucosa and are difficult to remove endoscopically; however, this may be reasonable in a last-ditch effort.

17. **The answer is A.** (Chapter 196) The toxidrome of bradycardia, pinpoint pupils, and altered mental status raises several diagnostic possibilities. The administration of properly-dosed naloxone should help to exclude the possibility of opiates/opioids. Although some opiates/opioids may require larger or repeated doses of naloxone, they typically do not present with initial hypertension. Clonidine is an alpha-2-adrenergic and imidazoline agonist. The central alpha-2 stimulation results in sympatholysis as well as decreased heart rate and blood pressure. In massive overdose, there is stimulation of the peripheral post-synaptic alpha-2 receptors which can produce vasoconstriction and hypertension. Neither beta- nor calcium channel blockers typically present with these symptoms.

18. **The answer is C.** (Chapter 177) This electrocardiogram shows findings associated with cyclic antidepressant toxicity. The findings of tachycardia, a right bundle branch block pattern, and a tall "terminal R wave" in lead aVR suggest the diagnosis. Cyclic antidepressants were a significant source of overdose several decades ago; however, a 2013 study showed that cyclic antidepressants were still the most common antidepressant associated with overdose death. They are currently prescribed for a myriad of conditions aside from depression including headache prophylaxis, neuropathic pain, and enuresis. Cyclic antidepressants have multiple mechanisms of action including sodium and potassium channel blockade, antihistaminic and antimuscarinic effects, inhibition of alpha-adrenergic receptors, and inhibition of biogenic amine reuptake. Treatment is primarily aimed at these drugs' sodium channel blockade. Sodium bicarbonate administration treats cardiac conduction abnormalities, ventricular dysrhythmias, and neurologic manifestations. Hemodialysis

should not be considered before maximizing medical therapies. Normal saline infusion may be beneficial in the setting of hypotension, but is not the best initial treatment. Synchronized cardioversion may be attempted, but not before bicarbonate administration.

19. **The answer is D.** (Chapter 178) This patient demonstrates classic findings of serotonin syndrome including hyperthermia, tachycardia, hypertension, altered mental status, and hyperreflexia in the lower extremities greater than upper extremities. The likely etiology of his presentation is the combination of dextromethorphan-containing cough medicine with his citalopram, another serotonergic medication. Treatment includes intravenous fluids to prevent acute tubular necrosis and rhabdomyolysis; additionally, aggressive control of hyperthermia and agitation are paramount. Antimuscarinic (anticholinergic) toxicity typically exhibits diffuse hyperreflexia/clonus and responds to benzodiazepines. Ethanol intoxication does not fit this clinical scenario. Neuroleptic malignant syndrome is typically characterized by altered mental status with a rather insidious onset in the setting of exposure to a dopamine antagonist or the rapid withdrawal of a dopamine agonist.

20. **The answer is D.** (Chapter 185) Isopropanol ingestion results in inebriation and "ketosis without acidosis." Isopropanol is a colorless, volatile liquid found in household products like rubbing alcohol and hand sanitizer, and is more potent than ethanol as an intoxicating agent. Isopropanol is metabolized by alcohol dehydrogenase to acetone (a ketone) but cannot be further oxidized by aldehyde dehydrogenase to a carboxylic acid. This results in "ketosis without acidosis." Supportive care and watchful waiting is the best answer in this scenario. Fomepizole, while not necessarily harmful in this situation, will prolong the patient's inebriation and will not be effective in preventing untoward effects. CT scan of the head may be obtained; however, this patient's altered mental status is secondary to inebriation rather than intracranial pathology. Hemodialysis is unnecessary in this scenario.

21. **The answer is C.** (Chapter 189) Salicylate toxicity is classically associated with the triple acid-base disturbance of respiratory alkalosis and metabolic acidosis which subsequently transitions to respiratory acidosis. This patient was exposed to oil of wintergreen, a minty-smelling liniment containing methyl salicylate (a particularly concentrated form of salicylate). Methyl salicylate contains approximately 1.4 g of salicylate per mL of liquid (7 g/ tsp). Severe toxicity typically occurs in the 500 mg/kg range. This child weighs 12 kg, meaning a potential fatal dose could be less than a single teaspoon. Acetaminophen is an extremely common household ingestion; however,

it is unlikely to result in this constellation of symptoms. Isopropanol or "rubbing alcohol" will result in ketosis without acidosis. Caustics such as sodium hydroxide may cause significant mucosal injury but are unlikely to be sedating.

22. **The answer is A.** (Chapter 192) Liquid nicotine is an increasing toxicologic threat with the advent of electronic cigarettes, vaporizing pens, and other alternatives to "traditional" cigarettes. Liquid nicotine concentrations are varied and the listed concentration is often much lower than actual amount contained in the solution. A 1.8% solution contains 18 mg of nicotine per mL. Toxic doses in children have been shown to be as low as 0.1 mg/kg and a mouthful of swallowed solution may be fatal. Nicotine is absorbed through the gastrointestinal tract and will bind to acetylcholine receptors throughout the body. Initially there can be a stimulatory effect heralded by hypertension, tachycardia, and dizziness. At higher doses—such as those seen with pesticides, patches, and concentrated liquid solutions—acetylcholine will bind both muscarinic and nicotinic receptors. Bradycardia, decreased mental status, seizure, and respiratory failure have been described in addition to the classic findings of cholinergic excess. Atropine, an antimuscarinic agent, will only reverse the symptoms of muscarinic cholinergic crisis and treat bradycardia. Atropine will not be effective in treating the hypotension, wheezing, or diaphragm paralysis.

23. **The answer is C.** (Chapter 199) This man is likely the victim of "sudden sniffing death syndrome." This is the result of "huffing" a halogenated or aromatic hydrocarbon solvent, which in turn results in a "sensitized" myocardium via a complex mechanism. If this sensitization is followed by a catecholamine surge (seen with startling or sudden exertion), there is concern for QTc prolongation and subsequent development of torsades de pointes. Paradoxically, the treatment of choice in these cases is to terminate the reentrant rhythm. The ultra-short-acting beta-blocker esmolol is an excellent choice; propranolol, lidocaine, or a class 1b antidysrhythmic are also acceptable options. The other choices listed are likely to be ineffective in treatment of the patient's reentrant rhythm.

24. **The answer is D.** (Chapter 206) The anti-malarial quinine has a very narrow therapeutic window. Multiple organ systems may be affected with overdose. It has both pro- and antidysrhythmic effects by inhibiting sodium and potassium channels. This may cause both QRS widening and QTc prolongation. Early symptoms occur within a few hours and usually effect the gastrointestinal tract. Significant overdose will typically be heralded by both central nervous system and cardiac toxicity. One

source lists the average oral lethal dose at 8 g, but death has been described in as little as 1.5 g. Hypoglycemia may result from increased release of insulin. Quinine is one of the drugs in which multi-dose activated charcoal has been useful in treating toxicity by decreasing enterohepatic recirculation. Amiodarone is unlikely to be of benefit in this scenario, and may prolong the patient's QTc. Hemodialysis is unlikely to be of assistance given this drug's high degree of protein binding and large volume of distribution. High-dose diazepam has been used to treat the dysrhythmias associated with chloroquine toxicity.

25. **The answer is B.** (Chapter 187) The constellation of symptoms including severe hypertension, tachycardia, anxiety, diaphoresis, chest pain, and abdominal pain is suggestive of sympathomimetic effects. This patient traveling solo along with her current symptoms and radiologic findings should prompt a consideration of body packing, which is the process of swallowing or rectally inserting many well-sealed packets of drugs to elude detection (often while smuggling). The patient here is likely smuggling cocaine or another sympathomimetic and one or more of the packets unfortunately ruptured. This patient's severe abdominal pain may indicate that she is experiencing bowel ischemia from drug-induced local vasoconstriction. She will require emergent laparotomy to ensure there is no area of ischemic bowel, and resection of such if it is present. Administration of benzodiazepines may help treat the patient's sympathetic symptoms, but it will be inadequate definitive care for the underlying process. Whole bowel irrigation is a reasonable choice for those who are asymptomatic; however, this patient is severely ill and requires emergent intervention. Supportive care is not sufficient in this symptomatic patient.

26. **The answer is C.** (Chapter 203) This patient has been poisoned with thallium. Thallium is odorless and colorless and was formerly used as a rodenticide. It has been a reported cause of homicide throughout the world. Many of the effects of thallium poisoning are nonspecific and occur over days to weeks, making diagnosis and detection difficult. Alopecia with ascending painful peripheral neuropathy are classic findings in toxicity. Early symptoms include nausea, vomiting, and abdominal pain; the typical absence of diarrhea is somewhat unique among metal poisoning. Gastrointestinal symptoms will often fade by the time the intermediate effects are observed. Pleuritic chest pain along with alopecia are seen within this intermediate phase. Persistent tachycardia often portends a poor prognosis. Death is usually a result of respiratory failure, coma, and cardiac arrest. The treatment of choice for thallium toxicity is the ion exchange resin Prussian blue. Calcium disodium ethylenediamine tetraacetic acid (EDTA)

is employed for lead encephalopathy. Dimercaprol is used in conjunction with calcium disodium EDTA in the treatment of severe lead toxicity. Succimer is used in the chelation of lead, cadmium, arsenic, and mercury.

27. **The answer is C.** (Chapter 204) This patient was exposed to the "rapid knockdown gas" and known suicide agent hydrogen sulfide. Hydrogen sulfide smells of "rotten eggs" and is a strong oxidizing agent; hence, the discolored coins were found in his pocket during decontamination. Other clinical findings may include mucous membrane and ocular irritation (often termed "gas eye"), nausea and vomiting, corneal ulceration, and severe shortness of breath with acute respiratory distress syndrome. Initial treatment should include removal from the source, decontamination, and high-flow oxygen administration. Those with altered mental status should receive sodium nitrate which has been shown to produce rapid improvement. There is no role for hyperbaric oxygen therapy as it is equivalent to atmospheric oxygen for preventing delayed neurological sequelae. Hydroxocobalamin and thiosulfate seem to be of limited benefit when analyzing existing literature.

28. **The answer is B.** (Chapter 176) Blood and countercurrent dialysate fluids are separated by a semi-porous membrane which allow xenobiotics to diffuse across the membrane into the dialysate fluid based on concentration gradients. Common xenobiotics amenable to hemodialysis are lithium, salicylate, ethylene glycol, methanol, and theophylline. Low protein binding, a small volume of distribution, and a relatively small molecular weights are all conducive to removal via hemodialysis.

29. **The answer is B.** (Chapter 188) Several species of Bufo toad are considered hallucinogenic. In the United States, B. alveris and B. marinus contain 5-methoxydimethyltryptamine and bufotenine, which are both psychedelic. In addition to the psychoactive substances, venom also contains catecholamines (epinephrine and norepinephrine), non-cardiac sterols (cholesterol), and cardioactive steroids. Cardioactive steroids such as bufagins and bufadienolides produce digoxin-like toxicity. Acute digoxin toxicity is hallmarked by hyperkalemia, bradycardia, nausea, and vomiting. In the setting of cardiac glycoside toxicity, digoxin assays may be positive but should only be used qualitatively and not quantitatively. Alpha-2 agonists, lithium-like substances, and opioid-like substances are not known to be present in the venom of these species.

30. **The answer is C.** (Chapter 186) This toddler was likely exposed to methadone, which is a long-acting opioid that is used in the treatment of chronic pain or replacement

therapy in opioid-dependent individuals. The half-life is thought to be between 33 and 46 hours. This patient displays the classic opiate/opioid toxidrome with somnolence, miosis, and respiratory depression. He initially responds to naloxone; however, his symptoms return because naloxone's duration of action is much shorter than methadone's half-life. QTc prolongation in methadone overdose was noted to be as high as 25% in one case series of poisoned children. Treatment after multiple doses of naloxone should include initiation of a naloxone infusion and admission to the PICU. Activated charcoal administration to a patient with decreased mental status and unprotected airway may result in charcoal aspiration and subsequent pneumonitis, and should be avoided. Awaiting sobriety in the emergency department would take an inappropriate amount of time and patient would best be served by admission. An abdominal radiograph is unlikely to be of any diagnostic benefit in this case.

Environmental Injuries

14

QUESTIONS

1. A 38-year-old man with a history of schizophrenia and homelessness presents to the emergency department with pain in his feet. He complains of altered sensation and burning pain in both feet for the last few days. On examination, he is unkempt and his feet are pale, mottled, and cold. He has difficulty moving them. Dorsalis pedis pulses are not palpable immediately but are detected by Doppler ultrasound. Rewarming does not immediately improve his symptoms. Which of the following is the MOST APPROPRIATE NEXT step in management?
   (A) Broad-spectrum parenteral antibiotics and medicine admission
   (B) Dry rewarming, dressing changes, elevation, and observation for development of infection
   (C) Heparin infusion and vascular surgery consultation
   (D) Surgical consultation for emergent debridement

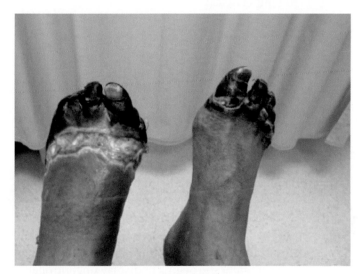

FIGURE 14.1 Photo contributed by Edward Lew, MD.

2. A 45-year-old man with a history of alcoholism is brought to the emergency department by EMS after being found unconscious in the snow. He arrives drowsy and complaining of severe pain in his feet. See image of his feet in Figure 14.1. What is the MOST APPROPRIATE emergency department management of this patient's injuries?

   (A) Broad-spectrum parenteral antibiotics
   (B) Emergent debridement of the devitalized tissue
   (C) Rapid rewarming, tetanus vaccination and parenteral opioids for pain management
   (D) Tissue plasminogen activator administration and vascular surgery consultation

3. A 27-year-old woman is brought to the emergency department in cardiac arrest. Prior to arrival, she had fallen through and become trapped underneath ice on a lake for a nearly an hour before being rescued by first responders. On arrival to the emergency department, she is pulseless and has a core temperature of 29°C. High-quality cardiopulmonary resuscitation (CPR) is ongoing. Which of the following is NOT an indication for termination of resuscitation?
   (A) Airway packed with snow
   (B) Body is frozen solid
   (C) Fixed and dilated pupils
   (D) Serum potassium >12 mmol/L

4. Which of the following patients is NOT at increased risk for development of heat stroke or other heat-related emergencies?
   (A) A 16-year-old boy with a history of asthma
   (B) A 28-year-old woman long-distance runner
   (C) A 44-year-old man with a history of schizophrenia
   (D) A 74-year-old woman with Parkinson disease

5. An otherwise healthy 7-year-old girl is brought to the emergency department by her parents for evaluation after being stung by a scorpion. Parents state that about 2 hours ago the patient began to scream and cry in pain after being stung on her foot by a scorpion found while putting on her shoes. On examination, she is tachycardic, diaphoretic, tremulous, and in acute discomfort. The plantar aspect of her right foot is erythematous and extremely tender. While in the emergency department she begins to display uncontrollable jerking motion of the extremities. Which is the MOST APPROPRIATE NEXT step in management?
   (A) Antivenom, benzodiazepines, and preparation for orotracheal intubation
   (B) Blood pressure control with prazosin
   (C) Repeated intravenous atropine administration
   (D) Tourniquet application to the right lower extremity and local wound care

6. Which of the following features is MOST consistent with a brown recluse spider bite?
   (A) Painful, 1 to 2 cm target lesion
   (B) Painless, firm, and erythematous lesion progressing to local hemorrhagic blister or dermatonecrosis
   (C) Painful, local erythema, and edema
   (D) Severely painful, erythematous wheal

7. Which of the following is an indicated first-aid measure for management of pit viper envenomation?

(A) Immobilization of the extremity in a neutral position below the level of the heart
(B) Incision and drainage
(C) Suction the bite site either by mouth or with snake bite kit
(D) Tourniquet application proximal to the bite site

8. A 31-year-old man comes to the emergency department complaining of severe pain in his leg. He states that while snorkeling off a coral reef he felt sudden onset stinging pain in his left calf. Shortly after arrival he begins to complain of chest tightness. In addition to supportive measures, which of the following is the BEST INITIAL management of his skin lesion (Figure 14.2)?

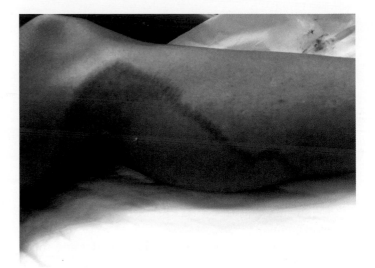

FIGURE 14.2 Photo contributed by Sittidet Toonpirom, MD, and Rittirak Othong, MD.

(A) Cold water immersion
(B) Irrigation with acetic acid
(C) Irrigation with normal saline and hot water immersion
(D) Tourniquet application

9. A 28-year-old male SCUBA diver arrives to your medical center for hyperbaric oxygen therapy after developing cough, hemoptysis, and shortness of breath during a deep, "no-stop" dive. On arrival to the emergency department, he is tachypneic but hemodynamically stable. Neurologic examination is normal. Which of the following types of decompression sickness is MOST consistent with these symptoms?
   (A) Arterial gas embolism
   (B) The "bends"
   (C) The "chokes"
   (D) The "staggers"

10. A 16-year-old boy is brought to the emergency department by EMS after a drowning incident. He was walking along a riverbed when he slipped and fell in. Friends rescued him downriver after an estimated submersion time of 15 minutes. On arrival to the emergency department, the patient is awake, tachypneic, and hypoxic requiring 4L NC. He has rales on examination. Chest x-ray shows bibasilar infiltrates. Supportive measures are initiated. Which of the following is the MOST APPROPRIATE disposition for this patient?
    (A) Admission to the hospital for laboratory evaluation and supportive care
    (B) Discharge home with close primary care follow-up
    (C) Emergent endotracheal intubation for anticipated respiratory failure
    (D) Observe in the emergency department for 4 to 6 hours and discharge home if symptoms improve

11. Which of the following is NOT an indication for transfer to a burn center?
    (A) Full thickness burns to the forearm <2% BSA
    (B) Inhalational injury
    (C) Oral burn injury in a 7-year-old boy who bit an electrical cable
    (D) Superficial partial-thickness burn overlying an open tibia/fibula fracture incurred during a house fire

12. A 44-year-old male construction worker arrives to your emergency department with a burn injury to his leg. He was preparing cement when he accidentally spilled it on his leg (Figure 14.3). Which of the following is the BEST INITIAL management of this type of injury?

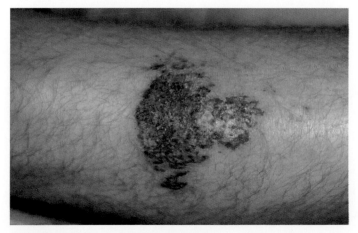

FIGURE 14.3 Photo contributed by Dr. Larry Stack

(A) Brushing off remaining particles from the wound then copious irrigation with saline
(B) Copious irrigation with saline
(C) Measurement of compartment pressures and fasciotomy
(D) Neutralization with a dilute acidic solution

13. A 2-year-old boy presents to the emergency department after biting an electrical cord. His injury is shown in Figure 14.4. Over the next few weeks, the child should be monitored for which feared complication of this injury?

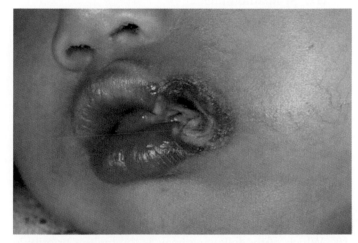

FIGURE 14.4 Reproduced with permission from Shah BR, Lucchesi M: Atlas of Pediatric Emergency Medicine. © 2006 by McGraw-Hill, Inc., New York.

(A) Cardiac dysrhythmia
(B) Labial artery hemorrhage
(C) Orofacial cellulitis
(D) Rhabdomyolysis

14. A 5-year-old otherwise healthy girl is brought to the emergency department by her parents for nausea and vomiting developed after eating a mushroom while camping about 4 hours prior to presentation. If delayed toxicity develops, the patient is at risk for which feared complication?
    (A) Acute renal failure
    (B) Autonomic disruption and cardiac dysrhythmia
    (C) Fulminant hepatic failure
    (D) Fungemia and cardiovascular collapse from septic shock

15. The toxic agent in poison hemlock is structurally MOST similar to which substance?
    (A) Acetylcholine
    (B) Histamine
    (C) Nicotine
    (D) Norepinephrine

16. Which toxidrome would be expected in an ingestion of deadly nightshade?
    (A) Antimuscarinic
    (B) Cholinergic
    (C) Sedative-hypnotic
    (D) Sympathomimetic

17. A 29-year-old male mountain climber develops exertional dyspnea that progresses to dyspnea at rest during an expedition to the peak of Mt. Everest. On examination, he has diffuse rales and is in obvious distress. Which of the following medications is NOT useful in the acute management of this patient's condition?
    (A) Acetazolamide
    (B) Dexamethasone
    (C) Nifedipine
    (D) Supplemental oxygen

18. Which of the following goals is the highest priority in treatment of patients with high-altitude cerebral edema?
    (A) Control of intracranial pressure
    (B) Emergent recompression therapy
    (C) Immediate descent
    (D) Prevention of hypotension

19. Which of the following is an indication for hyperbaric oxygen therapy in acute carbon monoxide poisoning?
    (A) Acute carbon monoxide poisoning with headache and vomiting that resolves over 4 to 6 hours
    (B) Carboxyhemoglobin level >20%
    (C) Carboxyhemoglobin level >25%
    (D) Pregnancy with carboxyhemoglobin level >20%

20. A 47-year-old man comes to your emergency department from home with his wife and son for evaluation of headache. He began to experience a mild, throbbing headache this morning that gradually worsened despite taking Tylenol. His symptoms worsened throughout the evening and he developed nausea. His wife and 11-year-old son began to experience similar headaches as well, prompting emergency department presentation. On arrival to the emergency department, the patient's headache has partially improved. Vital signs and neurologic examination are normal. Which of the following is the appropriate disposition for this patient?
    (A) Discharge home
    (B) Emergency department observation for 4 to 6 hours and discharge home
    (C) Emergency department observation for 4 to 6 hours, supplemental oxygen therapy, verification of home safety, and discharge home
    (D) Hospital admission with consideration for hyperbaric oxygen therapy

ANSWERS

1. **The answer is B.** (Chapter 208) The patient is most likely suffering from trench foot. On initial examination, the foot is pale, mottled, anesthetic, and immobile, with no immediate change after rewarming. Assessment of peripheral pulses may be obscured by soft tissue changes, but this does not necessarily suggest arterial occlusion, especially bilaterally. Sensory and motor symptoms are likely secondary to direct peripheral nerve injury by sustained cold and wet conditions. In the emergency department, feet should be kept clean, warm, dryly bandaged, elevated, and closely monitored for early signs of infection. In the absence of these, empiric therapy with IV antibiotics is not necessary. Severe cases progress to desquamation, skin sloughing, and gangrene development. There is no role for early debridement in the emergency department.

2. **The answer is C.** (Chapter 208) The patient is suffering from frostbite, specifically, the third and fourth degree frostbite, characterized by full thickness skin destruction and hemorrhagic blisters. Microvascular thrombosis is known to play a role in advanced frostbite and retrospective studies suggest reduced risk of digit amputations with thrombolysis. However, evidence for this is limited. The decision to administer tissue plasminogen activator (TPA) should be made with consideration of bleeding risk and in consultation with a vascular surgeon, rather than administering empiric thrombolysis. Immediate debridement of devitalized tissue is contraindicated in the emergency department because it may take days to weeks before margins of devitalized tissue become clearly demarcated and may lead to premature loss of tissue that may otherwise be viable later. The role of prophylactic parenteral antibiotics is unclear and topical antibiotics, such as bacitracin, appear to be beneficial. However, the initial edema present during the first few days of frostbite does not appear to predispose to infection. Core management of frostbite is aimed at rapid rewarming of the affected parts with warm water immersion (37–39°C), parenteral narcotics for pain management, meticulous local wound care, delayed soft tissue debridement, and tetanus immunization if required.

3. **The answer is C.** (Chapter 209) The adage "the patient is not dead until he is warm and dead" is well known to emergency physicians. However, management of patients with out-of-hospital cardiac arrest and stage IV hypothermia is controversial. Reliable indicators of poor prognosis and, therefore, indications for early termination of resuscitative efforts without rewarming include when the body is frozen solid (and therefore not compressible), prolonged burial (as in avalanches) with airway packed with snow

and serum potassium >12 mmol/L. Fixed and dilated pupils are not specific to hypothermia-induced cardiac arrest and should not be used to determine whether early termination of resuscitation is indicated. The physician must depend on the initial history and physical examination to determine whether patients will benefit from prolonged resuscitation. Refer to Figure 14.5 for a triage tool for hypothermic patients.

4. **The answer is A.** (Chapter 209) Special populations at increased risk of developing heat emergencies include the elderly, young children, persons with limited mobility, alcoholic individuals, and people taking antipsychotics, major tranquilizers, anticholinergics and antiparkinsonian agents, and athletes. Other risk factors for exertional heat emergencies include obesity, dehydration, and vigorous exertion in the heat without proper training and acclimatization.

5. **The answer is A.** (Chapter 211) Multiple toxins are present within scorpion venom but the most dangerous of these causes prolonged and excessive depolarization of neuronal sodium channels. Patients displaying neuromuscular excitation (cranial nerve dysfunction, myoclonic jerks), hypersalivation, or loss of pharyngeal muscle control are at increased risk for airway obstruction, respiratory compromise and rapid deterioration, mandating antivenom administration and airway protection. Additionally, benzodiazepines may be administered for muscle spasms and uncoordinated neuromuscular activity. Early, local toxicity may be treated with nonsteroidal anti-inflammatory drugs (NSAIDs) and local anesthetic administration, but there is no role for tourniquet application. Cholinergic effects may be seen in scorpion stings and may be treated with atropine. However, this patient does not display signs of this like hypotension, bronchorrhea, or bradycardia, arguing against atropine administration. Catecholaminergic surge can be caused by scorpion venom, resulting in high sympathetic outflow (hypertension, mydriasis, and tachycardia). While prazosin may be of use to blunt these effects, patients with scorpion stings and autonomic hyperactivity should also receive antivenom.

6. **The answer is B.** (Chapter 211) Brown recluse spider bite lesions are painless with surrounding erythema and result in local soft tissue injury and systemic toxicity is rare. Treatment is largely supportive, including pain medication and local wound care. Antibiotics are indicated if signs of infection exist, but these are rare. If ulceration or

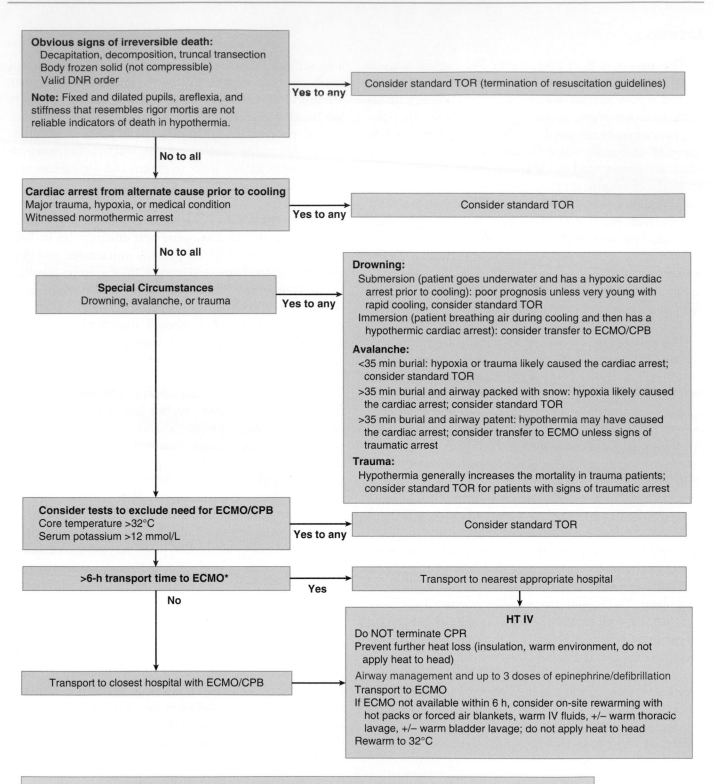

*Geographic location, vehicle/aircraft availability, and weather and road conditions will all impact transport time. In exceptional cases, >6-h transport time may be considered.

FIGURE 14.5 Reproduced with permission from Doug Brown, MD, FRCPC.

necrosis develops, surgical debridement is delayed until clear margins are established, often weeks after the bite. No treatment for these bites has been robustly validated. Small, often subcentimeter bites are most consistent with the bites of black widow spiders, which may be accompanied by severe muscle cramps of the abdomen and back. Antivenom and liberal benzodiazepine administrations are the mainstays of therapy. A severe painful, erythematous wheal is most consistent with funnel-web spider bites, found in Australia. Tarantulas are known to cause painful area of erythema and edema.

7. **The answer is A.** (Chapter 212) First-aid measures for snake bites should never substitute for, nor delay definitive management. All patients bitten by pit vipers should have their affected extremity immobilized and taken to a healthcare facility as soon as possible. Many proposed first-aid measures are dangerous and contraindicated. Suctioning apparatus in kits like the "snake bite kit" often provides poor seals and is ineffective at decreasing systemic spread of venom. Incision and drainage increases risk of damage to nearby arteries, nerves, and veins. Tourniquet application is contraindicated because of obstruction of arterial flow, which complicates envenomation by local tissue ischemia. Extremities that are bitten should be immobilized in a neutral position below the level of the heart. Constriction bands may be helpful in decreasing venous return from the bite site. They should be applied snugly but not so much that they obstruct arterial flow.

8. **The answer is C.** (Chapter 213) The patient is likely stung by a jellyfish, specifically, the box jellyfish. Known as one of the most venomous creatures on the planet, it uses nematocysts to discharge its highly potent toxin subcutaneously. Early effects include local skin irritation and tenderness, but delayed effects include cardiotoxicity and respiratory failure. First-aid measures include irrigation with sea water or normal saline and warm to hot water immersion to deactivate nematocysts. Irrigation with acetic acid is controversial and has shown variable success in nematocyst deactivation. Cold water immersion does not help in box jellyfish envenomations. Similarly, tourniquet application has no role in preventing the spread of the toxin and may worsen outcomes due to local limb ischemia.

9. **The answer is C.** (Chapter 214) The patient is most likely experiencing the "chokes," or respiratory symptoms caused by a large number of pulmonary artery bubbles that develop while breathing under pressure. The "bends" is a type of "pain only" decompression sickness characterized by arthralgias that are not worsened with movement and sometimes skin mottling and pruritic. It is caused by lymphatic obstruction by air bubbles that develop under pressure. Typically, only one joint is involved. The "staggers" refers to the development of vertigo, hearing loss, tinnitus, and disequilibrium caused by the precipitation of air bubbles into the central nervous system (CNS). Arterial gas embolisms can cause chest pain, dyspnea, and a variety of stroke symptoms that develop rapidly on surfacing. These result when air enters the left side of the vascular system. Management of arterial gas embolism involves rapid recompression therapy, 100% oxygen administration, IV fluid administration, and supine positioning.

10. **The answer is A.** (Chapter 215) The patient arrives to the emergency department after a near-drowning. Prognostication of patients who were submerged is challenging but is closely tied to the history of injury and initial presentation. Patients who needed bystander cardiopulmonary resuscitation (CPR) at the scene, CPR in the emergency department, or develop asystole after rewarming have a poor prognosis. Patients in the emergency department who have a short duration of submersion and arrive asymptomatic to the emergency department may be observed for 4 to 6 hours and considered for discharge home if they remain asymptomatic. If decompensation is going to occur, it will within the 4- to 6-hour observation period. This patient, however, arrives tachypneic, hypoxic, and with pulmonary findings on examination, warranting further supportive measures and inpatient monitoring. While drowning victims are at risk for respiratory compromise, this patient's mental status is reassuring and while he displays increased work of breathing, is not distressed, arguing against immediate need for intubation. Discharge home without a period of observation is not indicated in drowning victims.

11. **The answer is A.** (Chapter 217) Full-thickness burns less than 2% body surface area (BSA) are classified as minor burns and may treated on an outpatient basis. According to the American Burn Association, major burns mandate transfer to a burn center for evaluation (Table 14.1).

12. **The answer is A.** (Chapter 218) The patient has been exposed to lime (calcium oxide), a common ingredient in cement. Lime converts to the calcium hydroxide, an alkali, on contact with water producing an exothermic reaction. Even small amounts of remaining particles can produce this reaction and cause worsening damage to the wound. For this reason, particles of remaining irritant should be brushed away before aggressive irrigation takes place. For the same reason, neutralization of the exposed area should be avoided. Compartment pressures are elevated in compartment syndrome, which is usually caused by

TABLE 14.1	Burn Depth Features: American Burn Association Burn Classification	
Burn Classification	Burn Characteristics	Disposition
Major burn	Partial-thickness >25% BSA, age 10–50 y	Burn center treatment
	Partial-thickness >20% BSA, age <10 y or >50 y	
	Full-thickness >10% BSA in anyone	
	Burns involving hands, face, feet, or perineum	
	Burns crossing major joints	
	Circumferential burns of an extremity	
	Burns complicated by inhalation injury	
	Electrical burns	
	Burns complicated by fracture or other trauma	
	Burns in high-risk patients	
Moderate burn	Partial-thickness 15%–25% BSA, age 10–50 y	Hospitalization
	Partial-thickness 10%–20% BSA, age <10 y or >50 y	
	Full-thickness burns ≤10% BSA in anyone	
	No major burn characteristics present	
Minor burn	Partial-thickness <15% BSA, age 10–50 y	Outpatient treatment
	Partial-thickness <10% BSA, age <10 y or >50 y	
	Full-thickness <2% in anyone	
	No major burn characteristics present	

Abbreviation: BSA = body surface area.

Reproduced with permission from J.E. Tintinalli, J.S. Stapczynski, O.J. Ma, D. Yealy, G.D. Meckler, D.M. Cline: Tintinalli's Emergency Medicine: A Comprehensive Study Guide, 9th Edition. McGraw-Hill Education; 2020.

crush injuries. Elevated compartment pressures can indicate need for fasciotomy, but this procedure is not indicated in alkali burns.

13. **The answer is B.** (Chapter 219) The patient presents with an oral/lip burn. Vascular injury to the labial artery is not immediately apparent due to vascular spasm and thrombosis. Eschar separation from the wound occurs after ~5 days and can result in severe labial artery hemorrhage in ~10% of cases. Delayed cardiac dysrhythmias are rare if not present on initial presentation and if the patient has a normal ECG on arrival. Systemic complications of this injury, such as rhabdomyolysis, are rare. While infection of the wound is a possibility, the most severe delayed complication is hemorrhagic, not infectious.

14. **The answer is C.** (Chapter 220) *Amanita* phalloides, or the death cap mushroom, accounts for the vast majority of mushroom-related deaths worldwide. Toxicity from mushroom ingestion can be divided into two categories. Initial symptom onset (0–4 hours) typically includes symptoms of gastrointestinal (GI) upset and usually indicates a benign course. Symptom onset over 6 to 24 hours post ingestion, however, includes similar symptoms but

also with jaundice, lethargy, elevated transaminases, and disseminated intravascular coagulation (DIC), followed 2 to 4 days later with multiorgan failure. Fungemia is not a common cause of death in mushroom ingestion, which is amatoxin mediated. End-organ damage resulting in acute renal failure is possible from profound dehydration in these ingestions and is a hallmark of amanita toxicity, but typically it does not occur without liver failure. Direct cardiac toxicity is not specific to amanita toxicity.

15. **The answer is C.** (Chapter 221) Poison hemlock contains alkaloids that are structurally similar to nicotine. Mild toxicity can result in tremulousness and anxiety from sympathomimetic stimulation. Late toxicity can result in paralysis from nicotinic receptor stimulation at the neuromuscular junction. The alkaloids of poison hemlock are not structurally related to norepinephrine, histamine, or acetylcholine.

16. **The answer is A.** (Chapter 221) Deadly nightshade (*Atropa belladonna*) contains atropine-like alkaloids that produce the antimuscarinic toxidrome in overdose. Expected signs/symptoms include tachycardia, hyperthermia, mydriasis, dry flushed skin, urinary retention, and altered mental status. Treatment is largely supportive. Benzodiazepines may be used for agitation. Physostigmine inhibits acetylcholinesterase and may be used for reversal of muscarinic symptoms. Both can be redosed as needed.

17. **The answer is A.** (Chapter 216) The patient is likely suffering from high-altitude pulmonary edema, a noncardiogenic, hydrostatic edema resulting from high microvascular pressure. Pulmonary hypertension is an essential component. Treatment includes immediate descent, nifedipine, supplemental oxygen therapy, dexamethasone if cerebral signs are present, and hyperbaric therapy if descent is not possible. Acetazolamide is useful for expediting acclimatization and prevention of acute mountain sickness but has questionable value in severe high-altitude illness.

18. **The answer is C.** (Chapter 216) High-altitude cerebral edema (HACE), like all other forms of high altitude illness, benefits from (1) immediate descent and (2) supplemental oxygen administration. Cerebral edema is vasogenic in nature, thus benefiting from steroid administration and potentially improving intracranial pressure. Prevention of hypotension is critical but not specific to management of HACE, which results from progression of poor acclimatization to hypoxia. Emergent recompression therapy is used but not widely available when immediate descent is not possible.

TABLE 14.2	Common Indications for Referral for Hyperbaric Oxygen Treatment	
Loss of consciousness/syncope		Acute myocardial ischemia
Altered mental status/confusion		Cardiovascular dysfunction/dysrhythmia
Seizure		Hypotension
Coma		Severe metabolic acidosis
Focal neurologic deficit		Carboxyhemoglobin level ≥25%
Pregnancy carboxyhemoglobin level ≥15%		

Reproduced with permission from J.E. Tintinalli, J.S. Stapczynski, O.J. Ma, D. Yealy, G.D. Meckler, D.M. Cline: Tintinalli's Emergency Medicine: A Comprehensive Study Guide, 9th Edition. McGraw-Hill Education; 2020.

19. **The answer is C.** (Chapter 222) Common indications for referral for hyperbaric oxygen therapy in acute carbon monoxide poisoning are noted in Table 14.2. The carboxyhemoglobin level that warrants hyperbaric oxygen therapy in pregnancy is greater than 15%, not 20%. Any carboxyhemoglobin level greater than 25% warrants consideration of hyperbaric oxygen therapy. Carbon monoxide poisoning resulting in symptoms like headache and vomiting that resolved during a period of observation (typically 4–6 hours) does not necessarily mandate hyperbaric oxygen therapy. High-risk symptoms associated with carbon monoxide poisoning include ataxia, seizure, syncope, chest pain, focal neurologic deficits, confusion, ECG changes, and dysrhythmias.

20. **The answer is C.** (Chapter 222) Management of carbon monoxide poisoning can be divided based on symptom severity. All patients should receive supplemental oxygen if carbon monoxide toxicity is strongly suspected. Patients with mild symptoms (i.e., nausea, self-limited, or improving headache) that improve after a period of observation may be discharged home if the exposure was not related to a suicide attempt and symptoms resolve. Fire department officials should be contacted to investigate whether ambient levels of carbon monoxide at the patient's home are safe before the patient is discharged. If carbon monoxide toxicity is being considered "discharge home" is not sufficient treatment without exploring the etiology. Patients with severe intoxication (i.e., with ataxia, persistent vomiting, dysrhythmia) should be considered for hospital admission and potentially transfer to the closest hyperbaric treatment center.

Endocrine, Metabolic, and Nutritional Disorders

15

QUESTIONS

1. Which of the following is TRUE about type 1 diabetes mellitus?
   - (A) Accounts for greater than 50% of all diabetes diagnosis
   - (B) β-cells are able to respond to insulinogenic stimuli
   - (C) Mostly diagnosed in adults
   - (D) There is almost no circulating endogenous insulin

2. Which of the following is NOT part of the diagnostic criteria for diabetes
   - (A) $A_{1C} \geq 6.5\%$
   - (B) 2-hour plasma glucose 200 mg/dL during oral glucose tolerance test
   - (C) Fasting plasma glucose ≥ 126 mg/dL
   - (D) Urine glucose test ≥ 10 mg/dL

3. A 22-year-old man with type 1 diabetes being treated with an insulin pump presents to the emergency department with altered mental status and blood glucose of 30 mg/dL. What should be done with the insulin pump while he is getting treated with IV glucose for hypoglycemia and what is the rationale?
   - (A) Disconnect the insulin pump and administer the standard dextrose dose
   - (B) Disconnect the insulin pump and administer double the standard dose of dextrose
   - (C) Do not disconnect the insulin pump and administer the standard dose of dextrose
   - (D) Do not disconnect the insulin pump and administer double the standard dose of dextrose

4. A 5-year-old boy with type 1 diabetes mellitus presents to the emergency department due to altered mental status. His diabetes is treated with an insulin pump. Vital signs are T 37.2°C, BP 112/72, HR 95, RR 14, and SpO_2 100% RA. Point-of-care glucose is 300 mg/dL. Arterial blood gas shows a pH of 7.12. Glucose and ketones are present in his urine dipstick. The patient has an anion gap of 16. What is the APPROPRIATE INITIAL STEP in the management for this patient?
   - (A) Bolus of insulin IV
   - (B) Disconnect the insulin pump
   - (C) Give bicarbonate
   - (D) Insulin SQ

5. A 45-year-old woman with no known medical problems presents to the emergency department with symptoms of blurry vision, polyuria, and polydipsia. Her plasma glucose level is 205 mg/dL. What is the MOST LIKELY underlying cause of this patient's condition?
   - (A) Decreased insulin sensitivity and excessive insulin secretion
   - (B) Decreased insulin sensitivity and impaired insulin secretion
   - (C) Increased insulin sensitivity and normal insulin secretion
   - (D) Increased insulin sensitivity and excessive insulin secretion

6. A 40-year-old woman presents to the emergency department with several weeks of blurry vision, polyuria, and polydipsia. Her plasma glucose on chemistry panel is 400 mg/dL. You would like to start her on metformin upon discharge. What lab value must you check before prescribing this medication?
   (A) Creatinine level
   (B) Magnesium level
   (C) Potassium level
   (D) Sodium level

7. A 70-year-old man is brought in by family members secondary to altered mental status. Blood glucose is 45 mg/dL and family members note that he recently started a new oral medication for diabetes but has had decreased oral intake for the last week. You treat the patient with IV dextrose for hypoglycemia and his mental status improves. Which of these oral medications MOST LIKELY has caused the patient's symptoms?
   (A) Glyburide
   (B) Miglitol
   (C) Metformin
   (D) Pioglitazone

8. A 30-year-old woman presents with polyuria, polydipsia, and fatigue. Vital signs are BP 93/56, HR 114, SpO_2 100% RA, and RR 25. Point of care test results are remarkable for a room air arterial blood gas with pH of 7.12, pCO_2 of 18 mm Hg, and bicarbonate of 5.8 mEq/L and serum glucose of 380 mg/dL. Urine dipstick is positive for ketones and glucose. While waiting on further results from the laboratory, the MOST APPROPRIATE NEXT step in management is administration of which of the following?
   (A) Insulin
   (B) Normal saline
   (C) Potassium
   (D) Sodium bicarbonate

9. A 16-year-old boy with type 1 diabetes presents with generalized weakness and polyuria. You notice a fruity odor to his breath during physical examination. Vital signs are BP 93/56, HR 114, SpO_2 100% RA, and RR 25. Chemistry panel reveals glucose of 400 mg/dL, BUN of 18 mg/dL, creatinine of 0.5 mg/dL, sodium of 139 mEq/L, chloride of 110 mEq/L, CO_2 of 13 mmol/L, and potassium of 5.0 mEq/L. Laboratory results are remarkable for a room air arterial blood gas with pH of 7.20, pCO_2 of 18 mm Hg, and bicarbonate of

5.8 mEq/L. Which additional test should you order to confirm the diagnosis?
   (A) Serum ketones
   (B) Serum osmolality
   (C) Serum magnesium
   (D) Serum thyroid stimulating hormone

10. A 50-year-old woman presents to the emergency department with nausea, vomiting, and mild abdominal discomfort upset. She reports binge drinking for the past week and stopped suddenly due to multiple episodes of vomiting. Her lab values are positive for serum ketones and an elevated blood urea nitrogen (BUN). Serum chemistry panel is MOST LIKELY to show which of the following?
    (A) Metabolic alkalosis
    (B) Normal gap metabolic acidosis
    (C) No acid base disturbance
    (D) Wide anion gap metabolic acidosis

11. A 25-year-old man presents to the emergency department 3 days after an episode of binge drinking. Over the past 2 days, he has had decreased oral intake due to persistent nausea and vomiting. Vital signs are BP 98/56, HR 105, SpO_2 100% RA, and RR 18. Serum lab values show glucose of 80 mg/dL, a wide anion gap metabolic acidosis, and positive serum ketones. In addition to administration of normal saline, what other treatment should be initiated?
    (A) Intravenous glucose
    (B) Intravenous insulin
    (C) Intravenous magnesium
    (D) Intravenous sodium bicarbonate

12. A 53-year-old woman with type 2 diabetes mellitus presents to the emergency department due to persistently high readings on her glucometer. She reports that her blood glucose values are generally well controlled with her usual medication regimen but she started taking a new medication for her blood pressure last month. Her lab values are glucose 650 mg/dL, plasma osmolality of 330 mOsm/kg, serum ketones negative, and arterial pH 7.40. You are concerned for hyperosmolar hyperglycemic state (HHS). Which of the following medications is MOST LIKELY to have predisposed this patient to develop HHS?
    (A) Hydralazine
    (B) Losartan
    (C) Lisinopril
    (D) Metoprolol

13. A 30-year-old woman presents to the emergency department with facial features as well as hair loss and weight gain (Figure 15.1). Which of the following would you also expect to find on physical examination?

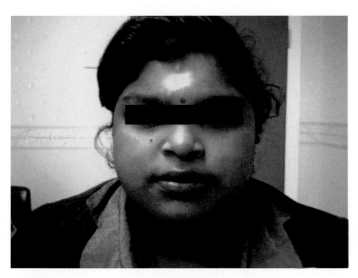

FIGURE 15.1 Image used with permission of Dr. Zanariah Hussein.

(A) Delayed relaxation of ankle jerks
(B) Fat accumulation on the back of the neck and upper back
(C) Increased skin pigmentation
(D) Pitting edema in bilateral lower extremities

14. A 86-year-old woman with a history of hypertension and coronary artery disease presents to the emergency department with altered mental status. She lives alone and appears unkempt. Her vital signs are T 35.3°C, HR 45, BP 87/56, and RR 7. Physical examination findings are notable for periorbital puffiness, nonpitting edema, and delayed relaxation of the ankle tendon reflex. Which of the following is the MOST APPROPRIATE initial pharmacotherapy for this condition?
(A) Propylthiouracil
(B) Radioactive iodine
(C) Thyroxine
(D) Triiodothyronine

15. Which of the following thyroid-stimulating hormone (TSH) and free thyroxine (FT$_4$) trends are classically associated with secondary hypothyroidism?
(A) TSH decreased and FT$_4$ decreased
(B) TSH decreased and FT$_4$ elevated
(C) TSH elevated and FT$_4$ decreased
(D) TSH elevated and FT$_4$ elevated

16. A 43-year-old woman presents to the emergency department for a prescription to help with insomnia. Upon further questioning, she also reports unexplained weight loss, persistent irritability, and frequent episodes of loose stools daily for the past 2 months. While speaking with you, you notice that the patient has exophthalmos, a neck mass seen in Figure 15.2 and a fine resting tremor in her hands. Thyroid function tests are ordered. Which thyroid function test values for thyroid-stimulating hormone (TSH) and free thyroxine (FT$_4$) are indicative of the patient's presentation?

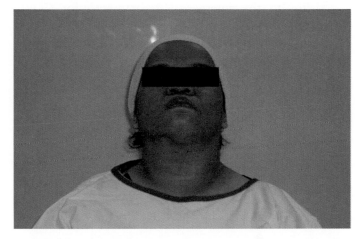

FIGURE 15.2 Reproduced with permission from J.E. Tintinalli, J.S. Stapczynski, O.J. Ma, D. Yealy, G.D. Meckler, D.M. Cline: Tintinalli's Emergency Medicine: A Comprehensive Study Guide, 9th Edition: Copyright Â© McGraw-Hill Education. All rights reserved.

(A) TSH decreased and FT$_4$ decreased
(B) TSH decreased and FT$_4$ elevated
(C) TSH elevated and FT$_4$ decreased
(D) TSH elevated and FT$_4$ elevated

17. A 34-year-old woman presents to the emergency department with diaphoresis, diarrhea, and palpitations. Vital signs are T 39.3°C, HR 128, BP 160/88, RR 22, and SpO$_2$ 100% RA. On physical examination, the patient has exophthalmos, palpable goiter, and pretibial myxedema. Her electrocardiogram shows sinus tachycardia. After providing supportive measures including intravenous fluids for hydration and antipyretics, which of the following medications although indicated for this condition should be administered NEXT?
(A) Esmolol
(B) Guanethidine
(C) Methimazole
(D) Propranolol

18. The use of methimazole for treatment of thyroid storm is contraindicated in which scenario?
    (A) A 16-year-old girl with amenorrhea
    (B) A 30-year-old woman with new onset atrial fibrillation and heart failure
    (C) A 32-year-old woman pregnant in her first trimester
    (D) A 50-year-old woman with diabetes

19. A 62-year-old man presents to the emergency department with hypotension, fever, and cough. He has a past medical history significant for chronic obstructive pulmonary disease (COPD). He is a frequent visitor to the emergency department for COPD exacerbations and was just discharged from the hospital last week. You diagnose him with pneumonia and arrange admission to the hospital. The patient is febrile and persistently hypotensive despite two fluid boluses and timely initiation of antibiotics. Which of the following medications may improve the patient's blood pressure?
    (A) Albuterol
    (B) Glucagon
    (C) Hydrocortisone
    (D) Methimazole

20. A 40-year-old man with lymphoma, who is currently undergoing chemotherapy, is sent to the emergency department for persistent hypotension. He otherwise feels well and denies fever, cough, or dysuria. The patient's oncologist is concerned about primary adrenal insufficiency. What values on the serum chemistry panel are consistent with this diagnosis?
    (A) Hyperkalemia and hyponatremia
    (B) Hyperkalemia and Hypernatremia
    (C) Hypokalemia and hyponatremia
    (D) Hypokalemia and hypernatremia

ANSWERS

1. **The answer is D.** (Chapter 223) Type 1 diabetes mellitus (T1DM) is characterized by almost no circulating insulin and the failure of β-cells to respond to insulinogenic stimuli. T1DM accounts for only 5% to 10% of all cases of diabetes. Diagnosis peaks before school age and at puberty and is mostly diagnosed in children and young adults.

2. **The answer is D.** (Chapter 223) The American Diabetes Association Criteria for the diagnosis of diabetes is shown in Table 15.1.

3. **The answer is C.** (Chapter 223) Hypoglycemia in patients using insulin pumps should be treated the same way as hypoglycemia in patients without pumps. Do not disconnect the insulin pump since this can precipitate diabetic ketoacidosis. Changing the dosage of dextrose administered is also not necessary. Give the standard dosage of 15 to 20 g IV and then recheck this value in 15 minutes and repeat if necessary.

4. **The answer is B.** (Chapters 223 and 225) If a patient with an insulin pump presents in diabetic ketoacidosis, assume there is a pump malfunction and disconnect the pump. The onset of diabetes ketoacidosis can be very rapid after insulin pump failure. An IV infusion of insulin should be started after fluid hydration has been initiated. A bolus of IV insulin has no clinical benefit and is not recommended in children. An alternative insulin regimen includes IM insulin. Bicarbonate is recommended when pH is less than 6.9.

5. **The answer is B.** (Chapter 224) Decreased insulin sensitivity (insulin resistance) and impaired insulin secretion are the two most important pathophysiologic features of type 2 diabetes mellitus. Insulin resistance is defined as, "the diminished tissue response to insulin at one or more sites in the complex pathways of hormone action and higher than normal plasma insulin levels are required to maintain normoglycemia." Additionally, insulin secretion is insufficient to compensate for insulin resistance.

6. **The answer is A.** (Chapter 224) Renal excretion is the major route for metformin elimination. Following oral intake, approximately 90% of the absorbed drug is eliminated via the kidneys in the first 24 hours. The guidelines for metformin prescription The U.S. Food and Drug Administration lists serum creatinine concentration is ≥1.4 mg/dL as a contraindication to administration.

7. **The answer is A.** (Chapter 224) Hypoglycemia is a major adverse effect of sulfonylureas. Glyburide belongs to the sulfonylurea class of drugs that bind to the sulfonylurea receptor on the plasma membrane of pancreatic β-cells to stimulate insulin release. Miglitol acts by competitively inhibiting the final step of carbohydrate digestion of intestinal epithelium. The most common side effect is flatulence and the advantage is that this medication does not increase hypoglycemic risk. Metformin belongs to the biguanide class of drugs and its precise mechanism is unknown. The rare side effect is lactic acidosis that occurs in patients with renal insufficiency. Pioglitazone works by improving insulin sensitivity and reducing level of free-fatty acids. Liver function should be assessed and is contraindicated in patients with unexplained serum alanine aminotransferase levels >2.5 times the upper limit of normal. Side effects include weight gain and fluid retention.

TABLE 15.1	American Diabetes Association Criteria for the Diagnosis of Diabetes
A₁c ≥6.5%*	The test should be performed in a laboratory using a method that is NGSP certified and standardized to the DCCT assay.
Or Fasting plasma glucose ≥126 mg/dL (7.0 mmol/L)*	Fasting is defined as no caloric intake for at least 8 h.
Or Casual plasma glucose ≥200 mg/dL (11.1 mmol/L) and symptoms of hyperglycemia or hyperglycemic crisis	Classic symptoms of hyperglycemia include polyuria and polydipsia.
Or 2-h plasma glucose ≥200 mg/dL (11.1 mmol/L) during an oral glucose tolerance test (OGTT)*	OGTT must be performed as described by the World Health Organization.

Abbreviations: A₁c = glycated hemoglobin; DCCT = Diabetes Control and Complications Trial; NGSP = National Glycohemoglobin Standardization Project.

*Should be confirmed by repeat testing unless unequivocal hyperglycemia is present.

Reproduced with permission from J.E. Tintinalli, J.S. Stapczynski, O.J. Ma, D. Yealy, G.D. Meckler, D.M. Cline: Tintinalli's Emergency Medicine: A Comprehensive Study Guide, 9th Edition. McGraw-Hill Education; 2020.

8. **The answer is B.** (Chapter 225) When treating diabetic ketoacidosis (DKA), the order of priorities for management is to correct volume first, second potassium deficits, and third is insulin administration. Refer to Figure 15.3

for timeline for DKA treatment guidelines. It is important to first treat volume depletion even prior to obtaining lab values when the diagnosis of DKA is suspected because fluid helps to restore intravascular volume, perfuse vital

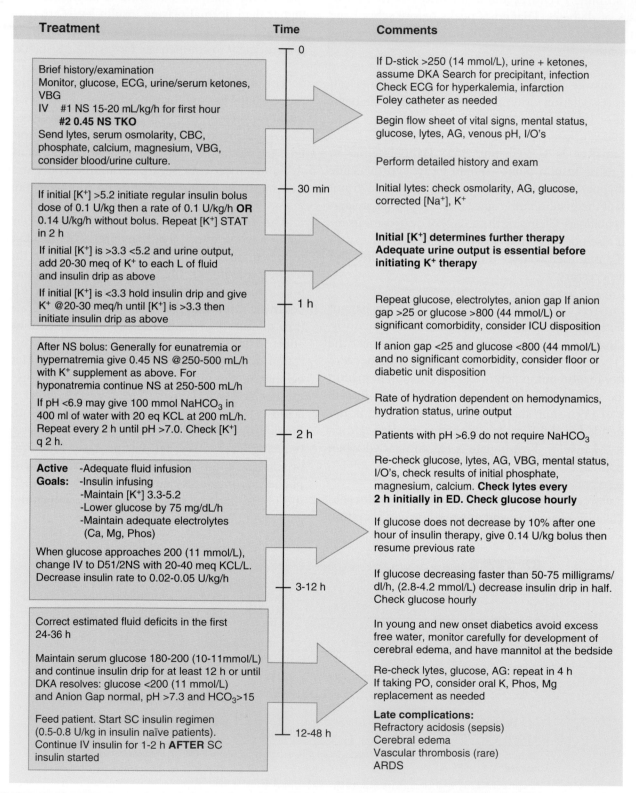

Treatment	Time	Comments
Brief history/examination Monitor, glucose, ECG, urine/serum ketones, VBG IV #1 NS 15-20 mL/kg/h for first hour **#2 0.45 NS TKO** Send lytes, serum osmolarity, CBC, phosphate, calcium, magnesium, VBG, consider blood/urine culture.	0	If D-stick >250 (14 mmol/L), urine + ketones, assume DKA Search for precipitant, infection Check ECG for hyperkalemia, infarction Foley catheter as needed Begin flow sheet of vital signs, mental status, glucose, lytes, AG, venous pH, I/O's Perform detailed history and exam
If initial [K⁺] >5.2 initiate regular insulin bolus dose of 0.1 U/kg then a rate of 0.1 U/kg/h **OR** 0.14 U/kg/h without bolus. Repeat [K⁺] STAT in 2 h If initial [K⁺] is >3.3 <5.2 and urine output, add 20-30 meq of K⁺ to each L of fluid and insulin drip as above If initial [K⁺] is <3.3 hold insulin drip and give K⁺ @20-30 meq/h until [K⁺] is >3.3 then initiate insulin drip as above	30 min 1 h	Initial lytes: check osmolarity, AG, glucose, corrected [Na⁺], K⁺ **Initial [K⁺] determines further therapy** **Adequate urine output is essential before initiating K⁺ therapy** Repeat glucose, electrolytes, anion gap If anion gap >25 or glucose >800 (44 mmol/L) or significant comorbidity, consider ICU disposition
After NS bolus: Generally for eunatremia or hypernatremia give 0.45 NS @250-500 mL/h with K⁺ supplement as above. For hyponatremia continue NS at 250-500 mL/h If pH <6.9 may give 100 mmol NaHCO₃ in 400 ml of water with 20 eq KCL at 200 mL/h. Repeat every 2 h until pH >7.0. Check [K⁺] q 2 h.	2 h	If anion gap <25 and glucose <800 (44 mmol/L) and no significant comorbidity, consider floor or diabetic unit disposition Rate of hydration dependent on hemodynamics, hydration status, urine output Patients with pH >6.9 do not require NaHCO₃
Active Goals: -Adequate fluid infusion -Insulin infusing -Maintain [K⁺] 3.3-5.2 -Lower glucose by 75 mg/dL/h -Maintain adequate electrolytes (Ca, Mg, Phos) When glucose approaches 200 (11 mmol/L), change IV to D51/2NS with 20-40 meq KCL/L. Decrease insulin rate to 0.02-0.05 U/kg/h	3-12 h	Re-check glucose, lytes, AG, VBG, mental status, I/O's, check results of initial phosphate, magnesium, calcium. **Check lytes every 2 h initially in ED. Check glucose hourly** If glucose does not decrease by 10% after one hour of insulin therapy, give 0.14 U/kg bolus then resume previous rate If glucose decreasing faster than 50-75 milligrams/dl/h, (2.8-4.2 mmol/L) decrease insulin drip in half. Check glucose hourly
Correct estimated fluid deficits in the first 24-36 h Maintain serum glucose 180-200 (10-11mmol/L) and continue insulin drip for at least 12 h or until DKA resolves: glucose <200 (11 mmol/L) and Anion Gap normal, pH >7.3 and HCO₃>15 Feed patient. Start SC insulin regimen (0.5-0.8 U/kg in insulin naïve patients). Continue IV insulin for 1-2 h **AFTER** SC insulin started	12-48 h	In young and new onset diabetics avoid excess free water, monitor carefully for development of cerebral edema, and have mannitol at the bedside Re-check lytes, glucose, AG: repeat in 4 h If taking PO, consider oral K, Phos, Mg replacement as needed **Late complications:** Refractory acidosis (sepsis) Cerebral edema Vascular thrombosis (rare) ARDS

FIGURE 15.3 Reproduced with permission from J.E. Tintinalli, J.S. Stapczynski, O.J. Ma, D. Yealy, G.D. Meckler, D.M. Cline: Tintinalli's Emergency Medicine: A Comprehensive Study Guide, 9th Edition. McGraw-Hill Education; 2020.

organs, and lowers serum glucose and ketone levels. Reversing dehydration also leads to improved response to insulin therapy at lower doses.

9. **The answer is A.** (Chapter 225) The diagnosis of diabetic ketoacidosis (DKA) is defined as a blood glucose level >250 mg/dL, an anion gap >10 mEq/L, a bicarbonate level <15 mEq/L, and pH <7.3 with moderate ketonuria or ketonemia. Serum ketones should be ordered to confirm the diagnosis of DKA.

10. **The answer is D.** (Chapter 226) The patient is presenting with alcoholic ketoacidosis. Alcoholic ketoacidosis results in a wide anion gap metabolic acidosis due to elevated ketoacid levels caused by alcohol metabolism combined with minimal glycogen reserves.

11. **The answer is A.** (Chapter 226) Fluids should be administered with supplemental glucose when treating alcoholic ketoacidosis. Administering fluids alone corrects the ketoacidosis more slowly. Glucose also stops ketone production by increasing oxidation of NADH to NAD. Administering insulin has no proven benefit, especially in patients with low glucose levels. Sodium bicarbonate is not indicated unless patients have pH <7.0. Administration of magnesium sulfate is based on laboratory results.

12. **The answer is D.** (Chapter 227) Refer to Table 15.2 for a list of drugs that may predispose individuals to

TABLE 15.2   Some Drugs That May Predispose Individuals to the Development of HHS

- Diuretics
- Statins
- β-Blockers
- Chlorpromazine
- Cimetidine
- Glucocorticoids
- β-Agonists
- Antipsychotics
- Antidepressants
- Phenytoin
- Calcium channel blockers
- Pentamidine
- Immunosuppressive drugs (tacrolimus, cyclosporine)
- Diazoxide
- L-asparaginase
- Protease inhibitors
- Nicotinic acid
- Nucleoside reverse transcriptase inhibitors
- Interferons

Reproduced with permission from J.E. Tintinalli, J.S. Stapczynski, O.J. Ma, D. Yealy, G.D. Meckler, D.M. Cline: Tintinalli's Emergency Medicine: A Comprehensive Study Guide, 9th Edition. McGraw-Hill Education; 2020.

TABLE 15.3   Clinical Differentiation of Primary and Secondary Hypothyroidism

Features	Primary Hypothyroidism	Secondary Hypothyroidism
Previous thyroid operation	Yes	None
Obese	More obese	Less obese
Hypothermia	More common	Less common
Voice	Coarse	Less coarse
Pubic hair	Present	Absent
Skin	Dry and coarse	Fine and soft
Heart size	Increased	Normal
Menses and lactation	Normal	No lactation, amenorrhea
Sella turcica size	Normal	May be increased
Serum TSH	Increased	Decreased
Plasma cortisol	Normal	Decreased
Response to TSH	None	Good
Response to levothyroxine without steroids	Good	Poor response

Abbreviation: TSH = thyroid-stimulating hormone.

Reproduced with permission from J.E. Tintinalli, J.S. Stapczynski, O.J. Ma, D. Yealy, G.D. Meckler, D.M. Cline: Tintinalli's Emergency Medicine: A Comprehensive Study Guide, 9th Edition. McGraw-Hill Education; 2020.

development of hyperosmolar hyperglycemic state (HHS). Beta-blockers and calcium channel blockers can predispose development of HHS. Of the list of antihypertensives given, metoprolol is a beta-blocker. All of the other medications are not known to cause hyperglycemia or precipitate HHS.

13. **The answer is A.** (Chapter 228) Facial swelling is one of the physical examination findings of hypothyroidism. Table 15.3 in Tintinalli lists other common features of hypothyroidism. Delayed relaxation of ankle jerks is the correct answer from the list. Fat accumulation in the back of the neck and upper back is a type of lipodystrophy, sometimes referred to as a "buffalo hump" and is a symptom of excessive glucocorticoid or cortisol hormones. Increased skin pigmentation is a finding of Addison's disease that is primary dysfunction of the adrenal gland. Hypothyroidism causes nonpitting edema.

14. **The answer is C.** (Chapter 228) Propylthiouracil and radioactive iodine are treatments for hyperthyroidism. The patient in this vignette is presenting in myxedema crisis, a severe presentation of hypothyroidism. In addition, she is elderly and has a history of a cardiac condition. Given this patient profile, the correct choice is to treat this patient with thyroxine. The onset of action for IV thyroxine is 6 to 8 hours. While this onset is slower than triiodothyronine, it has an advantage of widespread availability and smooth and steady onset of action. Triiodothyronine is contraindicated in patients who are elderly with cardiac conditions.

15. **The answer is A.** (Chapter 228) Secondary hypothyroidism results from a hypothalamus-pituitary etiology with a normal functioning thyroid gland. Therefore, thyroid-stimulating hormone (TSH) and free thyroxine (FT_4) are both decreased from baseline.

16. **The answer is B.** (Chapter 229) This patient presents with signs and symptoms of hyperthyroidism. Excess production of thyroid hormones from the thyroid glands causes primary hyperthyroidism. Excess production of thyroid-releasing hormones or thyroid-stimulating hormones (TSH) in the hypothalamus and pituitary gland causes secondary hyperthyroidism. The patient in this picture has a diffuse goiter and a clinical presentation suggestive of hyperthyroidism. In this situation, primary hyperthyroidism is the cause and thyroid panel should show decreased TSH and elevated free thyroxine.

17. **The answer is C.** (Chapter 229) This patient is in thyroid storm. After supportive care measures, administration of beta-adrenergic receptor blockade medications and inhibition of new thyroid hormone synthesis with either propranolol, esmolol, reserpine, or guanethidine should begin (Table 15.4). An hour should pass prior to administering medications that inhibit thyroid hormone release such as methimazole or propylthiouracil. Administering medications to prevent the peripheral conversion of thyroxine to triiodothyronine is also an important step in management. Throughout this process, a search for the precipitating event must occur.

18. **The answer is C.** (Chapter 229) The main contraindication for methimazole usage is first trimester pregnancy due to concern for teratogenicity.

TABLE 15.4	Differential Diagnosis for Thyroid Storm
Infection and sepsis
Sympathomimetic ingestion (e.g., cocaine, amphetamine, ketamine drug use)
Heat exhaustion
Heat stroke
Delirium tremens
Malignant hyperthermia
Malignant neuroleptic syndrome
Hypothalamic stroke
Pheochromocytoma
Medication withdrawal (e.g., cocaine, opioids)
Psychosis
Organophosphate poisoning

Reproduced with permission from J.E. Tintinalli, J.S. Stapczynski, O.J. Ma, D. Yealy, G.D. Meckler, D.M. Cline: Tintinalli's Emergency Medicine: A Comprehensive Study Guide, 9th Edition. McGraw-Hill Education; 2020.

19. **The answer is C.** (Chapter 230) The patient is being treated for sepsis but has persistent hypotension in the setting of adequate fluid resuscitation. Prior to starting vasopressors to improve hypotension, treat the patient for adrenal crisis with hydrocortisone given that he is most likely on chronic steroid treatment for his condition.

20. **The answer is A.** (Chapter 230) Patients with primary adrenal insufficiency have a deficiency in aldosterone (mineralocorticoid). This condition is classically characterized by hyperkalemia and hyponatremia.

Hematologic Disorders

QUESTIONS

1. Which of the following conditions might be expected to cause a decreased mean corpuscular volume (MCV) in an emergency department patient?
   (A) Alcohol abuse with cirrhosis
   (B) Iron deficiency
   (C) Penetrating gunshot wound to the abdomen
   (D) Ruptured ectopic pregnancy

2. A patient presents with hypotension after vomiting copious amounts of coffee ground emesis. Which physiologic change in addition to hypotension might you predict in this patient?
   (A) Decreased cardiac output
   (B) Initial vasoconstriction of the central vasculature
   (C) Increased systemic vascular resistance
   (D) Tachycardia

3. Which one of these factors will make the symptoms of anemia worse?
   (A) Chronic blood loss
   (B) Multiple comorbid conditions
   (C) Small volume of blood lost
   (D) Young age

4. An otherwise healthy 25-year-old woman has a chief complaint of fatigue and lightheadedness. A review of systems reveals heavy vaginal bleeding during her menstrual periods. She has normal vital signs but conjunctival pallor on her examination (Figure 16.1). Her hemoglobin is 6.4 g/dL. You suspect chronic blood loss anemia. Which red blood cell measurement would best support your diagnosis?

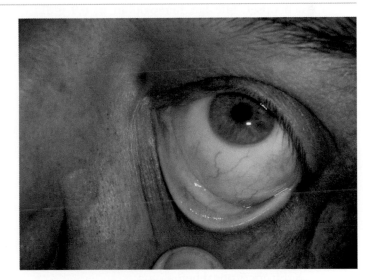

FIGURE 16.1 Image used with permission of J. Stephan Stapczynski, MD.

   (A) Decreased mean corpuscular volume (MCV)
   (B) Decreased red cell distribution width (RDW)
   (C) Normal mean corpuscular hemoglobin concentration (MCHC)
   (D) Normal reticulocyte count

5. A 75-year-old man presents to the emergency department with 2 days of melena. He has a history of coronary artery disease for which he is on clopidogrel. He noticed fatigue about 3 days ago. Which other symptom would be MOST concerning for clinically significant anemia?
   (A) Mild epistaxis
   (B) New-onset chest pain on exertion
   (C) Occasional hematuria
   (D) Peripheral neuropathy

6. The 75-year-old patient in the above question has a blood pressure of 90/50 and a hemoglobin of 7.5 g/dL. Which of the following would be the MOST APPROPRIATE initial management?
   (A) IV fluids and vasopressors
   (B) IV fluids while preparing for a blood transfusion
   (C) Vasopressors only
   (D) Watchful waiting and cessation of his clopidogrel

7. Which of these emergency department patients could potentially be discharged to home?
   (A) A patient who had a nosebleed for 2 hours, which has now stopped. His hemoglobin is 8.0 g/dL and platelets are 20,000/mm^3.
   (B) A patient who stopped taking her iron supplements months ago because they made her stomach upset. She has hemoglobin of 8.0 g/dL, is mildly fatigued, and promises to start her supplements again.
   (C) A patient with known coronary artery disease, mild dyspnea on exertion, and ECG changes. His hemoglobin is 8.0 g/dL.
   (D) A patient with sickle cell disease who presents with joint pain typical of her usual sickle cell crisis. Her hemoglobin is 8.0 g/dL, which is about her baseline. Her white blood cell (WBC) count is 35,000/mm^3.

8. Which site of bleeding is MOST LIKELY to result from a coagulation factor deficiency than a platelet disorder?
   (A) A retroperitoneal hematoma
   (B) Epistaxis
   (C) Menstrual bleeding
   (D) Petechiae

9. A patient accidentally cut his finger on a broken glass while washing dishes. He put direct pressure on it, and it stopped bleeding within a short while. The formation of this patient's platelet plug through primary hemostasis required collagen, platelets, fibrinogen, and which other component?
   (A) Factor V
   (B) Factor VII
   (C) Prothrombin
   (D) Von Willebrand factor

10. A 27-year-old, otherwise healthy patient presents to the emergency department with this rash (Figure 16.2) on his lower extremities. He is otherwise asymptomatic. He does not take any medication on a regular basis. His physical examination is otherwise normal. His complete blood cell count (CBC) is normal other than a platelet count of 24,000/mm^3. His peripheral smear shows large, well-granulated platelets. What is first-line treatment for this patient?

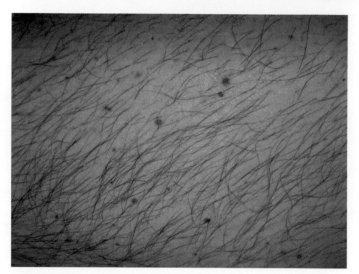

FIGURE 16.2 Image used with permission of J. Stephan Stapczynski, MD.

   (A) A 4-week course of corticosteroids
   (B) A platelet transfusion
   (C) A splenectomy
   (D) Watchful waiting and anticipatory guidance

11. Which of the following is an example of an immune-mediated cause of thrombocytopenia?
   (A) Drug-induced thrombocytopenia in a patient 1 week after starting quinine
   (B) Hemolytic uremic syndrome in a child with *Escherichia coli* diarrhea.
   (C) Splenic sequestration in a patient with sickle cell disease
   (D) Thrombocytopenia in a chronic alcoholic

12. Which of the following patients with thrombocytopenia is MOST LIKELY to have normally functioning platelets?
   (A) A dialysis patient with uremia
   (B) A patient who takes aspirin daily
   (C) A patient with chronic myeloid leukemia
   (D) A patient with drug-induced thrombocytopenia

13. A patient with severe liver disease from primary biliary cirrhosis has known esophageal varices. He presents to your emergency department with brisk upper gastrointestinal bleeding. He will need stabilization and emergent endoscopy. Which of the following statements is TRUE regarding the coagulation defects associated with this patient's liver disease?
    (A) Four-factor prothrombin complex concentrate and vitamin K will be helpful in stopping this patient's bleeding.
    (B) The patient has decreased synthesis of coagulation factors that will most likely cause less clotting than a normal patient.
    (C) The prothrombin time is a good test for predicting severity of bleeding during an invasive procedure.
    (D) The treatment for heavy bleeding in this patient should include fresh frozen plasma.

14. A renal dialysis patient presents at 2 AM with continuous oozing around a new dialysis catheter site in her upper chest wall. The catheter was placed 1 day ago, but she has not been dialyzed for 3 days. She otherwise looks well and is stable. Which of the following is the fastest and BEST INITIAL treatment to stop the bleeding quickly?
    (A) Cryoprecipitate
    (B) Desmopressin
    (C) Hemodialysis
    (D) Platelet transfusion

15. Your elderly patient has a history of frequent urinary tract infections and appears to have urosepsis. His last documented urine culture grew *E. coli*. You notice purpura on his extremities and are concerned that he may be developing disseminated intravascular coagulation (DIC). Which statement about DIC in this patient is TRUE?
    (A) His fibrinogen level will be normal or low in early DIC.
    (B) His levels of fibrin degradation products will be elevated.
    (C) Hyperfibrinolysis will be the dominant effect of DIC in this patient.
    (D) Worsening thrombocytopenia is specific for DIC.

16. A 34-year-old woman presents with a swollen and painful leg. She does not recall any trauma, she has not had any periods of immobility, and she is not on any oral contraceptives. She notes that her uncle died of a pulmonary embolus. You suspect that she has a deep venous thrombosis and that she may be hypercoagulable at baseline. What is TRUE about the evaluation and treatment of suspected venous thrombotic disease in patients with hypercoagulable states?
    (A) D-dimer testing is a reliable and validated test in patients with known hypercoagulable disorders.
    (B) Laboratory testing should be started in the emergency department for suspected hypercoagulable conditions such as protein C and S deficiency and factor V Leiden mutation.
    (C) The duration of anticoagulation for a patient with a hypercoagulable state is the same as that of a patient without a hypercoagulable state.
    (D) The emergency department evaluation and treatment of patients with a hypercoagulable state is the same as that of patients without a hypercoagulable state.

17. Which of the following statements about the causes of hypercoagulable states is TRUE?
    (A) Antiphospholipid syndrome is due solely to antibodies that target the phospholipids on vascular endothelium.
    (B) Factor V Leiden mutation causes factor Va to be less resistant to inhibition by activated protein C.
    (C) Heparin-induced thrombocytopenia is due to antibodies against a complex of heparin and antithrombin.
    (D) Transient hypercoagulability after starting warfarin is due to a decrease in protein C production.

18. A patient presents with a spontaneous nosebleed. On review of systems he notes that he does tend to bruise easily and his gums often bleed when he flosses. You order a complete blood cell (CBC) count that shows significant thrombocytopenia. Which other bleeding symptom is this patient MOST LIKELY to experience?
    (A) Hemarthrosis
    (B) Hematuria
    (C) Intracranial bleeding
    (D) Retroperitoneal bleeding

19. A teenager with known hemophilia A sprained his ankle while skateboarding. He has needed factor transfusions before. On examination he has mild swelling around his lateral malleolus, good pulses and sensation, and slightly diminished range of motion of his joint. He has no bruising at or near his ankle. What is the MOST APPROPRIATE initial treatment?
    (A) Consult orthopedics for splinting
    (B) Ice, rest, and elevation
    (C) Immediate treatment with factor VIII
    (D) Watchful waiting and treatment with factor if bruising appears

20. Which bleeding problem is matched with the CORRECT treatment?
    (A) An 8-year-old boy with moderate hemophilia A (factor activity 1%–5% of normal) who accidentally bit the inside of his cheek—desmopressin
    (B) An 18-year-old man with moderate hemophilia A who was struck in the flank during a lacrosse game—recombinant factor IX
    (C) A 23-year-old man with moderate hemophilia B who struck his head on a windshield during a minor motor vehicle crash—human plasma-derived factor VII concentrate.
    (D) A 43-year-old woman with mild von Willebrand disease and a nosebleed—cryoprecipitate

21. A 28-year-old woman with known sickle cell disease presents with hip pain and a low-grade fever typical of her usual sickle cell crises. Which of the following should prompt consideration for further testing and possible admission?
    (A) A hemoglobin of 8.2 g/dL
    (B) A white blood cell count of 12,500/mm^3
    (C) Localized pain to one hip and difficulty walking
    (D) Pain requiring two rounds of morphine to alleviate

22. An adult man with sickle cell disease presents to the emergency department shortly after discharge from the hospital for sickle cell pain. He has a cough, a fever of 38.9°C, and a new infiltrate on chest x-ray. Which of the following statements about his condition is TRUE?
    (A) Aggressive hydration does not worsen this condition.
    (B) Clinical severity of this condition correlates well with chest radiographs.
    (C) Fat emboli can precipitate this condition.
    (D) The most common pathogen that causes it is *Streptococcus pneumoniae*.

23. Which of these laboratory findings would be consistent with splenic sequestration in a patient with sickle cell disease?
    (A) Hemoglobin at baseline, reticulocyte count low, elevated bilirubin
    (B) Hemoglobin lower than baseline, reticulocyte count elevated, elevated bilirubin, normal platelet count
    (C) Hemoglobin lower than baseline, reticulocyte count elevated, moderate thrombocytopenia
    (D) Hemoglobin lower than baseline, reticulocyte count low, normal bilirubin

24. Which of the following statements about glucose-6-phosphate dehydrogenase (G6PD) deficiency is TRUE?
    (A) In this condition, oxidative stress can cause hemoglobin to precipitate within red blood cells, forming Heinz bodies.
    (B) Nitrofurantoin would be a good choice for an uncomplicated urinary tract infection in a patient with G6PD deficiency.
    (C) The clinical expression of G6PD deficiency shows little variability.
    (D) Sulfamethoxazole should be avoided in G6PD-deficient patients.

25. A 65-year-old woman with chronic lymphocytic leukemia presents with fatigue and dyspnea on exertion. On examination she is pale with mild tachycardia. Her laboratory studies show a new anemia with schistocytes and spherocytes, elevated bilirubin, and an elevated reticulocyte count. Which condition is MOST LIKELY in this patient?
    (A) Autoimmune hemolytic anemia
    (B) Gastrointestinal bleeding
    (C) Hereditary spherocytosis
    (D) Sickle cell disease

26. A 10-year-old boy presents with fatigue after 1 week of bloody diarrhea. On examination, he has pallor and trace pedal edema. Laboratory tests show anemia, elevated bilirubin, thrombocytopenia, and renal failure. He has normal coagulation studies. He has no rash or confusion. Which is the MOST LIKELY cause of this patient's condition?
    (A) Disseminated intravascular coagulation
    (B) Hemolytic uremic syndrome
    (C) Macrovascular hemolysis
    (D) Thrombotic thrombocytopenic purpura

27. Which statement regarding blood transfusions is TRUE?
    (A) A single unit of packed red blood cells will raise the hemoglobin by about 1 g/dL in adults.
    (B) A stable patient should not need a transfusion until their hemoglobin is 7 g/dL or less.
    (C) A unit of packed red blood cells should never be transfused in less than 1 hour.
    (D) For patients with active bleeding, transfusion needs should be based on hemoglobin levels.

28. Which statement regarding fresh frozen plasma (FFP) is TRUE?
    (A) FFP can be given in a 1:1:1 ratio with packed red blood cells and platelets for patients needing massive transfusions.
    (B) FFP can be used for reversal of dabigatran.
    (C) FFP is the preferred reversal agent for patients on warfarin with severe bleeding.
    (D) Type O is the universal donor type for FFP.

29. Your patient is starting a blood transfusion in the emergency department when they develop fever, chills, and dyspnea. What is the FIRST STEP in their management?
    (A) Administer acetaminophen
    (B) Administer normal saline intravenously
    (C) Repeat the type and crossmatch
    (D) Stop the transfusion

30. Which of the following statements about blood transfusions is TRUE?
    (A) An acute intravascular hemolytic reaction, a febrile nonhemolytic transfusion reaction, and a severe allergic reaction may all present in a similar fashion.
    (B) Massive transfusions can cause hypercalcemia.
    (C) Patients who have had a severe transfusion reaction should not receive future blood products.
    (D) Premedication with acetaminophen and diphenhydramine is recommended as routine prophylaxis for all patients who will be receiving a transfusion.

31. A 47-year-old woman on warfarin for a deep venous thrombosis was prescribed trimethoprim-sulfamethoxazole 1 week ago for a urinary tract infection. Her international normalized ratio (INR) at that time was 2.5. An urgent care center advised her to go to the emergency department today because her INR is 5.5. She has no headache, abdominal pain, melena, fatigue, or deep bruising. She is otherwise healthy and not at high risk for bleeding. Her complete blood cell (CBC) count is normal. What is the appropriate treatment for her elevated INR?
    (A) Administer vitamin K intravenously
    (B) Administer vitamin K orally
    (C) Advise her to hold one to two doses of warfarin and recheck her INR as an outpatient
    (D) Stop warfarin and start a factor Xa inhibitor

32. An elderly woman fell and struck her head on her bedside table at home. She is on warfarin for atrial fibrillation and also has a history of congestive heart failure. She was found a few hours later by her son. She arrives with a headache and altered mental status. She has pedal edema and some crackles at her lung bases. A head CT shows a large subdural hematoma and her international normalized ratio (INR) is 6.5. What is the MOST APPROPRIATE initial treatment for this patient in addition to prompt neurosurgical consult?
    (A) Administer IV vitamin K and an appropriate weight-based dose of prothrombin complex concentrate
    (B) Administer IV vitamin K and fresh frozen plasma.
    (C) Administer oral vitamin K and an appropriate weight-based dose of prothrombin complex concentrate
    (D) Administer oral vitamin K and fresh frozen plasma

33. Which statement about the factor Xa inhibitors rivaroxaban and apixaban is TRUE?
    (A) Drug and food interactions can affect their efficacy, similar to warfarin.
    (B) Overdoses of these agents can be treated with hemodialysis.
    (C) Prothrombin time is a reliable measure of the effect on blood clotting.
    (D) They have an elimination half-life of about 12 hours in healthy individuals.

34. Which of the following statements about unfractionated heparin (UFH) and low-molecular-weight heparin (LMWH) is TRUE?
    (A) Both can be completely reversed by protamine.
    (B) Subcutaneous UFH can be used for the treatment of a deep vein thrombosis.
    (C) The incidence of heparin-induced thrombocytopenia is approximately the same for both UFH and LMWH.
    (D) The plasma half-life of LMWH is longer than that of UFH.

35. Which of the following is an absolute contraindication to tissue plasminogen activator for an ischemic stroke?
    (A) A prior hemorrhagic stroke
    (B) Active peptic ulcer disease
    (C) Hemorrhagic diabetic retinopathy
    (D) Insertion of an internal jugular vein catheter 5 days ago

36. A 73-year-old man with a history of lung cancer presents with 1 week of progressively worsening midthoracic back pain. It is worse when he is sleeping at night but not with movement. He has noticed some increasing weakness in his legs. Based on this history, the MOST worrisome condition in your differential is
    (A) Malignant spinal cord compression
    (B) Metastasis to his thoracic spine
    (C) Muscle soreness
    (D) Pathologic vertebral compression fracture

37. A woman who is undergoing chemotherapy for breast cancer presents with confusion, poor appetite, nausea, and constipation. Her electrolytes show a calcium of 15 mg/dL. She has no history of cardiac or renal insufficiency. What is the MOST APPROPRIATE initial treatment in the emergency department?

    (A) A 1-L bolus of normal saline followed by an infusion.
    (B) Bisphosphonate therapy.
    (C) Furosemide.
    (D) No treatment is needed at this time.

38. A woman with acute lymphocytic leukemia presents shortly after a round of chemotherapy with the complaint of feeling unwell. She has a history of tumor lysis syndrome with previous chemotherapy, and you suspect that she may have this again. What is the MOST life-threatening abnormality that you might find on her laboratory studies?
    (A) Hyperkalemia
    (B) Hyperphosphatemia
    (C) Hypocalcemia
    (D) Renal failure

39. A man presents with a fever of 38.1°C that lasted for 90 minutes. He has prostate cancer and his last round of chemotherapy was one week ago. He looks otherwise well, and you cannot find a source for his fever on examination. You have carefully checked his port site and his dentition and looked at his perianal area. His white blood cell count is 2,400/mm^3 with 15% neutrophils and 5% bands on his differential, for an absolute neutrophil count of 480/mm^3. Which of the following is TRUE about this patient?
    (A) Empiric antibiotics should be started immediately.
    (B) He might be able to be discharged to home without antibiotics and with close follow-up.
    (C) He will require dual antibiotic therapy.
    (D) His temperature peak and duration do not technically count as a fever.

ANSWERS

1. **The answer is B.** (Chapter 231) An iron deficiency will impair red blood cell (RBC) production and cause a decreased mean corpuscular volume (MCV). Chronic alcohol abuse will often cause an increased MCV. Acute blood loss anemia is the result of the other two conditions if left untreated. These will result in the acute loss of red blood cells and, ultimately, a decrease in the patient's hemoglobin without necessarily changing RBC indices.

2. **The answer is D.** (Chapter 231) This patient is experiencing acute intravascular blood loss. They will exhibit tachycardia if their blood loss is severe enough, which will help to increase their cardiac output. Initially their central blood vessels will vasodilate and their peripheral vessels will constrict, but as blood loss worsens, small blood vessels will also dilate, resulting in a decrease in systemic vascular resistance.

3. **The answer is B.** (Chapter 231) Elderly or chronically ill patients with poor reserve will have an earlier symptomatic response to anemia, whereas children and young adults may tolerate blood loss surprisingly well until they decompensate and become hypotensive. Patients with acute loss or large volume loss will have more severe signs and symptoms. Patients with chronic loss may be asymptomatic even with hemoglobin levels below 7 g/dL.

4. **The answer is A.** (Chapter 231) This patient most likely has iron deficiency anemia from her chronic blood loss. This would result in a normal or low mean corpuscular volume with a low mean corpuscular hemoglobin concentration. Her red cell distribution width might be high in early iron deficiency anemia. Her reticulocyte count would tend to be low, reflecting the bone marrow's inability to produce red blood cells secondary to the iron deficiency.

5. **The answer is B.** (Chapter 231) This patient's use of clopidogrel puts him at increased risk of bleeding. His fatigue suggests that he has anemia. Although epistaxis and hematuria might be causes of anemia, the chest pain on exertion suggests that his anemia is severe enough to affect blood flow to his heart; this patient's new gastrointestinal bleeding is acutely worsening his already poor cardiac reserve. Peripheral neuropathy might suggest a nutritional deficiency, but this would most likely cause a chronic and well-tolerated anemia.

6. **The answer is B.** (Chapter 231) This patient has symptomatic hypotension in the setting of an acute gastrointestinal bleed. His age, underlying cardiac disease, and likelihood of further bleeding indicate that he would benefit from a transfusion at this level of anemia. He will need an IV fluid bolus to expand his intravascular volume and raise his blood pressure. Vasopressors should generally not be used until intravascular volume is repleted, and since this patient's symptoms are caused by anemia, transfusion will be a better option to correct his hypotension. All patients with anemia and ongoing blood loss should have a type and crossmatch drawn in case they require transfusion.

7. **The answer is B.** (Chapter 231) Treatment for a nutritional deficiency (iron, B_{12}, or folate) will produce a reticulocyte response by about 1 week. Since the patient is mildly symptomatic from what is most likely a chronic anemia, she will not need admission. The patient with epistaxis might be a candidate for discharge except for his significant thrombocytopenia. The patient with coronary artery disease has symptomatic anemia with ECG evidence of cardiac strain and would probably benefit from admission and a transfusion. The patient with sickle cell disease has chronic and probably well-tolerated anemia, but her white blood cell (WBC) count suggests an infection that may need further investigation.

8. **The answer is A.** (Chapter 232) Hemarthroses, retroperitoneal bleeds, and bleeding between fascial planes are more likely to be associated with coagulation factor deficiencies such as hemophilia. Petechia, epistaxis, menstrual bleeding, and gastrointestinal (GI) or genitourinary (GU) bleeding are more likely to be associated with platelet abnormalities or a deficiency of von Willebrand factor.

9. **The answer is D.** (Chapter 232) von Willebrand factor is needed to link platelets to damaged vascular endothelium, which is why a deficiency leads to symptoms similar to those of platelet disorders. The other factors are involved with the process of secondary hemostasis, which stabilizes the initial platelet plug by converting fibrinogen to fibrin. Secondary hemostasis can be triggered by either the contact activation pathway (also known as the intrinsic pathway and measured by the partial thromboplastin time) or the tissue factor pathway (also known as the extrinsic pathway, measured by prothrombin time).

10. **The answer is A.** (Chapter 233) This patient has idiopathic thrombocytopenic purpura. Most serious bleeding complications occur at a platelet count of less than

$30,000/mm^3$, so this patient would qualify for treatment. Watchful waiting and anticipatory guidance to avoid contact sports, falls, or head injuries could be considered for higher counts or in children. Initial treatment for primary immune thrombocytopenia (ITP) is corticosteroids at this platelet count. Platelet transfusion would be considered prophylactically at counts below 10,000 to $20,000/mm^3$ to prevent bleeding complications, and at higher levels if actively bleeding or in need of an invasive procedure. Splenectomy is considered only in refractory cases or for life-threatening bleeding that does not respond to other treatments such as IV immunoglobulin.

11. **The answer is A.** (Chapter 233) Drug-induced thrombocytopenia is immune-mediated and has been linked to hundreds of drugs, including heparin, quinine, sulfa drugs, and phenytoin. It usually occurs within 2 weeks of starting a drug. A careful medication history is necessary for all patients with a new onset of thrombocytopenia. Hemolytic uremic syndrome results in consumption of platelets in small vessel thrombi but is not immune-mediated. Thrombocytopenia in alcoholics can be multifactorial, including poor production from nutritional deficiencies, hepatitis, or portal hypertension. In children with sickle cell disease, splenic sequestration can also cause anemia.

12. **The answer is D.** (Chapter 233) Drug-induced thrombocytopenia is the result of immune-mediated suppression of platelet production or increased platelet destruction. The remaining platelets function normally. Platelet counts will normalize after the drug is stopped. The other conditions all have abnormal platelet function and an increased bleeding time. The platelet dysfunction of uremia might be treatable with desmopressin. Aspirin causes irreversible platelet impairment. Patients with myeloproliferative diseases may have dysfunctional platelets even if their platelet counts are normal.

13. **The answer is D.** (Chapter 233) Fresh frozen plasma will reverse the patient's coagulation factor deficits and should be used in addition to standard packed red blood cell and platelet transfusion. Treatment with four-factor complex concentrate and vitamin K has not been shown to be effective for the cessation of bleeding. Patients with liver disease have decreased production of all coagulation factors and regulatory proteins except for factor VII and von Willebrand factor. Many may also have malabsorption of vitamin K resulting in a prolonged prothrombin time. Despite this, there is usually also a decrease in the anticoagulant proteins like protein C and antithrombin, so that the prothrombin time does not accurately reflect their potential for bleeding. These patients actually have a

higher chance than average of thrombotic complications like deep venous thrombosis and portal vein thrombosis.

14. **The answer is B.** (Chapter 233) Patients with uremia have platelet dysfunction that interferes with the platelets' ability to bind to vascular endothelium. This will cause an increased bleeding time, though other measures of coagulation available in the emergency department such as prothrombin time and activated partial thromboplastin time may be normal. Desmopressin will increase the amount of circulating von Willebrand factor and promote platelet aggregation. Cryoprecipitate should be reserved for life-threatening bleeding. Hemodialysis will be effective but will most likely take some time to coordinate. Platelet transfusion will not be effective because the donor platelets will also be affected by the uremic toxins in the patient's blood.

15. **The answer is B.** (Chapter 233) Fibrin-related markers like fibrin degradation products and d-dimer will be elevated. Gram-negative sepsis is the most common cause of disseminated intravascular coagulation though trauma, pregnancy, pancreatitis, snake envenomation, and leukemia can also trigger the inappropriate activation of coagulation that is the first step in disseminated intravascular coagulation (DIC). Widespread coagulation consumes clotting factors and platelets and also activates the fibrinolytic system, leading to bleeding. Hypercoagulation may predominate in sepsis, causing thrombotic purpura or gangrene. Hyperfibrinolysis may predominate in DIC from other causes, leading to petechiae and oozing from minor wounds. Thrombocytopenia is quite sensitive but not specific for DIC, and in early DIC fibrinogen levels may actually be elevated, though they will eventually drop if the DIC worsens. Prothrombin time will also be high.

16. **The answer is D.** (Chapter 234) The initial testing and treatment of a known or suspected hypercoagulable patient will not differ from that of a normally coagulable patient. The use of d-dimer to exclude thrombus in patients with known hypercoagulable states has not been validated. Testing for hypercoagulable conditions is not helpful in the emergency department, as protein C and S levels may be abnormal in the face of a large clot. If an emergency physician suspects a hypercoagulable state, the patient should be referred for outpatient testing. The duration of anticoagulation will most likely be longer than a patient without a known thrombophilia.

17. **The answer is D.** (Chapter 234) Warfarin causes a decrease in all vitamin K–dependent coagulation factors and proteins. This includes factors II, VII, IX, X, and proteins C and S. Protein C levels decrease before most of the

other factors, leading to a relative protein C deficiency that can cause hypercoagulability. This is why patients who are started on warfarin are usually bridged with heparin until their international normalized ratio (INR) becomes therapeutic. Antiphospholipid syndrome can also be due to proteins that interact with the phospholipids, which are usually on platelet membranes. Heparin-induced thrombocytopenia is actually due to antibodies against the heparin and platelet factor 4 complex. The combination of antibodies, heparin, and platelet factor binds to platelets, activates them, and causes diffuse clots to form and resulting in thrombocytopenia from consumption of the platelets. Despite this, patients are actually hypercoagulable because the same complex can stimulate the release of tissue factor and activation of the extrinsic coagulation cascade. Factor V Leiden mutation causes factor Va to be more resistant to inhibition by activated protein C, leading to uninhibited clotting.

18. **The answer is B.** (Chapter 235) His easy bruising, gingival bleeding, and thrombocytopenia suggest a problem with platelet dysfunction or deficiency. This would also predispose to hematuria, gastrointestinal (GI) bleeding, or heavy menses. Patients with a coagulation factor deficiency tend to have deep bruising, hemarthrosis, retroperitoneal bleeding, or intracranial bleeding without significant trauma, although they may have hematuria as well.

19. **The answer is C.** (Chapter 235) Prompt treatment of hemarthroses can prevent later complications, so do not wait for signs of bruising to appear before starting factor replacement. Patients with hemophilia can reliably report when they are bleeding. For patients with moderate to severe hemophilia, factor replacement, preferably with the same product that they use at home, is indicated for anything more than abrasions and superficial lacerations. Consult their hematologist for appropriate dosing. Orthopedics can be consulted for large hemarthroses or if there is concern for compartment syndrome.

20. **The answer is A.** (Chapter 235) Desmopressin is the treatment for mild (type 1) von Willebrand disease but can also be used for hemophilia A patients with minor injuries. This is because von Willebrand factor (vWF) is a carrier protein for factor VIII. Desmopressin causes an increase in the amount of circulating vWF, resulting in a subsequent increase in factor VIII level. The 18-year-old with a flank injury and hemophilia A will need either recombinant or plasma derived factor VIII, while the hemophilia B patient will need factor IX. A factor VIII concentrate that also contains vWF would be preferable to cryoprecipitate for patients with von Willebrand disease who continue to bleed despite the first-line treatment of desmopressin.

21. **The answer is C.** (Chapter 236) Unilateral hip pain and difficulty ambulating are warning signs for aseptic necrosis of the femoral head. Osteomyelitis and a joint effusion would also be in the differential. An MRI or radionuclide study would be helpful in differentiating osteomyelitis from aseptic necrosis. Many patients with sickle cell disease are chronically anemic, and hemoglobin of 8.2 mg/dL alone would not be an indication for transfusion or admission. It is also not uncommon to have a low-grade fever and a mild to moderately elevated leukocyte count. A white blood cell count over $20,000/mm^3$ is suggestive of an infection. Pain that can be controlled in the emergency department with a few doses of medication does not necessitate admission.

22. **The answer is C.** (Chapter 235) This patient has acute chest syndrome, which classically presents 1 to 3 days after hospitalization for an acute pain crisis. It is this leading cause of death in the United States for patients with sickle cell disease. Precipitants include pulmonary infections, fat emboli, and rib infarction. The most common infectious organisms in acute chest syndrome are *Chlamydia pneumoniae* and *Mycoplasma pneumoniae*. It is thought that reduced blood flow to bone marrow during a vaso-occlusive crisis can cause necrosis and embolization of marrow fat that lodge in the pulmonary vasculature. Pain and excessive opioid use can cause hypoventilation, which can cause atelectasis and further hypoxia. Excessive hydration can cause edema and hypoxia. Hypoxia causes sickling of the red blood cells, with resultant further infarction in a vicious circle. Radiographic changes of acute chest syndrome can lag behind the clinical picture, so that clinical severity of disease may not correlate well with imaging.

23. **The answer is C.** (Chapter 236) Splenic sequestration usually presents in children. On physical exam you may find pallor, left upper quadrant pain, and an enlarged spleen. Both platelets and red blood cells may be sequestered, causing anemia and thrombocytopenia. Since the bone marrow is not affected, production of red blood cells as indicated by the reticulocyte count should not be affected and should remain high to compensate. In aplastic crisis (choice D), the bone marrow is affected, causing a rapid decrease in the hemoglobin level without the ability to produce more red blood cells. There is no increased hemolysis in splenic sequestration as there would be in hemolytic anemia.

24. **The answer is A.** (Chapter 236) Oxidative stress can also damage the red blood cell membrane, causing hemolysis and resultant jaundice. Nitrofurantoin is one of seven medications that can cause acute hemolysis in patients with glucose-6-phosphate dehydrogenase (G6PD)

deficiency. The others are dapsone, phenazopyridine, primaquine, rasburicase, methylene blue, and toluidine blue. G6PD expression is widely variable, ranging from severe enzyme deficiency that causes chronic hemolytic anemia to increased enzyme activity that is clinically silent. The most prevalent severity causes a moderate enzyme deficiency with self-limited hemolysis that is precipitated by stressors such as infections and drugs. Sulfamethoxazole may cause precipitation of hemoglobin in hemoglobin H disease, but should not in G6PD patients.

25. **The answer is A.** (Chapter 237) Autoimmune hemolytic anemia (AIHA) is a condition in which the patient forms autoantibodies to their own red blood cells, causing either intravascular or extravascular hemolysis. Intravascular hemolysis can cause schistocytes from shearing of red blood cells. Extravascular phagocytosis of red blood cells produces spherocytes. AIHA can be divided into primary (idiopathic) and secondary disease as well as into warm, cold, or mixed type AIHA based on which temperature the autoantibodies adhere most strongly to the red blood cells. Some causes of AIHA include lymphoproliferative disorders, respiratory infections like *Mycoplasma pneumoniae* and influenza, and autoimmune disorders like lupus and Sjögren's syndrome. Gastrointestinal bleeding would not be expected to show schistocytes or spherocytes. Hereditary spherocytosis does have spherocytes but would most likely be detected at an earlier age since it is a congenital condition, as is sickle cell anemia.

26. **The answer is B.** (Chapter 237) Typical hemolytic uremic syndrome is caused by Shiga toxin-producing *Escherichia coli*, usually serotype O157:H7 in North America. The toxin has greatest affinity to receptors on renal epithelial and endothelial cells, causing platelet aggregation in the microvascular circulation, mostly of the kidneys. Disseminated intravascular coagulation does present with thrombocytopenia but would have an abnormal prothrombin time secondary to consumption of coagulation factors. Macrovascular hemolysis would be more common in patients with prosthetic heart valves, ventricular assist devices, hemodialysis, or similar conditions that could cause shearing of red blood cells in larger blood vessels. Thrombotic thrombocytopenic purpura can present with similar symptoms and laboratory abnormalities to hemolytic uremic syndrome but is more common in adults and its microangiopathy is less confined to the renal vasculature.

27. **The answer is A.** (Chapter 238) A single unit of packed red blood cells will increase the hemoglobin by about 1 g/dL (or the hematocrit by about 3%) in adults. A transfusion of 10 to 15 mL/kg of packed red blood cells in children will raise the hemoglobin level by about 2–3 g/dL and the hematocrit by 6% to 9%. The transfusion threshold depends on a patient's age and underlying comorbidities, such as cardiac disease, and there is not one universal threshold. A unit of packed red blood cells may be transfused more rapidly than over one hour in patients that are unstable or experiencing rapid blood loss. For actively bleeding patients, transfusion needs should be based on estimated blood loss rather than hemoglobin levels because the drop in hemoglobin will lag behind the clinical signs of blood loss.

28. **The answer is A.** (Chapter 238) Although the optimal ratio is debated, fresh frozen plasma, platelets, and red blood cells can be given in a 1:1:1 ratio in patients with massive bleeding to replace platelets and coagulation factors that are being lost in addition to red blood cells. Fresh frozen plasma will not reverse dabigatran; four-factor prothrombin complex concentrate (PCC) or hemodialysis are effective. It is also not the preferred agent for emergent warfarin reversal; four-factor PCC is also more effective for warfarin reversal. Type AB is the universal donor for fresh frozen plasma since it will not contain antibodies to types A and B blood group antigens.

29. **The answer is D.** (Chapter 238) All of these steps should be considered, but stopping the transfusion should be the first intervention. You should also call the blood bank and send samples of the patient's blood and the donor blood. Give acetaminophen for fever and use IV hydration to maintain intravascular volume.

30. **The answer is A.** (Chapter 238) These blood transfusion reactions may be difficult to differentiate clinically. Massive transfusions have the potential to cause hypocalcemia because the citrate preservative chelates calcium. This is not usually a problem in patients with normal hepatic function and smaller amounts of transfused blood. Patients who have had a severe reaction to a blood product may safely receive future transfusions as long as the blood products are appropriately matched to the patient. Routine premedication with acetaminophen and diphenhydramine is not recommended but may be used for patients with previous febrile or allergic reactions to transfusion.

31. **The answer is C.** (Chapter 239) Drugs that interfere with vitamin K absorption, reduce gut bacteria (like antibiotics), or alter warfarin's metabolism by cytochrome P-450 can all increase international normalized ratio (INR). For an asymptomatic patient with no active bleeding and an INR between 4.5 and 10.0, holding one to two doses and monitoring the INR may be appropriate.

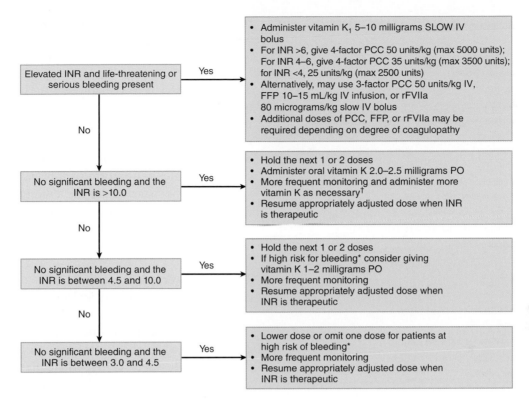

FIGURE 16.3 Reproduced with permission from J.E. Tintinalli, J.S. Stapczynski, O.J. Ma, D. Yealy, G.D. Meckler, D.M. Cline: Tintinalli's Emergency Medicine: A Comprehensive Study Guide, 9th Edition. McGraw-Hill Education; 2020.

Oral vitamin K can be given for asymptomatic patients with an INR over 10.0, or an INR between 4.5 and 10.0 that are at high risk for bleeding. IV vitamin K is generally used only in patients with an elevated INR and dangerous bleeding, such as brisk gastrointestinal (GI) bleeding or intracranial bleeding (Figure 16.3).

32. **The answer is A.** (Chapter 239) This patient has a life-threatening hemorrhage and her warfarin needs to be reversed immediately. IV vitamin K would be indicated in this patient. The onset of vitamin K takes about 2 hours, while prothrombin complex concentrates reverse the international normalized ratio (INR) within 30 minutes. Four-factor prothrombin complex concentrate is preferred over the three-factor concentrate. Both of these are generally preferred over fresh frozen plasma, which could also cause fluid overload in this patient with congestive heart failure.

33. **The answer is D.** (Chapter 239) These factor Xa inhibitors have a half-life of about 12 hours, and invasive procedures can be done 24 hours or more after the last dose a patient has taken. The half-life may be longer in elderly patients or those with decreased renal function. FXa inhibitors are not affected as warfarin is by drug and food interactions. They also do not require laboratory monitoring. Overdoses of these agents are treated with prothrombin complex concentrate, fresh frozen plasma, or activated factor VII. Since FXa inhibitors are highly protein bound, hemodialysis will not be effective. (Dabigatran, on the other hand, is a direct thrombin inhibitor that can be removed by dialysis. Prothrombin complex concentrate will also work for dabigatran, but fresh frozen plasma will not.) Prothrombin time and activated partial thromboplastin time are not reliable measures of their effects.

34. **The answer is D.** (Chapter 239) Since the plasma life of low-molecular-weight heparin (LMWH) is longer than that of unfractionated heparin (UFH), it can be administered once or twice daily, instead of more frequently. Aside for the need for more frequent dosing, unfractionated heparin is also not appropriate for treatment for a venous thrombus because of inconsistent bioavailability, although it can be used for venous thromboembolism prophylaxis. Only unfractionated heparin can be fully reversed by protamine. The incidence of heparin-induced thrombocytopenia is 10 times greater for unfractionated heparin than for low molecular weight heparin.

35. **The answer is A.** (Chapter 239) There are multiple absolute contraindications to fibrinolytic therapy

TABLE 16.1	General Contraindications to Fibrinolytic Therapy

Absolute
- Active or recent (<14 d) internal bleeding
- Ischemic stroke within the past 2-6 mo
- Any prior hemorrhagic stroke
- Intracranial or intraspinal surgery or trauma within the past 2 mo
- Intracranial or intraspinal neoplasm, aneurysm, or arteriovenous malformation
- Known severe bleeding diathesis
- Current anticoagulant treatment (e.g., warfarin with INR >1.7 or heparin with increased activated PTT)
- Current use of a direct thrombin inhibitor or direct factor Xa inhibitor with evidence of anticoagulant effect by laboratory tests
- Platelet count <100,000/mm^3 (<100 × 10^9/L)
- Uncontrolled hypertension (i.e., blood pressure >185/110 mm Hg)
- Suspected aortic dissection or pericarditis
- Pregnancy

Relative*
- Active peptic ulcer disease
- Cardiopulmonary resuscitation for longer than 10 min
- Hemorrhagic ophthalmic conditions
- Puncture of noncompressible vessel within the past 10 d
- Significant trauma or major surgery within the past 2 wk to 2 mo
- Advanced renal or hepatic disease

*Concurrent menses is not a contraindication.

Reproduced with permission from J.E. Tintinalli, J.S. Stapczynski, O.J. Ma, D. Yealy, G.D. Meckler, D.M. Cline: Tintinalli's Emergency Medicine: A Comprehensive Study Guide, 9th Edition. McGraw-Hill Education; 2020.

(Table 16.1). Prior hemorrhagic stroke is one, as are uncontrolled hypertension (over 185/110 mm Hg), current treatment with warfarin and an international normalized ratio (INR) over 1.7, and pregnancy. Peptic ulcer disease, hemorrhagic ophthalmic conditions, and puncture of a noncompressible vessel within the past 10 days are relative contraindications.

36. **The answer is A.** (Chapter 240) The combination of worsening pain and extremity weakness is concerning for malignant spinal cord compression. An MRI would be the best imaging choice for this patient and it would not be unreasonable to image the entire spine because of the potential for malignant involvement at multiple levels. If left untreated, cord compression may progress to anesthesia below the involved cord level, urinary retention, and paralysis. Bony metastases will present with localized pain and might lead to a fracture, but neither will be as likely

to cause paralysis. Muscle soreness will generally be worse with movement and better with rest, so this diagnosis is less likely, as well as the least likely to cause complications.

37. **The answer is A.** (Chapter 240) The patient is symptomatic so will require therapy. In the emergency department the most appropriate initial treatment is volume repletion, which can best be accomplished by a 1- to 2-L bolus followed by an infusion. Bisphosphonates could be considered after restoration of intravascular volume but are usually not started in the emergency department. Furosemide could be used in patients with heart failure or renal insufficiency in addition to the fluids, but is not needed in this patient.

38. **The answer is A.** (Chapter 240) You might expect to find all of these abnormalities on her laboratory studies, but severe hyperkalemia would be the most life-threatening because it can cause cardiac arrest due to dysrhythmia. If there is a delay in getting lab results back, an ECG might detect the peaked T waves of hyperkalemia faster. Treatment would involve dextrose and insulin therapy, beta-adrenergic agents, and consideration of calcium administration. Hypocalcemia may present with tetany and seizures. Renal failure is caused by precipitation of uric acid and calcium phosphate in the renal tubules and is generally treated with fluids.

39. **The answer is A.** (Chapter 240) This patient meets the criteria for fever in this case, which is a temperature of 38.0°C that lasts for over one hour or a single temperature of 38.3°C or greater. His absolute neutrophil count (ANC) is calculated as WBC count in thousands × (neutrophil % + band%). An ANC of less than 500/mm^3 is severe neutropenia, and empiric antibiotic administration is recommended even in the absence of a source on examination. Monotherapy with broad spectrum antibiotics like cefepime or piperacillin/tazobactam is considered to be as good as dual therapy in many cases. Your institution may recommend specific antibiotics or combinations of antibiotics. Patients with an ANC over 1000/mm^3 might be able to be discharged to home without antibiotics but this will require discussion with their oncologist and the ability for close follow-up.

Eye, Ear, Nose, Throat, and Oral Disorders

17

QUESTIONS

1. A 24-year-old man presents with redness, "irritation," and tearing from his eye. Examination demonstrates erythematous, edematous eyelids, and significant chemosis with papillae on the inferior conjunctival fornix. A fluorescein examination of the eye is normal. What is the appropriate treatment?
   - (A) Discharge home with artificial tears and a topical antihistamine
   - (B) Discharge home with cool compresses, artificial tears, and ocular decongestants
   - (C) Discharge home with topical steroids and artificial tears
   - (D) Discharge home with trimethoprim-polymyxin B four times daily for 5 days

2. A 36-year-old woman presents with a foreign body sensation of her left eye after "something got stuck in it" while weeding her plants. Her fluorescein examination is shown in Figure 17.1. What are the appropriate NEXT steps?

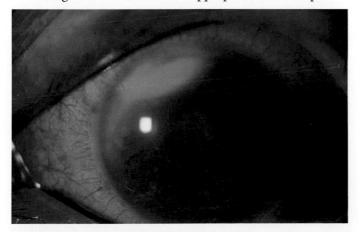

FIGURE 17.1 Reproduced with permission from Knoop K, Stack L, Storrow A: Atlas of Emergency Medicine, 2nd ed. © 2002, McGraw-Hill, New York.

   - (A) Computed tomography to evaluate for ocular foreign body
   - (B) Discharge home with topical antibiotics, cycloplegics, a topical anti-inflammatory, and eye patching for comfort at the patient's discretion
   - (C) Discharge home with topical antibiotics, cycloplegics, and a topical anesthetic
   - (D) Emergent ophthalmology consult for open globe injury

3. A 40-year-old man presents with acute onset of severe eye pain after walking into an underground parking garage at the hospital. His examination shows a fixed pupil in midposition, extremely injected conjunctiva, and cloudy appearance of his cornea. What is the underlying mechanism of this disorder?
   - (A) Inflammation of medium and large arteries
   - (B) Inflammation of the optic nerve
   - (C) Obstruction of ocular aqueous humor outflow
   - (D) Obstruction of the central retinal artery

4. A 23-year old man with sickle cell disease presents with a spontaneous hyphema. Which treatment is contraindicated in this patient?
   - (A) Acetazolamide
   - (B) Cycloplegics
   - (C) Topical beta-blockers
   - (D) Topical steroids

5. A 32-year-old man presents with an eye injury after he was assaulted with a broken bottle. Examination reveals significant eyelid edema and ecchymosis surrounding the eye. The extraocular movements and pupillary response are normal. The lower eyelid has an approximately 3-mm laceration at the lid edge. Which of the following require emergent ophthalmologist consultation for evaluation and closure?
   (A) Corneal abrasion
   (B) Corneal foreign body
   (C) Eyelid margin laceration >1 mm
   (D) Lacerations within 15 mm of the medial canthus

6. A 63-year-old diabetic woman presents to the emergency department with painless loss of vision in her left eye. She describes the vision loss as a dark curtain in her visual field with associated "flashers." An ultrasound image is shown in Figure 17.2. What is the diagnosis?

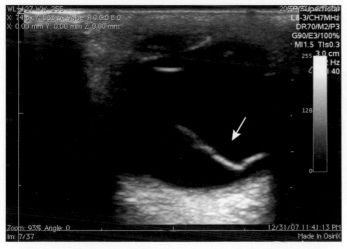

FIGURE 17.2 Courtesy of D. Chandwani and Allen R. Katz, Department of Ophthalmology, University of Nebraska Medical Center.

   (A) Central retinal artery occlusion
   (B) Central retinal vein occlusion
   (C) Retinal detachment
   (D) Vitreous hemorrhage

7. A 43-year-old woman with a history of diabetes presents with gradual onset of right eye pain, redness, and swelling. This was preceded by a recent upper respiratory infection. On examination, she is febrile and tachycardic, with noted scleral injection and chemosis, painful eye movements, and limited rightward gaze. What are the MOST APPROPRIATE NEXT steps for this patient?
   (A) Computed tomography scan of the orbits with intravenous contrast, initiation of broad-spectrum intravenous antibiotics, emergent ophthalmology consultation, and admission to the hospital

   (B) Computed tomography scan of the orbits without contrast, initiation of broad-spectrum intravenous antibiotics, emergent ophthalmology consultation, and admission to the hospital
   (C) Discharge home with erythromycin ointment, amoxicillin/clavulanic acid, hot packs, and follow-up the next day
   (D) Emergent ophthalmology consult for aspiration of the vitreous and administration of intravitreal antibiotics and steroids, intravenous antibiotics, and admission to the hospital

8. In the event of blunt auricular trauma, damage to which structure results in auricular necrosis and asymmetric formation of new cartilage known as "cauliflower ear"?
   (A) Auricular cartilage
   (B) Perichondrial blood vessels
   (C) Skin blood vessels
   (D) Subcutaneous adipose tissue

9. A 43-year-old woman with a past medical history of diabetes presents with severe right ear pain for 2 to 3 days. On examination, her right external auditory canal is erythematous, with significant edema and otorrhea that obstructs further view to the tympanic membrane. She is afebrile and clinically well appearing. Her neurologic examination is normal. What is the appropriate treatment?
   (A) Admission to the hospital and initiation of intravenous imipenem
   (B) Admission to the hospital and initiation of cefepime and ciprofloxacin
   (C) Cleansing with hydrogen peroxide or saline and administration of acetic acid 1%/hydrocortisone 2% drops
   (D) Cleansing with hydrogen peroxide or saline and administration of ofloxacin 0.3% drops

10. A 33-year-old man presents with ear pain and sudden loss of hearing after assault with blunt force to his head. What is the MOST APPROPRIATE treatment for his injury?
   (A) Discharge home with referral to audiology for audiogram as soon as possible
   (B) Initiation of oral antibiotics and discharge home with referral for audiogram as soon as possible
   (C) Initiation of topical antibiotics and discharge home with referral for audiogram as soon as possible
   (D) Referral to otolaryngology within 24 hours

11. A 2-year-old boy is brought by his mother with concern for fever and lethargy. He is complaining of ear pain after a recent upper respiratory infection but became acutely worse today. External physical examination of his left ear is shown in Figure 17.3. What is the MOST APPROPRIATE treatment for this patient?

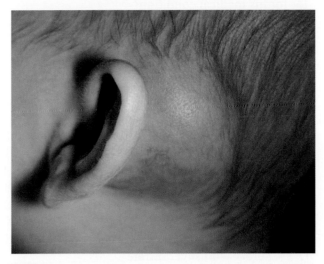

FIGURE 17.3 Photo contributor: Lawrence B. Stack, MD. Reproduced with permission from K.J. Knoop, L.B. Stack, A.B. Storrow, R.J.Thurman: The Atlas of Emergency Medicine, 4th ed. Copyright @McGraw-Hill Education, All rights reserved.

   (A) Initiation of intravenous ceftriaxone and admission for tympanocentesis and myringotomy
   (B) Initiation of intravenous vancomycin and admission for tympanocentesis and myringotomy
   (C) Initiation of oral antibiotics and discharge home with follow-up for a recheck tomorrow
   (D) Local anesthesia and incision and drainage

12. What is the MOST APPROPRIATE treatment for a patient who presents with this facial infection (Figure 17.4)?

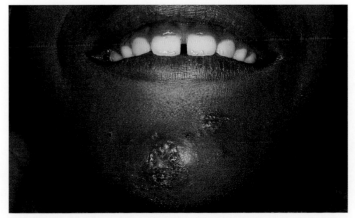

FIGURE 17.4 Photo contributed by Michael J. Nowicki, MD. Reproduced with permission from Knoop K, Stack L, Storrow A, Thurman RJ: Atlas of Emergency Medicine,3rd ed. © 2010, McGraw-Hill, New York.

   (A) Intravenous clindamycin
   (B) Oral cephalexin
   (C) Oral penicillin
   (D) Topical mupirocin ointment

13. A 23-year-old hockey player presents with pain and swelling around his jaw on the left side. This was preceded by 3 days of fever, malaise, and body aches. Several of his teammates have similar symptoms. What complications are associated with this illness?
   (A) Orchitis
   (B) Renal failure
   (C) Salivary duct stricture
   (D) Sialolithiasis of Stensen duct

14. A patient presents with a spontaneous, atraumatic anterior jaw dislocation with yawning. What is the best method to reduce the dislocation?
   (A) The patient is seated; the provider induces the gag reflex while assisting the patient by applying downward pressure on the mandible.
   (B) The patient is seated; the provider places thumbs over the mentum and fingers over the mandible and applies downward force in both locations.
   (C) The patient is seated; the provider places thumbs over the molars and applies downward and backward pressure.
   (D) The patient is supine; the provider places the thumbs over the molars and applies upward and backward pressure.

15. A 43-year-old woman presents to the emergency department with severe pain in her right face. It is intermittent, sharp/stabbing pain that lasts only a few seconds. What is the underlying cause of her pain?
   (A) Collagen vascular disease
   (B) Inflammation of the temporal artery
   (C) Mastoiditis
   (D) Unknown

16. A 68-year-old woman presents to the emergency department with right-sided facial weakness. Her examination shows paralysis of the entire right side of her face, including flattening of the forehead and nasolabial fold. Which of the following treatments has ONLY modest effect?
   (A) Ocular lubricants
   (B) Oral antivirals
   (C) Oral steroids
   (D) Taping the patient's eyelid closed for sleep

17. A 64-year-old man presents with a nosebleed that he has been unable to control at home with direct pressure. Which of the following would be an acceptable FIRST STEP in controlling the bleeding?
    (A) Apply silver nitrate chemical cauterization to the bleeding on both sides of the septum
    (B) Clear the nose, apply oxymetazoline, and hold direct pressure on the nose for 15 minutes
    (C) Clear the nose, then use electrical cautery applied just proximal to the identified bleeding source within the nose
    (D) Pack the nose with a commercially available balloon or nasal tampon/sponge

18. A 34-year-old woman presents with 5 days of nasal congestion, rhinorrhea, facial pain, and sinus pressure. Her examination shows tenderness to palpation over the frontal sinuses. What is the MOST APPROPRIATE NEXT step?
    (A) Antibiotic therapy with amoxicillin
    (B) Antibiotic therapy with high dose amoxicillin/clavulanate
    (C) Computed tomography of the sinuses prior to initiation of treatment to confirm the diagnosis
    (D) Supportive care with nasal saline irrigation, nasal decongestants, and topical nasal corticosteroids

19. A 6-year-old girl presents with pain and swelling to the nose after falling from a swing. She cried immediately and has significant deformity of her nose. What is the MOST APPROPRIATE NEXT step in treatment?
    (A) Computed tomography to evaluate naso-orbital-ethmoid injury
    (B) Plain radiographs to confirm fracture
    (C) Referral to otolaryngology for reduction
    (D) Ultrasound of the nose to confirm fracture

20. Which of the following statements about nasal septal hematoma is MOST ACCURATE?
    (A) After incision and drainage, nasal packing should be placed on the side of the incision only.
    (B) Incision and drainage should be performed within 1 week of injury.
    (C) Incision and drainage will help avoid ischemic necrosis, saddle deformity, and infection.
    (D) Infection of nasal septal hematoma is self-limited and can be treated as an outpatient.

21. A 28-year-old man presents to the emergency department with a complaint of oral pain, a foul metallic taste in his mouth, and poor breath. His physical examination is most notable for gingival bleeding, "punched-out" interdental papillae, fever, and mobile teeth. What is the MOST significant predisposing factor for his medical condition?
    (A) Alcohol abuse
    (B) Caucasian descent
    (C) Human immunodeficiency virus infection
    (D) Tobacco use

22. A 19-year-old woman presents to an urgent care with concern for continued bleeding after having a wisdom tooth extraction earlier the same day. The patient called the nurse line and was told to try to hold pressure with gauze at the site of bleeding for 20 minutes. After this did not work, the patient decided to come in for evaluation. What is the NEXT STEP in controlling postdental extraction bleeding?
    (A) Cautery with silver nitrate
    (B) Gelatin sponge placed in the socket
    (C) Lidocaine with epinephrine injection
    (D) Tight suture of the gingival flap

23. When performing an inferior alveolar block, what anatomical landmark should the needle touch to ensure correct placement of the anesthetic medication?
    (A) Condylar process
    (B) Coronoid process
    (C) Lingula
    (D) Mylohyoid line

24. A patient presents with a dental abscess to the labial surface of tooth number 8. If this goes untreated, what life-threatening condition may occur?
    (A) Cavernous sinus thrombosis
    (B) Ludwig's angina
    (C) Parotitis
    (D) Retropharyngeal abscess

25. An alcohol-intoxicated patient is seen in the emergency department and is noted to have bleeding coming from the mouth. On further evaluation, you notice a linear 0.5-cm laceration to the central dorsal surface of his tongue and no other oral or facial trauma. The patient is able to converse with you and consents to medical interventions. After irrigation, what should be done for treatment of this patient's laceration?
    (A) Laceration repair with absorbable sutures that include the muscle and superficial mucosal layers of the tongue
    (B) No indication for suture placement, provide instruction for several daily chlorhexidine mouth rinses
    (C) Placement of nonabsorbable sutures with loose approximation of the muscle and superficial mucosal layers
    (D) Placement of sutures for tight approximation of the laceration edges

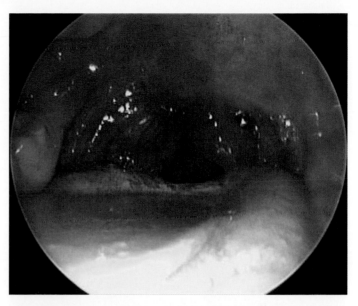

26. A 62-year-old man presents with painful swelling in his right lateral neck for many weeks prior to presentation. He came today at his wife's prompting. He denies difficulty breathing or swallowing. Which element this patient's presentation is concerning for a malignancy?
    (A) Age more than 40
    (B) Intact airway and swallowing
    (C) Male gender
    (D) Pain on presentation

27. A 26-year-old man presents with sore throat. He denies cough or other upper respiratory symptoms. His examination shows bilateral tonsillar exudates and tender cervical lymphadenopathy. What is the MOST APPROPRIATE NEXT step?
    (A) Obtain a rapid strep test and treat based on these results
    (B) Symptomatic treatment with oral analgesics, fluids, and rest
    (C) Treat with oral cephalexin for 10 days
    (D) Treat with oral penicillin VK for 10 days

28. A 34-year-old woman presents with severe sore throat. Her examination is shown in Figure 17.5. What is the correct diagnosis?

    (A) Epiglottitis
    (B) Peritonsillar abscess
    (C) Quincke's edema
    (D) Retropharyngeal abscess

29. What is the FIRST PRIORITY in treatment of Ludwig angina?
    (A) Computed tomography to establish extent of disease
    (B) Control of the airway
    (C) Intravenous antibiotics
    (D) Otolaryngology consultation for surgical debridement

30. What percentage of posttonsillectomy bleeding requires surgical intervention?
    (A) 5%
    (B) 10%
    (C) 25%
    (D) 50%

31. A long-term care facility patient with a chronic tracheostomy tube presents to the emergency department with increased work of breathing that began during bathing. An x-ray was obtained (Figure 17.6). What is the BEST course of action for this patient?

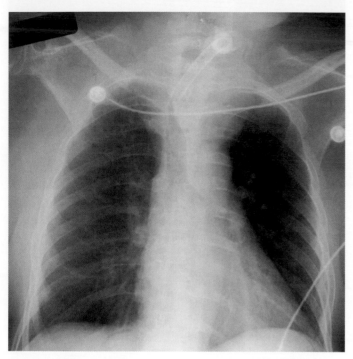

FIGURE 17.6 J.E. Tintinalli, J.S. Stapczynski, O.J. Ma, D. Yearly, G.D. Meckler, D.M. Cline: Tintinalli's Emergency Medicine: A Comprehensive Study Guide, 9th Edition: Copyright © McGraw-Hill Education. All rights reserved.

(A) Pass a suction catheter through the tracheostomy tube
(B) Perform a needle decompression of the chest
(C) Remove the entire tracheostomy tube
(D) Remove the inner cannula to allow for clearing of adherent debris

32. What are the appropriate steps in assessing a patient with a tracheostomy tube presenting in respiratory distress?
(A) Bring intubation/tracheostomy/suction equipment to the bedside, oxygenate the patient with 100% oxygen, remove the inner cannula, remove the tracheostomy tube, and suction the stoma
(B) Bring intubation/tracheostomy/suction equipment to the bedside, remove the inner cannula, oxygenate the patient with 100% oxygen, perform saline irrigation of the tracheostomy, remove the tracheostomy tube, and suction the stoma
(C) Oxygenate the patient with 100% oxygen, bring intubation/tracheostomy/suction equipment to the bedside, remove the inner cannula, remove the tracheostomy tube, and suction the stoma

(D) Oxygenate the patient with 100% oxygen, bring intubation/tracheostomy/suction equipment to the bedside, suction through the inner cannula, remove the inner cannula, perform saline irrigation of the tracheostomy, remove the tracheostomy tube, and suction the stoma

33. A patient presents to the emergency department with a nonfunctioning tracheostomy tube. Basic maneuvers to troubleshoot the tracheostomy tube are not successful and the decision is made for oral intubation. Which patient is NEVER a candidate for oral endotracheal intubation?
(A) A patient with a history of laryngectomy
(B) A patient with large volume airway bleeding
(C) A patient with a tracheostomy placed less than 10 days ago
(D) A patient ≤12 years

34. A 65-year-old man underwent tracheostomy 7 days ago after a prolonged intensive care unit stay. He is brought into the emergency department for accidental dislodgement of his tracheostomy tube secondary to his grandchild jumping up to give him a hug. The patient is in no respiratory distress and vital signs are stable. What is the BEST approach to replace the tracheostomy tube?
(A) Consultation with a surgeon to evaluate the patient in the emergency department
(B) Replace the same tube that was accidentally removed
(C) Use a bougie and a modified Seldinger technique to thread a fresh tracheostomy tube
(D) Use an obturator inside of the outer cannula of a fresh tracheostomy tube to aid in replacement

35. A patient with a tracheostomy is brought in by ambulance in hemorrhagic shock, with significant bleeding noted from her tracheostomy site. The staff is obtaining intravenous access, placing the patient on the monitor, and obtaining O-negative blood for rapid infusion. What is the BEST first step to control the airway with massive bleeding from a tracheostomy site?
(A) Digital pressure of the innominate artery against the manubrium
(B) Hyperinflate the cuff of the current tracheostomy tube while planning for operative intervention
(C) Place an endotracheal tube orally and inflate the tube distal to the tracheoinnominate artery
(D) Slowly withdraw the tracheostomy tube with pressure placed against the anterior trachea

ANSWERS

1. **The answer is A.** (Chapter 241) This patient presents with chemosis and "papillae," which are irregular heaped-up tissue which can be seen with allergic conjunctivitis. The appropriate initial treatment is artificial tears and topical antihistamines. Ocular decongestants have been shown to be beneficial for viral conjunctivitis, which is characterized by associated upper respiratory infection, mild to moderate clear discharge, conjunctival injection, chemosis, and preauricular lymphadenopathy. Topical antibiotics should be reserved for suspected bacterial infection, which is characterized by mucopurulent discharge, adherence of the eyelids on wakening, conjunctival injection, and chemosis, typically without preauricular lymphadenopathy. All of these will have a normal fluorescein examination, which is of utmost importance to rule out herpes keratitis and corneal ulcer. Topical steroids are not appropriate first-line treatment for any of these and should always be prescribed in conjunction with an ophthalmologist.

2. **The answer is B.** (Chapter 241) This patient has a corneal abrasion as noted on fluorescein examination. Given the likely low-velocity foreign body contact, computed tomography for ocular foreign body is not indicated. There is no Seidel's sign or indication of open globe injury, so emergent ophthalmologic consultation is not necessary. As this is a simple corneal abrasion, discharge home with topical antibiotics, cycloplegics, and topical-anti-inflammatory medications is appropriate. Eye patches are optional, but some patients have perceived improved comfort with an eye patch in place. Topical anesthetics inhibit corneal healing and suppress the normal protective blinking response of the eye and should not be prescribed.

3. **The answer is C.** (Chapter 241) This patient has a classic presentation for acute angle closure glaucoma, which is caused by aqueous humor outflow obstruction in which the lens or peripheral iris blocks the trabecular meshwork of the eye and block flow. A shallow anterior chamber is a risk factor for this, but with age the lens becomes less elastic and thicker and cataracts develop, which can increase the risk of acute angle closure. Temporal arteritis results from inflammation of the medium and large arteries and would present more insidiously in a patient older than 50 years, and with a more prominent headache and systemic symptoms. Optic neuritis progresses over hours to days and may present without pain or alterations in color vision and field deficits. Central retinal artery and vein occlusion are painless.

4. **The answer is A.** (Chapter 241) Carbonic anhydrase inhibitors such as acetazolamide are contraindicated for the control of intraocular pressure and hyphema in sickle cell patients because they lower the pH in the anterior chamber. This acidic environment causes the red blood cells to sickle and clog the outflow to the trabecular network, which results in worsening intraocular pressure.

5. **The answer is C.** (Chapter 241) Emergent specialty consultation for evaluation and repair is warranted for the following eyelid lacerations: those that include eyelid lacerations involving >1 mm of the lid margin, lacerations within 6 to 9 mm of the medial canthus or those that involve the lacrimal duct or sac, lacerations involving the inner surface of the lid, the tarsal plate or levator palpebrae muscle, and any laceration with associated ptosis or protruding orbital fat. Ptosis and orbital fat indicate a breach in the septum.

6. **The answer is C.** (Chapter 241) This patient presents with painless loss of vision. Her ultrasound is consistent with retinal detachment, in which the detached retina is seen as a thin, white line superficial to the posterior part of the eye on ocular ultrasound. Vitreous hemorrhage would appear as scattered white echoes in the posterior chamber on ocular ultrasound. Central retinal artery occlusion is characterized by a "cherry red" spot on the macula on fundoscopy, and central retinal vein occlusion is characterized by visualization of a "blood and thunder" appearance on fundoscopy. Neither central retinal artery nor vein occlusion is diagnosed by ultrasound.

7. **The answer is A.** (Chapter 241) This patient presents with classic signs of orbital cellulitis such as insidious onset of eye redness, swelling, and pain in the setting of an upper respiratory infection. Painful extraocular movements differentiate this from a simple preseptal cellulitis. Her examination finding of a sixth nerve palsy raises the suspicion for the associated complication of cavernous sinus thrombosis. Her systemic inflammatory responses (fever, tachycardia) are additional clues to a more sinister diagnosis. As such, computed tomography with contrast, intravenous antibiotics, emergent ophthalmology consultation, and admission are appropriate. Discharge home is only appropriate for a simple preseptal cellulitis, and oral antibiotics are adequate treatment. Topical antibiotics are not indicated. Vitreous aspiration and antibiotic administration would be appropriate for endophthalmitis, which would be indicated by hypopyon on examination.

8. **The answer is B.** (Chapter 242) Blunt trauma to the auricle results in shearing forces to the perichondrial blood vessels as the perichondrium tears from the cartilage.

As the underlying cartilage depends exclusively on this blood supply, disruption results in necrosis. Additionally, a subperichondrial fluid collection can stimulate the overlying perichondrium, resulting in abnormal growth and the classic "cauliflower ear." For this reason, it is imperative to recognize auricular hematomas, incise, and drain them, and provide an appropriate dressing to avoid these complications.

9. **The answer is D.** (Chapter 242) This patient has a history and examination most consistent with acute diffuse otitis externa. Treatment consists of cleansing with hydrogen peroxide or saline, often with application of a wick, and antibiotic drops that cover the most commonly implicated organism, pseudomonas. Normal treatment may consist of acetic acid or neomycin/polymyxin B/hydrocortisone ear drops. However, because the integrity of the tympanic membrane is unknown in this patient, antibiotic drops that are not ototoxic must be administered, such as ofloxacin or ciprofloxacin. Given the short time course and her overall well appearance, malignant otitis externa is less likely. This develops from the spread of simple otitis externa to the deeper structures in and surrounding the ear. These patients present after 2 to 3 weeks of symptoms and may have involvement of the parotid, masseter, or temporomandibular joint. Cranial nerve involvement indicates a severe infection.

10. **The answer is A.** (Chapter 242) This patient's history is most consistent with a tympanic membrane perforation secondary to blunt force trauma. In this case, no antibiotics are indicated, and the patient should get a referral for an audiogram as soon as possible. Topical and systemic antibiotics are not indicated unless there is suspicion of persistent foreign material in the ear. Immediate referral to otolaryngology is appropriate when there is concern for damage to the ossicular chain, which is more typical with penetrating trauma as these perforations tend to be in the posteriorsuperior quadrant where this chain lies. All patients should be instructed to not allow water to enter their ear canal.

11. **The answer is A.** (Chapter 242) This patient presents with acute mastoiditis, a complication of acute otitis media in which infection in the middle ear spreads to the mastoid air cells via the aditus ad antrum. Diagnosis can be confirmed on CT scan, after which initiation of intravenous antibiotics and admission for tympanocentesis and myringotomy should occur. For a first time occurrence, intravenous ceftriaxone is adequate treatment in most cases to cover the most common pathogens (*Streptococcus pneumoniae*, *Streptococcus pyogenes*, and *Pseudomonas aeruginosa*). Intravenous

vancomycin, piperacillin-tazobactam, and imipenem should be reserved for recurrent episodes. Incision and drainage of subperiosteal abscess or mastoidectomy may be required as an inpatient, but bedside incision and drainage should never be performed.

12. **The answer is D.** (Chapter 243) This image shows the classic amber colored crusts of impetigo, caused most commonly by *Streptococcus aureus* or *S. pyogenes*. Topical mupirocin or retapamulin ointment are often adequate treatment alone but can be combined with oral therapy of dicloxacillin, amoxicillin-clavulanate, or cephalexin. Oral penicillin, dicloxacillin, amoxicillin-clavulanate, or a cephalosporin are all options for erysipelas, which is characterized more typically by bright red cellulitis with a sharp demarcation. It is caused by nasopharyngeal bacteria, typically *S. pyogenes* or *S. aureus*. Intravenous clindamycin is appropriate treatment for masticator space infections.

13. **The answer is A.** (Chapter 243) This patient presents with a classic presentation for mumps, or viral parotitis. The course typically progresses from a 3- to 5-day viral prodrome, followed by unilateral and then bilateral swelling of the parotid gland. It can cause outbreaks given it is transmitted by airborne droplets. Parotitis is most commonly caused by the paramyxovirus, and less commonly by influenza, parainfluenza, coxsackie, echovirus, lymphocytic choriomeningitis virus, or human immunodeficiency virus. Twenty to 30% of men will also suffer from associated orchitis. Other complications include mastitis, pancreatitis, aseptic meningitis, sensorineural hearing loss, myocarditis, polyarthritis, hemolytic anemia, and thrombocytopenia. It is not known to cause renal failure. Sialolithiasis and salivary duct stricture can result in bacterial parotitis, which has a more acute-onset and associated red, tender skin overlying the gland.

14. **The answer is C.** (Chapter 243) There are several methods available to attempt anterior jaw dislocation reduction. They all involve getting the condyle to return to its appropriate position behind the anterior eminence. With the patient seated, the provider should position themselves in front of the patient, elbows at the level of the jaw, place the thumbs on the molars, and apply gentle downward and backward pressure. When the patient is in the supine position, the provider stands above the head, still placing their thumbs on the molars and applying the same downward and backward pressure. The "wrist flip" approach positions the provider's thumbs on the mentum, applying upward force, while the fingers are applying downward force to the mandible, with a subsequent "wrist flip" motion, which

also attempts to push the condyle downward and backward. The gag reflex method entails simply inducing the gag response in the patient with a tongue blade or other similar tool, resulting in relaxation of the muscles and joint relocation. It does not require additional assistance from the provider.

15. **The answer is D.** (Chapters 38 and 245) This patient presents with classic symptoms of trigeminal neuralgia, sharp intermittent pain in the distribution of cranial nerve V. The cause of this disorder is unknown. There are some theories that it arises from a peripheral nerve injury, dysfunction of afferent nerve firing, or central nerve inhibition failure. Classic trigeminal neuralgia includes these idiopathic cases and those that are due to microvascular compression. Secondary trigeminal neuralgia includes cases due to tumor, multiple sclerosis, or structural abnormalities. Tegretol and baclofen have been found to be effective treatments.

16. **The answer is B.** (Chapter 172) Bell's palsy is the most common cause of unilateral facial paralysis. This patient's examination confirms the diagnosis, as it includes paralysis of the entire face, including flattening of the forehead and nasolabial fold. The American Academy of Neurology recommends initiating oral steroids within 72 hours, as it is highly effective in improving the chances of recovery of nerve function, as well as ocular lubricants and taping the patient's eyelid shut. Antivirals have shown a moderate effect at best.

17. **The answer is B.** (Chapter 244) When a patient presents with epistaxis, the first step in controlling the bleeding is to clear the nose and apply a vasoconstrictor, like oxymetazoline or phenylephrine topically, then hold steady direct pressure on the nose for 10 to 15 minutes. If this has failed, additional interventions may be attempted, such as chemical cautery with silver nitrate. Silver nitrate cautery must be performed in a dry field and to only one side of the septum to avoid perforation. If the above methods have failed, a trial of application of thrombogenic foam or gel should be attempted. If all of this has failed, nasal packing with a commercially available balloon, nasal tampon or sponge or layered ribbon gauze is a viable option. Electrical cautery is reserved for otolaryngology and should not be performed in the emergency department due to risk of perforation of the septum.

18. **The answer is D.** (Chapter 244) This patient presents with signs and symptoms of acute rhinosinusitis. Patients may also present with fever, tooth pain, or pain when changing head position. Acute rhinosinusitis can last 7 days to up to 4 weeks. This is most commonly of viral etiology, and initial treatment is supportive care with nasal saline irrigation, along with oral or topical nasal decongestants and topical steroids. Antibiotics may be beneficial in patients with symptoms lasting more than 7 days and are therefore not indicated in this patient. When the decision to provide antibiotics is made, amoxicillin is a first line therapy. High-dose amoxicillin clavulanate should be reserved for patients who have already taken antibiotics in the last 4 to 6 weeks. Computed tomography should be reserved for patients with subacute (4–12 weeks) or chronic (>12 weeks) rhinosinusitis and is not necessary for acute rhinosinusitis as this patient presents.

19. **The answer is C.** (Chapter 244) This child has a clinical nasal fracture. No further imaging is indicated to confirm the fracture, and computed tomography is only indicated if there is suspicion of other associated injuries like intracranial hemorrhage, basilar skull fracture, or other significant facial fractures. In adults, referral to otolaryngology for closed reduction is appropriate and can be done 6 to 10 days after the injury. Because of the more rapid healing of pediatric patients, they should be referred for reduction within 2 to 4 days.

20. **The answer is C.** (Chapter 244) Nasal septal hematoma is a complication of nasal fractures. The vascular supply of the septal cartilage runs through the perichondrium, so when a hematoma lifts this off of the cartilage, the blood flow is obstructed, resulting in ischemic necrosis. As such, an urgent incision and drainage is indicated, and this should be performed in the emergency department at the time of injury. A week later is too long. Left untreated, the patient runs the risk of developing to ischemic necrosis and resultant saddle deformity. An infected septal hematoma can spread to local structures resulting in osteomyelitis, meningitis, cavernous sinus thrombosis, or meningeal abscess. After careful incision and drainage with sterile technique, the bilateral nares should be packed to avoid reaccumulation of fluid.

21. **The answer is C.** (Chapter 245) Acute necrotizing ulcerative gingivitis (ANUG) is a disease spectrum ranging from localized ulceration to systemic illness that can be fatal. Human immunodeficiency virus infection is the most important predisposing patient factor for ANUG. The exact cause of the disease is poorly understood but appears to be an opportunistic infection in a host with a compromised immune system. The second predisposing factor is a previous episode of ANUG. Caucasian descent, tobacco use, alcohol abuse as well as, younger than 21 years,

poor socioeconomic status, recent illness, poor diet, and malnutrition are also risk factors, however, not the most important.

22. **The answer is B.** (Chapter 245) Postextraction bleeding control should be performed in a stepwise fashion. The first step is to hold pressure with gauze for 20 minutes. If this does not work, gelatin sponge, microfibrillar collagen, or regenerated cellulose product should be placed in the socket or loosely sutured in place. If this does not work, lidocaine with epinephrine injected into the surrounding tissue can be tried. If there is still bleeding, silver nitrite cautery can be attempted. If all of these options are unsuccessful, the emergency provider should contact oral maxillary facial surgeon or his/her hospital's equivalent consultant for definitive management. No tight sutures should ever be placed by the emergency department medical provider as this can lead to gingival flap necrosis.

23. **The answer is C.** (Chapter 245) To perform a successful inferior alveolar nerve block, have the patient open his/her mouth with the provider retracting the check away from the patient's dentition to relax the musculature. Palpation of the coronoid notch can aid in the needle direction. The physician should direct the needle from the contralateral premolar toward the direction of the coronoid notch. The needle should enter the patient's tissue on the lingual side about 1 to 1.5 cm above the mandibular plane and the needle should contact the bone above the lingua to ensure that the anesthetic will be delivered in a sufficient location. If the injection is given too low, the sphenomandibular ligament will impede delivery of the anesthetic to the inferior alveolar nerve.

24. **The answer is A.** (Chapter 245) A dental infection on the labial surface of tooth number 8 (a maxillary anterior tooth) can primarily involve the infraorbital space. This can lead to spread of infection in a retrograde fashion through the ophthalmic veins to the cavernous sinus, leading to a cavernous sinus thrombosis. Infections in the submandibular space and Ludwig's angina typically arise from dental infections from the second and third mandibular molars. Parotitis is not caused by the spread of a dental infection. Retropharyngeal abscess is usually caused by the spread of an infection from the tonsils, throat, or sinuses.

25. **The answer is B.** (Chapter 245) Linear lacerations less than 1 cm that are on the dorsal surface and involve the central portion of the tongue and are not gaping will heal without repair. Larger, gaping wounds, or partial amputations should be repaired. When repair is needed, an absorbable suture should be used, and the stitch should be placed such that the muscular layer and the superficial mucosal layers of the tongue will be brought back together. Laceration edges should be closed loosely and a minimum of four square knots should be placed to allow for swelling and constant tongue movement.

26. **The answer is A.** (Chapter 246) This patient presents with a neck mass concerning for malignancy. In adults more than 40 years, up to 80% of lateral neck masses that persist more than 6 weeks are malignant. Male gender, pain on presentation, and intact airway and swallowing do not indicate malignant etiology, but his age and the time course are concerning.

27. **The answer is A.** (Chapter 246) This patient has acute pharyngitis and meets all four of the Centor criteria. While previous recommendations were to treat empirically in this case, in 2012 the Centers for Disease Control and Prevention and the Infectious Diseases Society of North America changed their recommendation to test all patients with two or more Centor criteria and only treat those with positive results. Symptomatic treatment with oral analgesics, fluids, and rest would be appropriate for viral pharyngitis if the strep test is negative. First-line treatment for a positive test is penicillin VK. As group A beta-hemolytic *Streptococcus* has not been known to have any resistance to penicillin, cephalosporins should be reserved for patients with a penicillin allergy.

28. **The answer is B.** (Chapter 246) This patient has a peritonsillar abscess, as visualized in the image with displacement of the right tonsil medially and deviation of the uvula away from the affected side. Quincke's edema is uvular edema that can be idiopathic or associated with an upper respiratory infection, pharyngitis, epiglottitis, or peritonsillar abscess. Epiglottitis is not classically diagnosed by direct inspection of the oropharynx. These patients are typically ill appearing, sitting in the sniffing position with associated drooling and/or stridor. Definitive diagnosis of epiglottitis is established with a lateral neck radiograph or transnasal fiberoptic laryngoscopy. Retropharyngeal abscess is also not a diagnosis made by direct inspection of the oropharynx. Patients present with severe sore throat, neck pain, and dysphagia with or without stridor. They may have associated muffled voice. The diagnostic study of choice for retropharyngeal abscess is contrast-enhanced computed tomography.

29. **The answer is B.** (Chapter 246) These are all important components in the management of Ludwig's angina, but control of the airway remains the top priority because rapid deterioration of respiratory status presents the

greatest immediate life threat to these patients. This may include awake fiberoptic intubation or awake tracheostomy. Ludwig's angina is an infection of the submental, sublingual, and submandibular spaces, which can produce trismus and edema of the floor of the mouth on examination. As the disease progresses, the tongue is displaced posteriorly, creating a risk of obstruction that makes airway control essential. Intravenous antibiotics, advanced imaging, and specialty consultation are all additional steps in treatment that should be pursued once any immediate airway concerns are addressed.

30. **The answer is D.** (Chapter 246) Posttonsillectomy bleeding rates range from <1% to 15%. Half of these will require surgical intervention, so it is important to involve the otolaryngologist as soon as possible. Bleeding is most common in adults aged 21 to 30 and more than 70 and can occur many days after the procedure. In fact, the most serious hemorrhage occurs 5 to 10 days post operation. This bleeding can result in airway obstruction, hemorrhagic shock, and death, so prompt treatment is essential. While awaiting otolaryngologist arrival, the emergency physician can control hemorrhage with direct pressure using a tonsillar pack or 4 × 4 gauze on a long clamp, moistened with thrombin or lidocaine with epinephrine. Cauterization with silver nitrate can also be performed if the site of bleeding can be identified, after appropriate anesthesia. If using a pack, be sure to secure the pack with a suture taped to the patient's cheek to prevent aspiration. Nebulized epinephrine or tranexamic acid is another option for controlling bleeding.

31. **The answer is C.** (Chapter 247) The figure demonstrates a tracheostomy tube with the tube located outside of the trachea, resulting in compression of the tracheal wall. The accidental decannulation likely occurred during patient maneuvering for bathing. Regardless of the maturity of the tracheostomy tract, removal of the tracheostomy tube is the only appropriate course of action. Since this patient has had the tracheostomy for an extended period of time, a trial replacement of the tracheostomy tube is appropriate. If the tract has not matured, the patient should be orally intubated if needed for emergent airway control, or surgical consultation for replacement can be pursued if the patient is in no distress.

32. **The answer is D.** (Chapter 247) A step-by-step approach should be considered any time a patient with a tracheostomy tube presents in respiratory distress. Place all patients on 100% oxygen, obtain intravenous access if none has been established prior to arrival, place the patient on cardiac and pulse oximetry monitors, and obtain a one view chest x-ray. The chest x-ray may show

displacement requiring complete tracheostomy tube removal or demonstrate a possible etiology of the patient's distress that is not directly related to the tracheostomy, such as pneumothorax. The equipment listed above should be brought directly to the bedside as soon as possible, even prior to the patient's arrival if advance warning is given. A soft suction catheter should be inserted through the inner cannula to attempt clearing any debris. If no improvement, remove the inner cannula as debris can become cemented to the inner cannula and not easily removed with a suction catheter. If distress continues, suction through the tracheostomy tube with saline irrigation. If the suction catheter does not pass and/or distress continues, remove the tracheostomy tube and suction the stoma. If no improvement, a nasopharyngoscope or bronchoscope can be passed through the stoma to evaluate for other obstructive processes. Granulation tissue and thickened secretions can be removed with a hemostat. If bleeding is noted in the stoma, an attempt for control with silver nitrate is appropriate. Tracheal bleeding should be temporized with either an endotracheal tube placed through the stoma or orally with the cuff inflated at the site of bleeding to provide tamponade and ventilation while waiting for the emergent surgical consultant to arrive.

33. **The answer is A.** (Chapter 247) Patients who have undergone laryngectomy or who have tumors or scarring that occludes the upper airway cannot be orally intubated. Key information to obtain from a patient presenting with a tracheostomy are as follows: When and why was the procedure done? What type of tracheostomy tube does the patient have? Can the patient be intubated orally?

34. **The answer is A.** (Chapter 247) The patient above is in no distress with an immature tracheostomy tract. A surgical consultation should be obtained for evaluation in the emergency department. Manipulation of an immature tract can create false passages within the soft tissue of the neck. If the patient with an immature tract is in respiratory distress and the patient does not have a laryngectomy or a large upper airway mass, oral intubation should be attempted in conjunction with surgical consultation after the patient's airway is secured.

35. **The answer is B.** (Chapter 247) Brisk bleeding tends to occur from a tracheoinnominate artery fistula. Risk factors for a fistula to form include cuff pressure >25 mm Hg, tracheostomy below the third tracheal ring, or deformed neck or chest. The bleeding occurs from vessel erosion caused by either direct pressure at the top of the tracheal cannula against the artery or from a cuff with excessively high pressure. The first step in the scenario above is to hyperinflate the cuff of the current trache-

ostomy tube while consulting for surgical intervention. If this is insufficient, slowly withdraw the tube while placing pressure against the anterior trachea in order to exert pressure on the tracheoinnominate artery. If bleeding continues, use a bronchoscope or nasopharyngoscope to place a cuffed endotracheal tube from above and then with direct visualization, pass the endotracheal tube past the tracheoinnominate fistula, while an assistant withdraws the tracheostomy tube as the endotracheal tube is passed. Then control stomal hemorrhage with direct digital pressure of the innominate artery against the manubrium. Definitive management is in the operating room.

Dermatology

18

QUESTIONS

1. Which of the following is NOT a feature of erythema multiforme major?
   (A) Epidermal detachment greater than 30% of total body surface area
   (B) Erosions of the mucous membranes
   (C) Multisystem involvement
   (D) Widespread vesiculobullous lesions

2. Nikolsky sign is NOT present in which of the following dermatologic conditions?
   (A) Bullous pemphigoid
   (B) Pemphigus vulgaris
   (C) Staphylococcal scalded skin syndrome
   (D) Toxic epidermal necrolysis

3. A 40-year-old woman presents with a 10-day prodrome of malaise, arthralgias, anorexia, sore throat, runny nose, and a sensation of skin burning. On examination, she is noted to have widespread erythema of the skin involving 40% of total body surface area with areas of bullae formation, skin peeling, and a positive Nikolsky sign. What is the BEST disposition for this patient?
   (A) Consult the critical care intensivist for admission to intensive care unit
   (B) Consult the internal medicine hospitalist for inpatient admission
   (C) Discharge home with outpatient dermatology follow-up
   (D) Transfer to burn center

4. Bullous pemphigoid can be distinguished from pemphigus vulgaris by which of the following?

   (A) Greater toxicity with poorer outcomes
   (B) Mucous membrane involvement
   (C) The absence of Nikolsky sign
   (D) Younger age of onset

5. A 30-year-old man with a recent diagnosis of seizure disorder presents to the emergency department complaining of a 4-day history of a pruritic rash and fever. On examination he has a fever of 101.4°F, tender cervical lymphadenopathy, and a diffuse maculopapular rash (Figure 18.1). Labs are notable for eosinophilia and mild transaminitis. What is the MOST LIKELY diagnosis?

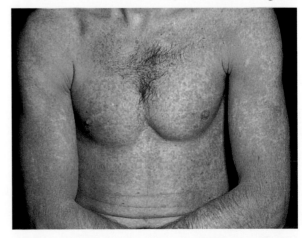

FIGURE 18.1 Reproduced with permission from J.E. Tintinalli, J.S. Stapczynski, O.J. Ma, D. Yealy, G.D. Meckler, D.M. Cline: Tintinalli's Emergency Medicine: A Comprehensive Study Guide, 9th Edition. Copyright © McGraw-Hill Education. All rights reserved.

   (A) Drug rash with eosinophilia and systemic symptoms (DRESS) syndrome
   (B) Exfoliative dermatitis
   (C) Urticaria
   (D) Viral exanthem

6. A 10-month-old infant is brought into the emergency department by a parent secondary to nasal congestion, poor oral intake, decreased energy, and fever to 103°F at home. On examination, the infant appears ill and is lethargic. She has poor capillary refill, tachycardia, and new skin lesions on her torso (Figure 18.2). What are the MOST APPROPRIATE NEXT steps in the emergency management of this infant?

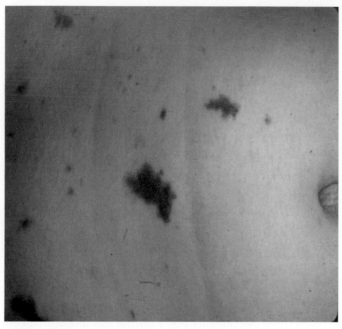

FIGURE 18.2 Photograph used with permission of Kenneth Greer, MD, University of Virginia Dermatology.

(A) Consult hematology
(B) Discharge home with good return precautions and close follow-up with their pediatrician
(C) Obtain blood cultures, administer IV ceftriaxone, and then perform a lumbar puncture
(D) Obtain blood cultures, perform a lumbar puncture and then administer Ceftriaxone

7. An elderly man presents to the emergency department with a rash on his face (Figure 18.3). Which of the following is he at risk for?
(A) Ramsay Hunt syndrome
(B) Recurrence of rash after repeat exposure to offending agent
(C) Recurrent painful vesicles at sight of primary infection
(D) Zoster ophthalmicus

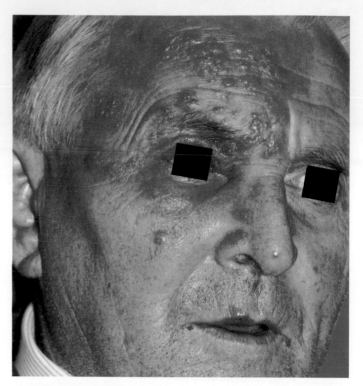

FIGURE 18.3 Reproduced with permission from Fleischer A Jr, Feldman S, McConnell C, et al: Emergency Dermatology: A Rapid Treatment Guide. New York: McGraw-Hill, Inc.; 2002.

8. A young boy presents with a low-grade fever, malaise, lymphadenopathy, and lesions on his mouth (Figure 18.4). What is the MOST LIKELY explanation?

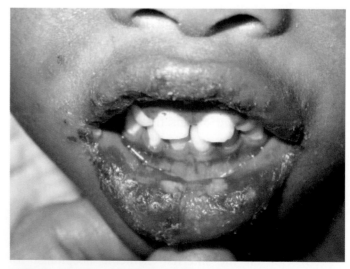

FIGURE 18.4 Photo contributed by University of North Carolina Department of Dermatology.

(A) Herpetic gingivostomatitis
(B) Herpes zoster
(C) Impetigo
(D) Recurrent oral trauma

9. What is the MOST APPROPRIATE treatment for the following condition (Figure 18.5)?

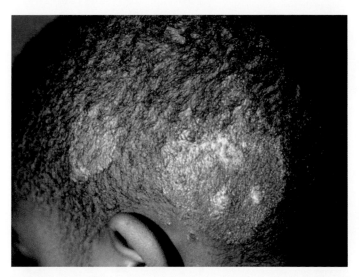

FIGURE 18.5 Photo contributed by University of North Carolina Department of Dermatology.

(A) Doxycycline orally
(B) Fluconazole topically
(C) Griseofulvin orally
(D) Hydrocortisone topically

10. A young girl is brought to the emergency department by her parents because of a pruritic rash on her face. She is well-appearing, afebrile, and does not have any other symptoms. On further questioning, the parents state that the family went camping in the woods in California about 10 days ago. What is the MOST LIKELY explanation for the girl's rash?
(A) Herpes zoster
(B) Impetigo
(C) Poison oak
(D) Seborrheic dermatitis

11. What condition should be considered in a patient with no known medical history, who presents with newly diagnosed severe seborrheic dermatitis?
(A) Hodgkin's lymphoma
(B) Human immunodeficiency virus
(C) Small cell carcinoma
(D) Systemic lupus erythematosus

12. A 39-year-old man with no medical history presents with the following rash on his trunk. The rash is itchy. This current rash was preceded by a single rash 2 weeks previous that was oval in shape, erythematous,

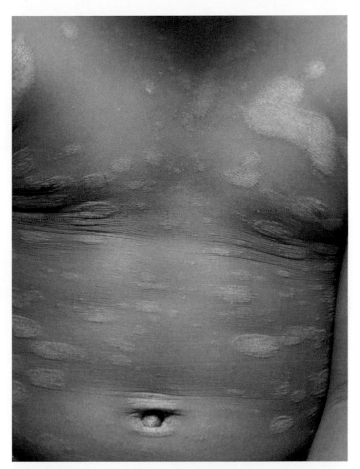

FIGURE 18.6 Photo contributed by University of North Carolina Department of Dermatology.

and scaly (Figure 18.6). What describes the BEST medical management for this rash?
(A) Fluconazole 200 mg oral
(B) Penicillin intramuscular 2.4 million units
(C) Permethrin 5% cream
(D) Triamcinolone 0.1% cream topical

13. Herpes zoster is a rash caused by reactivation of the latent varicella virus. What BEST describes the resulting rash at its onset?
(A) Beginning with a red macule or papule with slow expansion of nonscaling erythema occurring over 3 to 32 days, often becoming annular with central clearing
(B) Erythematous papules coalescing into plaques within a dermatome, followed by vesicles or bullae within 24 to 48 hours
(C) Evanescent macular rash lasting only a few hours or days of varying shades from light pink torso or brownish red
(D) Pruritic urticarial plaques and papules that evolve over weeks to months

14. A 23-year-old woman, 25 weeks pregnant presents with a rash with intense itching, particularly worse at night. This is an uncomplicated pregnancy thus far, and the patient is receiving prenatal care. On the physical examination, you note brown papules on the interdigital spaces of her hands bilaterally. What is the NEXT BEST step for management of this patient's rash?
    (A) Ceftriaxone intramuscular
    (B) Diphenhydramine orally
    (C) Ivermectin orally
    (D) Permethrin cream 5% topically

15. Which of the following is generally TRUE for this lesion (Figure 18.7)?

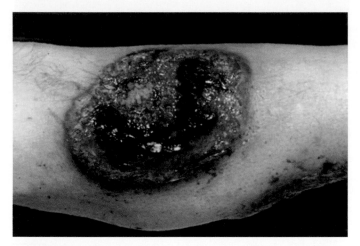

FIGURE 18.7 Reproduced with permission from Wolff KL, Johnson RA, Saavedra AP, Roh EK: Fitzpatrick's Color Atlas & Synopsis of Clinical Dermatology, 8th ed. 2017, McGraw-Hill, Inc., New York.

    (A) A CBC may demonstrate peripheral eosinophilia in an otherwise well-appearing patient.
    (B) It is often associated with underlying rheumatoid arthritis.
    (C) The classic lesion begins as tender, ill-defined erythematous nodules, most commonly seen on the pretibial area of the lower extremities.
    (D) Treatment modality is generally surgical debridement followed by 1 week of valacyclovir.

16. A 65-year-old woman presents with a spot on her lower leg that has been present for about 1 month. It was discovered incidentally when she was getting a pedicure, and she was urged to come to the emergency department by her manicurist (Figure 18.8). What is the NEXT BEST step in management?

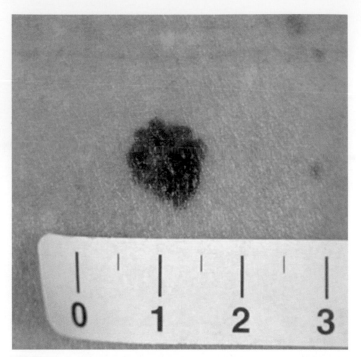

FIGURE 18.8 Reproduced with permission from Wolff KL, Johnson RA, Saavedra AP, Roh EK: Fitzpatrick's Color Atlas & Synopsis of Clinical Dermatology, 8th ed. 2017, McGraw-Hill, Inc., New York. Fig. 12-3.

    (A) Antibiotics
    (B) Antiviral
    (C) Incision and drainage
    (D) Refer to dermatology

17. A 25-year-old North Carolina man presents to the emergency department with a rash. Four days prior to noticing the rash, the patient had developed a fever, headache, and myalgias. The rash started on his wrists and ankles, and then spread toward his palms and soles. The rash appears as discrete macules that blanch with pressure, over time the rash appears as petechiae and involves the proximal extremities, trunk, and face. What is the responsible organism?
    (A) Borrelia burgdorferi
    (B) Hookworm larvae
    (C) Rickettsia rickettsii
    (D) Treponema pallidum

18. A 23-year-old college student presents to the emergency department after hiking in the local hills 3 days prior. She presents with an itchy rash that appears as linear streaks of erythematous papules and vesicles. Which of the following BEST describes the treatment modality for this rash?
    (A) High-dose oral prednisone
    (B) High-potency topical corticosteroids
    (C) Nonsteroidal anti-inflammatory drugs
    (D) Oral dapsone

19. A 9-month-old baby girl presents with a rash in the groin area that the mother noticed while changing her diaper. What is the etiology of this rash (Figure 18.9)?

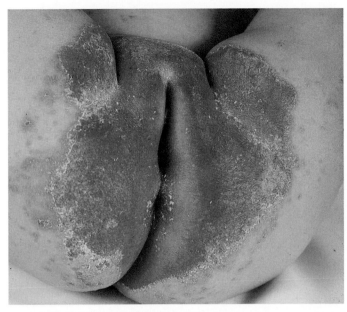

FIGURE 18.9 Reproduced with permission from Wolff KL, Johnson R, Suurmond R: Fitzpatrick's Color Atlas & Synopsis of Clinical Dermatology, 6th ed. © 2009, McGraw-Hill, Inc., New York.

(A) Cutaneous candidiasis
(B) Tinea cruris
(C) Scabies
(D) Seborrheic dermatitis

20. Which of the following is the best description for the rash associated with psoriasis?
    (A) Erythematous with well-marginated papules and plaques with silvery scale
    (B) Greasy, yellow scales
    (C) Macular erythema on trunk, abdomen, inner extremities; followed by papular or papulosquamous lesions
    (D) Purple, pruritic, polygonal, planar papules

ANSWERS

1. **The answer is A.** (Chapter 249) Erythema multiforme is a cutaneous reaction to drugs or infectious agents. Erythema multiforme minor is a localized papular eruption that classically manifests as target lesions involving the hands and extremities. Erythema multiforme major (Stevens-Johnson syndrome) is more severe with multisystem involvement, widespread vesiculobullous lesions, erosions of the mucous membranes, and epidermal detachment of less than 10% total body surface area. Toxic epidermal necrolysis presents with greater than 30% epidermal detachment. Erythema multiforme major (Stevens-Johnson syndrome) and toxic epidermal necrolysis can have an "overlap" presentation with 10% to 30% epidermal detachment.

2. **The answer is A.** (Chapter 249) Nikolsky sign is present if the epidermis separates from the dermis when a slight rubbing pressure is applied to the skin. It is associated with erythema major (Steven-Johnson syndrome), toxic epidermal necrolysis, staphylococcal scaled skin syndrome, and pemphigus vulgaris. It is absent in bullous pemphigus and can be used to clinically distinguish bullous pemphigus from pemphigus vulgaris.

3. **The answer is D.** (Chapter 249) The patient's presentation is most consistent with toxic epidermal necrolysis. Toxic epidermal necrolysis is a life-threatening skin condition characterized by tender erythema, bullae formation, mucous membrane lesions, and subsequent sheet-like skin and mucosal loss that typically involves greater than 30% of body surface area. Medications are the most common cause of toxic epidermal necrolysis. The mortality rate is as high as 30% and most often due to infection and dehydration with electrolyte abnormalities. Therefore, patients with toxic epidermal necrolysis are best managed in a burn unit.

4. **The answer is C.** (Chapter 249) Bullous pemphigoid presents similarly to pemphigus vulgaris but generally has an older average age of onset, larger blister size, lower rate of mucous membrane involvement, and an overall a better outcome. In contrast to pemphigus vulgaris, Nikolsky's sign is NOT present in bullous pemphigoid.

5. **The answer is A.** (Chapter 249) Drug rash with eosinophilia and systemic symptoms (DRESS) syndrome is a severe drug reaction that occurs within 8 weeks of starting a new medication. It is most associated with phenytoin, phenobarbital, allopurinol, and sulfa medications. However, several other medications can also cause DRESS syndrome. DRESS syndrome is characterized by fever, rash, and organ involvement (liver, kidneys, and hematologic system).

Treatment includes stopping the offending medication, systemic steroids in severe cases, supportive care, and hospital admission.

6. **The answer is C.** (Chapter 250) Given the fever, petechial rash, and lethargy, the most likely diagnosis is meningococcal infection due to *Neisseria meningitidis*. Patients with meningococcal infection can rapidly deteriorate and should be given prompt antibiotics and supportive care. Antibiotics should be given as soon as possible and usually right after blood cultures are obtained. Lumbar puncture should not delay the administration of antibiotics.

7. **The answer is D.** (Chapter 250) Herpes zoster (shingles) is a cutaneous reactivation of latent varicella-zoster virus infection. It will appear in a dermatomal distribution as painful, pruritic vesicles and pustules on an erythematous base. Zoster typically involves the thoracic and lumbar dermatomes, but lesions can also occur on the face. Herpes zoster ophthalmicus is of concern when zoster involves the ophthalmic branch of the trigeminal nerve and extends to the tip of the nose. Ramsay Hunt syndrome is manifest by painful vesicles in the external auditory canal due to reactivation of zoster in the geniculate ganglion. Herpes simplex can lead to recurrent painful vesicles at the site of primary infection.

8. **The answer is A.** (Chapter 250) Herpetic gingivostomatitis is caused by primary infection herpes simplex virus type 1. Children or adolescents with herpetic gingivostomatitis may presents with fever, malaise and herpetic lesions to the lips and mouth that can persist for weeks. Recurrences will occur along the lip margin and heal within 10 days. Treatment for primary herpetic gingivostomatitis is with oral acyclovir or valacyclovir for 7 to 10 days and treatment should ideally be initiated within the first 72 hours.

9. **The answer is C.** (Chapter 250) Tinea capitis is due to a fungal infection of the scalp and hair shaft. It will appear as a scaly patch of alopecia and broken hairs. The infection can cause an intense inflammatory response with the formation of a boggy, tender, indurated plaque with superficial pustules and overlying alopecia, known as a kerion. A kerion can result in permanent scarring and hair loss. First-line therapy is oral griseofulvin or terbinafine. Topical antifungals will not adequately treat tinea capitis.

10. **The answer is C.** (Chapter 250) Poison ivy/oak is a type of contact dermatitis caused by direct contact with the sap of the plant. Poison ivy is found East of the Rockies

while the poison oak is found West of the Rockies. Direct contact will lead to exposure to the toxic urushiols on surface of the plant. Patients will develop a rash 10 to 14 days after a first exposure, but the rash will appear earlier with subsequent exposures. Herpes zoster is a reactivation of varicella zoster virus and presents in a dermatomal distribution and is more common in adults and older people. Impetigo is a superficial bacterial infection usually caused by *Staphylococcus aureus* and characterized by pustules and honey-colored crusted lesions around the mouth and nose. Seborrheic dermatitis typically presents in infants as "cradle cap" and in adults as erythema and scaling to the face and facial skin folds.

11. **The answer is B.** (Chapter 251) Seborrheic dermatitis is a chronic inflammatory disease that manifests more often in areas of increased sebaceous gland activity. Severe involvement may occur in patients with Parkinson's disease, trisomy 21, HIV, or AIDS. A patient who is presenting with severe or new-onset seborrheic dermatitis should be worked up for HIV. Hodgkin's lymphoma, small cell carcinoma, and systemic lupus erythematosus are not otherwise associated with seborrheic dermatitis.

12. **The answer is D.** (Chapter 251) Triamcinolone 0.1% cream topical. The pathology described is pityriasis rosea, and the treatment is symptomatic. Oral antihistamines and topical steroid creams such as triamcinolone 0.1% cream with emollients can help alleviate pruritus. Fluconazole is indicated for fungal processes such as tinea corporis. Penicillin is indicated for treatment of syphilis. Permethrin 5% cream is the treatment modality for scabies.

13. **The answer is B.** (Chapter 251) Herpes zoster is a rash that manifests as erythematous papules coalescing into plaques within a dermatome, followed by vesicles or bullae within 24 to 48 hours. New lesions may develop for up to 1 week, and crusting of the lesions occurs within 7 to 10 days. Early Lyme disease begins with a red macule or papule at the site of the tick bite. Slow expansion of nonscaling erythema occurs over 3 to 32 days after the bite. It may become annular with central clearing around the bite site. Varying shades of red in concentric rings may be seen, and less commonly, the central portion may be indurated, blistering, or necrotic. Secondary syphilis exhibits skin manifestations in most patients and consists of early and later manifestations. The early eruption appears 2 to 10 weeks after the appearance of the primary chancre and is an evanescent macular rash lasting only a few hours or days. The macular erythema commonly appears on the sides of the trunk, midabdomen, and inner extremities. The discrete round macules are of varying shades from light pink torose or even brownish

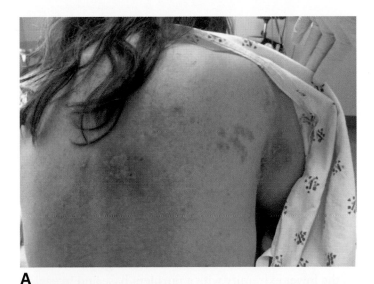

A

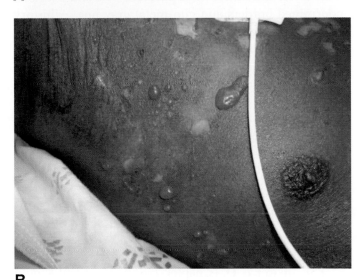

B

FIGURE 18.10 (A) Photo contributed by University of North Carolina Department of Dermatology. **(B)** University of North Carolina Department of Dermatology.

red. The macular eruption resolves spontaneously and may leave postinflammatory hyperpigmentation. Bullous pemphigoid often begins with pruritic urticarial plaques and papules. These are not transient like urticaria. Bullae evolve over weeks to months. The bullae are tense and firm-topped, appearing on normal or erythematous skin. They do not extend when lateral pressure is applied (Figure 18.10). Bullae eventually rupture, leaving a thin blister roof overlaying the lesion, crusts, and erosions.

14. **The answer is D.** (Chapter 252) This patient has scabies. To treat scabies, apply Permethrin cream 5% (Pregnancy Category B) from the neck down, leave on for 12 hours, and then bathe with soap and water. Repeat treatment in 1 week. Treat all resident family members and household and intimate contacts. Oral ivermectin can be used as an adjunct to permethrin for refractory cases

or in the setting of an immunocompromised or uncooperative patient, but it is contraindicated in pregnant and lactating women. Supportive care involves use of oral antihistamines and topical corticosteroids after use of the appropriate scabicidal agent. Ceftriaxone intramuscular is generally used in the management of infectious pathology, such as gonorrhea.

15. **The answer is B.** (Chapter 253) Pyoderma gangrenosum is a recurrent cutaneous, necrotizing, and noninfective ulceration of the skin. Most cases are associated with underlying disease, such as inflammatory bowel disease, rheumatoid arthritis, and myeloproliferative disorders. The classic lesion begins as a superficial pustule or erythematous nodule that expands into a large painful ulcer on the lower extremity with a purulent base and irregular, undermined borders and gun metal gray hue. A history of multiple surgical debridements with sterile cultures should suggest a potential diagnosis of pyoderma gangrenosum. Cutaneous larva migrans is a cutaneous eruption caused by the migration of hookworm larvae within the epidermis. A CBC may demonstrate peripheral eosinophilia; patients are otherwise well but will often complain of pruritus. Erythema nodosum is typically described as tender, arm ill-defined erythematous nodules, most commonly seen on the pretibial area of the lower extremities. Herpetic whitlow, caused by herpes simplex virus 1 or 2 (HSV-1 or -2), located on the distal finger or hand is treated with 1 week of valacyclovir. Surgical debridement is not indicated with herpetic whitlow.

16. **The answer is D.** (Chapter 253) This patient should be referred to dermatology. melanoma is a melanocytic tumor that most often originates in the skin and is most often caused by exposure to ultraviolet light. Involvement can also occur on oral, conjunctival, and vaginal surfaces, including the uveal tract of the eyes and leptomeninges. Clinical presentation includes brown to black tumors, attributed to melanin deposition whereas some are flesh colored to pink-red and termed amelanotic. One type of aggressive melanoma that occurs on hairless skin, such as under the nails and on palms or soles, and is more common in dark-skinned individuals is called acral lentiginous melanoma. Thus, any new or unusual spot on the body or extremities is worthy of dermatologic referral for definitive diagnosis.

17. **The answer is C.** (Chapter 253) Rocky Mountain spotted fever is a potentially fatal multisystem illness caused by *Rickettsia rickettsii*. Symptoms begin 2 to 14 days after an infected tickbite. The organism disseminates through the bloodstream and invades the vascular endothelium, causing a necrotizing vasculitis. Fever, headache, and myalgias

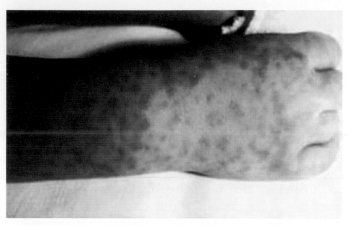

FIGURE 18.11 Centers for Disease Control and Prevention; National Center for Emerging and Zoonotic Infectious Diseases; Division of Vector-Borne Diseases: Rocky Mountain Spotted Fever. www.cdc.gov/rmsf/symptoms/. Updated September 5, 2013

develop about 1 week after exposure. The rash in classic Rocky Mountain spotted fever is evident 2 to 5 days after the onset of fever and other symptoms. In most patients, some type of rash develops during the illness, but about 10% never develop a rash. The rash first appears on the wrists and ankles and rapidly spreads to the palms and soles (Figure 18.11). As the rash moves centrally, the proximal extremities, trunk, and face become involved. The skin lesions at the onset are described as discrete macules or macular papules that blanch with pressure. The initial lesions evolve into petechiae over 2 to 4 days, fade slowly over 2 to 3 weeks, and heal occasionally with hyperpigmentation. Hookworm larvae is associated with a rash that shows the migratory pattern of the larvae. *Borrelia burgdorferi* causes Lyme disease and a rash known as erythema migrans. *Treponema pallidum* is the organism that causes syphilis, and a rash that manifests with secondary syphilis.

18. **The answer is A.** (Chapter 253) High-dose oral prednisone. The treatment modality for poison oak exposure is to remove contaminated clothing, wash with soap and water; for severe cases, oral prednisone starting at 60 mg for 5 to 7 days and then taper over 2 to 3 weeks. For milder cases oral antihistamines and topical steroids can be used. Contact dermatitis is best treated with removal of offending agent and high-potency topical corticosteroids. Erythema nodosum is a rash best treated with leg elevation and NSAIDs. Oral dapsone is the treatment for dermatitis herpetiformis.

19. **The answer is A.** (Chapter 252) Candidal infections of the skin favor moist, occluded areas of the body. Superficial *Candida* infections are commonly seen in the diaper area of infants, vulva and groin of women, glans penis (balanitis) of uncircumcised males, and inframammary

and pannus folds of obese patients. Antibiotic therapy, systemic corticosteroid therapy, urinary or fecal incontinence, immunocompromised states, poorly controlled diabetes mellitus, and obesity are predisposing factors. Women with vulvar or inner thigh involvement will often have vaginal candidiasis as well. Frequently, *Candida* infection may complicate other inflammatory intertriginous disorders. The typical presentation is erythema and maceration with peripheral small erythematous papules or satellite pustules. The rim of satellite pustules helps to distinguish *Candida* infection from other eruptions of the skinfolds. Tinea cruris is a fungal infection of the groin commonly called jock itch. It is very common in males, uncommon in females, and exceedingly rare in children. Lesions are characterized by symmetric erythema with a peripheral annular slightly scaly edge. Scabies is an infestation of the skin by *Sarcoptes scabiei*. The typical findings are slightly longitudinal erythematous or brown papules, predominantly on the lateral feet, wrists, ankles, and interdigital spaces of the fingers and toes. Involvement may be evident within the axillae, groin, and extensor extremities. Seborrheic dermatitis is one of the most common skin disorders. Seborrheic dermatitis of the scalp and skinfolds of the face presents as erythema with a greasy yellow scale.

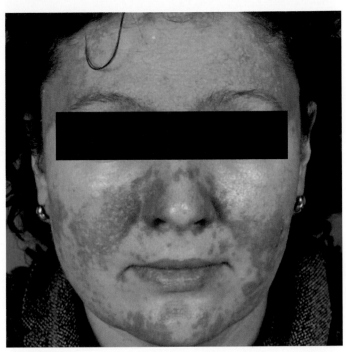

FIGURE 18.12 Reproduced with permission from Wolff K, Johnson R, Suurmond R: Fitzpatrick's Color Atlas & Synopsis of Clinical Dermatology, 5th ed. New York, McGraw Hill, Inc.; 2005:51.

20. **The answer is A.** (Chapter 251) Erythematous with well-marginated papules and plaques with silvery scale. Psoriasis rash is erythematous with well-marginated papules and plaques with silvery scale. The location of the rash is on the trunk, extensor surfaces, and scalp. Seborrheic dermatitis is described as greasy, yellow scales. Lichen planus is described as five Ps: purple, pruritic, polygonal, planar papules. Secondary syphilis is macular erythema on the trunk, abdomen, and inner extremities, followed by papular or papulosquamous lesions (Figure 18.12).

Traumatic Disorders

QUESTIONS

1. According to the American College of Surgeons, which of the following are level 1 trauma centers required to have?
   (A) 24-hour availability of surgeon in all subspecialties (including cardiac surgery/bypass capability)
   (B) 24-hour availability of trauma social worker
   (C) Helipad attached to the main hospital for air ambulance patients
   (D) Medical school affiliation with research program

2. EMS is called by the family of a 35-year-old man on warfarin for a mechanical heart valve after he fell off a 5-foot ladder in his kitchen, striking his head. He is confused, opens his eyes to speech, and localizes pain. His vital signs are BP 128/54, HR 60, SpO_2 99% on RA, RR 14, and his fingerstick glucose 89. A community hospital is 5 minutes away and a level 1 trauma center is 25 minutes away. Based on his presentation, which is the MOST APPROPRIATE?
   (A) Transfer to the community center due to concern for the patient's airway
   (B) Transfer to the community center due to the shorter transport time
   (C) Transfer to the trauma center due to mechanism of injury and anticoagulation status
   (D) Transfer to the trauma center due to physiologic criteria and anticoagulation status

3. EMS is called for a 22-year-old helmeted male motorcyclist who was traveling on a highway when he was sideswiped and crashed. On arrival he is comatose and has a Glasgow coma scale (GCS) of 3. His helmet was removed by EMS and he is brought to the nearest community hospital. His vital signs are BP 85/33, HR 140, SpO_2 89% on nonrebreather, and a RR 6. He has bilateral breath sounds. The NEXT BEST step in management for this patient is?
   (A) A FAST (focused assessment with sonography for trauma) examination should be performed.
   (B) An airway should be established with inline cervical spine stabilization.
   (C) Bilateral chest tubes should be inserted.
   (D) IV access with two large-bore IVs should be established.

4. A 47-year-old mechanic presents with a large laceration to the left antecubital fossa after a piece of metal he was hoisting fell onto him. He appears to have no other injuries and arrived by a private car from the garage holding pressure over the site with a piece of shirt. His vital signs are BP 115/74, HR 110, SpO_2 99% on RA, and a RR 14. Per his report, "there was a lot of blood on the ground." His primary survey notes no issues with airway or breathing, intravenous access is established in the right arm, and you are at a community hospital. He has diminished pulse with intact sensation and motor function. How would you proceed with evaluating the wound?
   (A) Consult general surgery to evaluate the wound
   (B) Remove the piece of clothing to examine the wound bed immediately
   (C) Tourniquet the arm proximal to injury until pulses are absent distally and examine the wound bed, marking the time of tourniquet
   (D) Transfer the patient for vascular surgery evaluation

5. During the evaluation of a 35-year-old woman who was the restrained driver in a rollover MVC, EMS established intravenous access and gave her 1 L of normal saline en route. Her vital signs on arrival are BP 87/45, HR 125, SpO$_2$ 99% on RA, and RR 16. She has a Glasgow coma scale (GCS) of 15 and bilateral breath sounds. She reports severe abdominal pain. She is at a trauma center. Her FAST (focused assessment with sonography for trauma) examination is positive. What is the NEXT BEST step for this patient?
   (A) CT scan of the abdomen and pelvis with IV contrast in radiology
   (B) Perform a diagnostic peritoneal lavage
   (C) Search for other causes of hypotension
   (D) Send the patient to the operating room for laparotomy

6. A 37-year-old woman is injured following an assault by her partner. She reports severe abdominal pain. A FAST (focused assessment with sonography for trauma) examination is positive. Her vital signs are BP 100/75, HR 110, SpO$_2$ 99% on RA, and a RR 15. What hemorrhage class is she currently exhibiting?
   (A) Class I
   (B) Class II
   (C) Class III
   (D) Class IV

7. A 78-year-old man presents after falling onto his right hip. No other injuries are noted, and the patient denies head strike, neck pain, chest, or abdominal pain. He reports pain with range of motion of the right hip. The right foot is neurovascularly intact and no deformity is noted. Plain films of the right hip are unremarkable. What is MOST sensitive and specific test to diagnose a hip fracture in this patient?
   (A) CT scan of the hip and pelvis
   (B) MRI of the hip
   (C) Nuclear medicine scintigraphy of the hip and pelvis
   (D) Repeat x-rays with stress views

8. A geriatric trauma patient is MORE LIKELY to have which of the following?
   (A) A lower mortality for similar injuries compared to young patients
   (B) Compensation from hypoperfusion of organs
   (C) Higher rate of epidural hematomas
   (D) Inability to tolerate large fluid boluses

9. A 72-year-old man with a history of atrial fibrillation on warfarin presents after a fall with head strike due to tripping on his dog's leash. He lives with his wife and has no other medical issues. His physical examination is notable only for a forehead abrasion. His international normalized ratio (INR) is 2.0, his Glasgow coma scale (GCS) is 15, and he ambulates without difficulty. His head CT is negative for acute hemorrhage. He reports that he feels safe going home. What is the NEXT BEST step?
   (A) Admission for observation for repeat head CT scan in 24 hours
   (B) Admission to the ICU for neuro checks
   (C) Consultation to neurosurgery for management
   (D) Discharge the patient with return precautions and discussion of delayed bleeding

10. A 97-year-old man presents after he was involved in a T-bone collision where he was struck on the driver's side. He reports severe chest pain. His physical examination is notable for left-sided chest wall tenderness. His only medication is lisinopril for hypertension. A chest x-ray shows a displaced posterior third right rib fracture. A chest CT reveals nondisplaced fractures of the second, fourth, and fifth ribs without pneumothorax or hemothorax. The patients' CT scans of his head, neck, abdomen, and pelvis reveal no other injuries. What is the NEXT BEST step in management for this patient?
   (A) Admission to the floor for pain control and incentive spirometry
   (B) Admission to the ICU for pain control and possible nerve blocks
   (C) Discharge home with oral pain medications and outpatient follow-up
   (D) Transfer to a skilled nursing facility for physical therapy

11. What is the MOST COMMON traumatic injury that leads to hospitalization in the elderly?
   (A) Arm fracture
   (B) Cervical spine fracture
   (C) Hip fracture
   (D) Traumatic brain injury

12. What is the MOST COMMON cause of blunt abdominal trauma in pregnancy?
   (A) Assault
   (B) Fall
   (C) Motor vehicle collision
   (D) Sporting accident

13. A 36-year-old woman, who is 36 weeks pregnant, presents after she was involved in a rollover motor vehicle collision. Another passenger in the compartment was killed. The patient is brought in on a backboard. EMS has established IV access and has administered 1 L of normal saline. Her vital signs are BP 75/63, HR 130, SpO_2 93% on RA, RR 20, and Glasgow coma scale (GCS) of 15. She has bilateral breath sounds. What is the NEXT BEST step in management?
    (A) Bilateral chest tubes
    (B) Initiate massive transfusion protocol and begin with 2 units of O-negatives packed red blood cells
    (C) Intubate and provide positive pressure ventilation
    (D) Place towel rolls under the right hip to tilt the patient 30 degrees to the left

14. What is the earliest age in weeks that a fetus is considered viable?
    (A) 16 weeks
    (B) 20 weeks
    (C) 24 weeks
    (D) 28 weeks

15. A 23-year-old woman, who is 30 weeks pregnant, presents after she fell onto her outstretched hand and lower abdomen. She reports mild abdominal cramping without bleeding. She is Rh positive. She reports no injuries to her head, neck, or chest. Her examination is notable only for mild fundal and suprapubic tenderness. An obstetrical ultrasound shows no placental abruption, no placenta previa, and fetal heart tones of 165. What is the NEXT BEST step?
    (A) Admit the patient to the trauma surgery service for observation
    (B) Admit the patient for cardiotocographic and fetal heart monitoring for 6 hours
    (C) Discharge the patient with close outpatient follow-up with her obstetrician
    (D) Discharge the patient with routine follow-up with her obstetrician

16. An 18-year-old woman presents after a high-speed motor vehicle collision with a seat belt sign and neck pain. Her vital signs are BP 100/70, HR 80, SpO_2 99% on RA, RR 16, and a Glasgow coma scale (GCS) of 15. A FAST (focused assessment with sonography for trauma) examination is negative, and after discussion with trauma surgery, the patient undergoes CT scans of the neck, chest, abdomen, and pelvis that are negative. It is discovered that she is pregnant with a quantitative beta-human chorionic gonadotropin (β-hCG) that is consistent with 7-week gestation and an intrauterine pregnancy is confirmed. What is the NEXT BEST for this patient?
    (A) Admit the patient for serial abdominal examinations
    (B) Discharge the patient with outpatient follow-up with obstetrics
    (C) Establish the Rh type of the patient
    (D) Perform a pelvic examination

17. A 33-year-old woman whose abdomen appears gravid presents after she was involved in a high-speed motor vehicle collision. She arrives via EMS in a cervical collar, intubated, with an IV established and 1 L of crystalloid administered prehospital. She is on a backboard but her uterus is being manually displaced to the left by a medic. Her vital signs are BP 80/55, HR 135, SpO_2 96% on 100 FiO_2, and mechanically ventilated with RR 18. She has a Glasgow coma scale (GCS) of 3T. She has bilateral breath sounds. The fundal height is noted to be 4 cm above the umbilicus. A FAST (focused assessment with sonography for trauma) examination is positive. A chest x-ray notes the tube in correct position with bilateral opacities. She is taken to a trauma center. An obstetric resident notes fetal heart tones of 80. What is the NEXT BEST step?
    (A) Admit the patient to the intensive care unit and resuscitate her with blood products
    (B) CT scanning of the patient with CT scanning of the head, neck, chest, abdomen, and pelvis
    (C) Have the obstetrics team perform an emergency cesarean section in the emergency department
    (D) Transfer the patient to the operating room for exploratory laparotomy with trauma surgery and obstetrics

18. A 28-year-old man is ejected from a car and is brought to the emergency department by EMS intubated with a Glasgow coma scale (GCS) of 3. A cervical collar is in place and the patient has bilateral breath sounds. What is your goal mean arterial pressure (MAP) for this patient?
    (A) 50 mm Hg
    (B) 65 mm Hg
    (C) 80 mm Hg
    (D) 125 mm Hg

19. Which injury is MOST LIKELY to require emergent neurosurgical intervention?
    (A) Diffuse axonal injury
    (B) Diffuse cerebral edema
    (C) Epidural hematoma
    (D) Subdural hematoma

20. A 22-year-old woman is thrown from the back of motorcycle without a helmet. Upon arrival EMS finds her to be comatose with agonal respirations and intubates her. En route she is noted to have a seizure and is given midazolam. On arrival in the emergency department, she has a Glasgow coma scale (GCS) of 3 and a fixed, dilated right pupil. This is MOST consistent with which type of herniation?
    (A) Central transtentorial herniation
    (B) Cerebellotonsillar herniation
    (C) Uncal herniation
    (D) Upward posterior fossa herniation

21. A 25-year-old man is assaulted in a bar fight and beaten by multiple people. When he arrives in the emergency department, he opens his eyes to pain, makes incomprehensible sounds, and withdraws from pain. What is his Glasgow coma scale score?
    (A) 3
    (B) 6
    (C) 8
    (D) 9

22. What does Figure 19.1 represent?

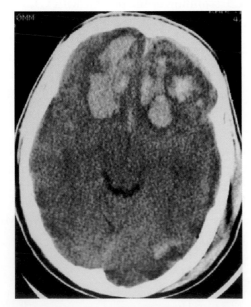

FIGURE 19.1 Image used with permission of Jack Fountain, Jr., MD, Emory University and Grady Memorial Hospital.

(A) Cerebral contusion with hemorrhagic progression
(B) Diffuse axonal injury
(C) Diffuse edema
(D) Subdural hematoma

23. An 18-year-old male football player is struck on the field while wearing his helmet and has loss of consciousness for 1 minute. After the event he vomits once. He has no other injuries. A CT scan of the head is ordered at triage and returns negative. The patient's Glasgow coma scale (GCS) is 15. His neurological examination is notable for slow responses. The patient asks if he can return to practice tomorrow. What is your response?
    (A) No, he cannot return until he is asymptomatic for 48 hours.
    (B) No, he cannot return until he is cleared by his primary care, neurology, or a sports medicine physician.
    (C) Yes, he can return tomorrow as long as he is symptom-free.
    (D) Yes, he can return tomorrow because the CT scan was negative.

24. Which of the following is an unstable injury of the cervical spine?
    (A) Anterior subluxation
    (B) Bilateral facet dislocation
    (C) Simple wedge compression fracture
    (D) Spinous process avulsion fracture

25. Which type of spinal fracture is associated with a flexion-distraction mechanism and is associated with seat-belt signs?
    (A) Burst fracture
    (B) Chance fracture
    (C) Fracture of the lateral mass
    (D) Unilateral facet dislocation

26. A 35-year-old man presents after he was involved in a high-speed motor vehicle collision. His physical examination is notable for 0/5 strength in his bilateral lower extremities, no sensation below his umbilicus, no rectal tone, and priapism. His presentation is MOST consistent with which syndrome?
    (A) Anterior cord syndrome
    (B) Brown-Sequard syndrome
    (C) Central cord syndrome
    (D) Cord transection syndrome

27. A 55-year-old man presents after he fell approximately 15 feet from a ladder onto both of his feet. He reports this occurred yesterday and since then he has been having severe back pain, difficulty with urinating, an episode of fecal incontinence, and increasing leg weakness. His physical examination is notable for 4/5 strength in bilateral lower extremities, decreased rectal tone, and diminished perineal sensation. What is the MOST LIKELY cause of this constellation of findings?
    (A) Anterior cord syndrome due to retropulsion of a fracture fragment
    (B) Ligamentous injury leading to disrupted blood flow to the spinal cord
    (C) Retropulsion of a fracture fragment causing compression of the cauda equina
    (D) Transection of the spinal cord

28. A 43-year-old man presents with severe mid back pain after being involved in a motor vehicle collision. His physical examination is notable for flaccid paralysis of both legs and decreased perception of temperature and light touch. He does have some sensation of the perineum and voluntary contraction of the external anal sphincter. What is the name of this clinical condition?
    (A) Brown-Sequard syndrome
    (B) Central cord syndrome
    (C) Neurogenic shock
    (D) Sacral sparing

29. A 23-year-old man presents with quadriplegia and decreased respiratory effort after diving head first into a swimming pool. He is intubated by EMS on scene. He is taken to a trauma center where he is noted to be hypotensive despite 2 L of fluid and 3 units of blood. CT scans of his head, neck, chest, abdomen, and pelvis reveal only a burst fracture at C3 with retropulsion. What is the BEST NEXT treatment for this patient's hypotension?
    (A) Atropine
    (B) Normal saline
    (C) Packed red blood cells
    (D) Phenylephrine

30. A 23-year-old man presents after he sustained multiple blows to the face during an altercation. He has a swollen right eye and blood from both nares. His triage vital signs are T 99.7°C, HR 80, BP 120/75, and RR 18 with SpO$_2$ 100%. His physical examination reveals no other injuries. He has a Glasgow coma scale (GCS) of 15, pupils are equal round and reactive to light, extraocular movements are intact, and he is conversant. His c-spine is nontender. What is the NEXT BEST step in management?
    (A) Assess visual acuity
    (B) CT of the brain
    (C) Maxillofacial CT scan
    (D) Plain films of the face

31. A 75-year-old man with atrial fibrillation on warfarin presents after he was the restrained driver involved in a motor vehicle collision at highway speed. The airbag deployed, striking him in the face, and he has a swollen right eye with a proptotic appearance. His vital signs are T 97.8°C, HR 80, BP 175/83, RR 16, and SpO$_2$ 98%. His physical examination reveals no other injuries. He has a Glasgow coma scale (GCS) of 15, pupils are equal, round, and reactive to light, and his extraocular movements are intact. Visual acuity is 20/20 in the left eye, but 20/200 in the right eye. His c-spine is nontender. A FAST (focused assessment with sonography for trauma) examination is normal. What is the NEXT BEST step in management?
    (A) CT of the face
    (B) Lateral canthotomy
    (C) Maxillofacial surgery consult
    (D) Ophthalmology consult

32. A 45-year-old man with no significant past medical history presents after an altercation where he sustained multiple blows to the face. He has a swollen left eye with a sunken appearance and blood from both nares. His triage vital signs are T 98.3°C, HR 105, BP 123/85, RR 16, and SpO$_2$ 97% on RA. His physical examination reveals no other obvious injuries. He has a Glasgow coma scale (GCS) of 15. Pupils are equal, round, and reactive to light. Extraocular movements are intact except he is unable perform upward deviation of the left eye. His visual acuity is 20/20 in both eyes. His cervical spine is nontender. What is the NEXT BEST step in management?
    (A) Maxillofacial CT scan
    (B) Maxillofacial surgery consult
    (C) Perform a lateral canthotomy
    (D) Ophthalmology consult

33. What does Figure 19.2 show?

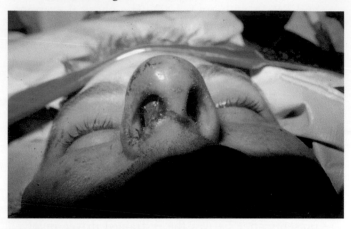

FIGURE 19.2 Reproduced with permission from Knoop K, Stack L, Storrow A, Thurman RJ: Atlas of Emergency Medicine, 3rd ed. 2010, McGraw-Hill, New York.

(A) LeFort fracture
(B) Nasal fracture
(C) Nasal laceration
(D) Septal hematoma

34. A patient presents after being struck in the face with a baseball bat. He has a step-off along the lower jaw with bleeding. The examiner is unable to break a tongue depressor, while the patient is biting down on it. What is the MOST LIKELY injury?
(A) Buccal laceration
(B) Open mandible fracture
(C) Open maxilla fracture
(D) Tooth fracture

35. What does Figure 19.3 demonstrate?

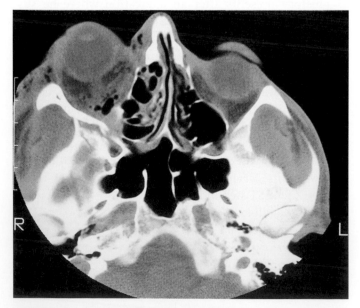

FIGURE 19.3 Reproduced with permission from Knoop K, Stack L, Storrow A, Thurman RJ: Atlas of Emergency Medicine, 3rd ed. 2010, McGraw-Hill, New York.

(A) Lens dislocation
(B) Maxillary fracture
(C) Retrobulbar hematoma
(D) Vomer fracture

36. Which of the following is NOT a hard sign of laryngotracheal injury in patients with neck trauma?
(A) Dysphonia
(B) Hemoptysis
(C) Stridor
(D) Tracheal deviation

37. What is the leading cause of mortality from penetrating neck trauma?
(A) Associated proximate injury
(B) Exsanguination from vascular injury
(C) Spinal cord injury
(D) Unstable airway

38. A 25-year-old baseball player was struck in the neck with a baseball. He presents with miosis and ptosis of the right eye. Which diagnostic modality should be utilized initially to screen this patient for his presumed injury?
(A) Diagnostic four-vessel cerebral angiography
(B) MDCTA (multidetector CT angiography)
(C) MRI (magnetic resonance imaging)
(D) Ultrasound

39. What is the MOST COMMON mechanism of death in strangulation injuries?
(A) Acute airway obstruction
(B) Bilateral vascular occlusion
(C) Carotid body mediated cardiac dysrhythmia
(D) Spinal cord transection

40. A 62-year-old man is involved in a motor vehicle crash at 35 mph. Glasgow coma scale (GCS) is 15. He is complaining of shortness of breath. He has a contusion, but no tenderness on palpation of the chest wall. He has no apparent distracting injuries. Why can't the NEXUS Rules for Chest Radiography be applied?
(A) Complaint of shortness of breath
(B) Patient's age
(C) Presence of chest wall contusion
(D) Speed of travel

41. A 30-year-old motorcycle driver was found unresponsive at the scene of a collision and brought to the emergency department. You intubated the patient without difficulty, but a few minutes after intubation the patient suffers a brady-asystolic arrest. Please refer to the postintubation chest x-ray that was obtained (Figure 19.4). What is the MOST APPROPRIATE NEXT course of action?

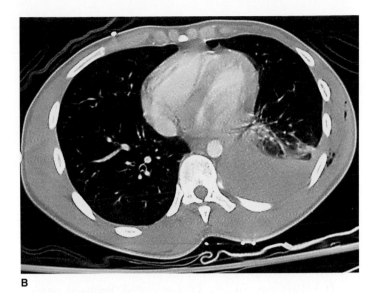

B

FIGURE 19.5 Reproduced with permission from Block J, Jordanov MI, Stack LB, Thurman RJ (eds): The Atlas of Emergency Radiology. McGraw-Hill, Inc., 2013.

(A) Blood continues to drain at 200 cc/h for 1 hour
(B) Greater than 1000 cc blood is evacuated immediately after the procedure
(C) Greater than 1500 cc blood is evacuated immediately after the procedure
(D) The patient is hemodynamically unstable requiring persistent blood product administration

43. A 48-year-old man was stabbed in the chest. His chest x-ray is negative for pneumothorax. He has no shortness of breath or chest pain other than at the site of the entrance wound. What is the MOST APPROPRIATE management?
(A) CT scan of the chest, and if negative discharge to home
(B) Discharge to home
(C) Repeat chest x-ray or bedside transthoracic ultrasound in 6 hours, and if negative discharge to home
(D) Transthoracic ultrasound, and if negative discharge to home

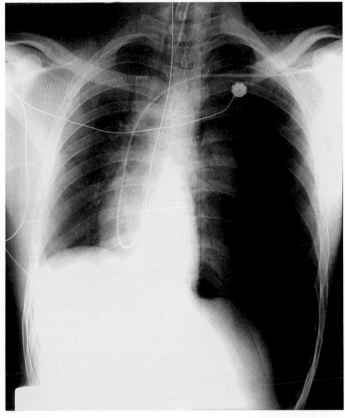

FIGURE 19.4 Reproduced with permission from Schwartz DT (ed): Emergency Radiology, Case Studies. 2008 McGraw-Hill Inc

(A) Perform immediate needle decompression
(B) Perform immediate transthoracic ultrasound
(C) Perform immediate tube thoracostomy
(D) Withdraw the endotracheal tube 3 cm

42. A 42-year-old man was stabbed in the chest and had the following CT finding. Tube thoracostomy was performed. Which of the following would NOT be an indication for surgical exploration (Figure 19.5)?

44. A 25-year-old man presents after falling off a horse onto his back. He has stable vital signs and decreased breath sounds on the left side on primary survey. What is the MOST APPROPRIATE NEXT step in the management of this patient?
(A) AP chest x-ray
(B) Bedside transthoracic ultrasound
(C) Immediate needle decompression of the chest
(D) Immediate tube thoracostomy

45. What is the MOST common structure injured in penetrating trauma to the heart?
    (A) Left atrium
    (B) Left ventricle
    (C) Right atrium
    (D) Right ventricle

46. A 30-year-old man presents with a penetrating left parasternal wound to community hospital. He is noted to have distended neck veins, with HR 102 and BP of 106/82. After assessing that the patient has a stable airway and IV access, what would the NEXT MOST APPROPRIATE course of action be?
    (A) Obtain a chest x-ray
    (B) Obtain a CT scan of the chest
    (C) Perform an eFAST (extended Focused assessment with sonography for trauma) examination
    (D) Transfer to a trauma center

47. What is the MOST COMMON mechanism of blunt cardiac injury?
    (A) Direct impact to the chest wall
    (B) Injury due to compression between the sternum and spine
    (C) Rapid changes in intrathoracic pressure
    (D) Rapid deceleration causing shearing injury at points of fixation (right atrium, vena cava)

48. Which of the following MOST accurately describes commotio cordis?
    (A) A result of structural damage to the chest wall
    (B) Asystole as a result of high-impact direct chest wall trauma
    (C) Ventricular fibrillation due to a congenital heart defect
    (D) Ventricular fibrillation induced by low-impact chest wall trauma at the time of ventricular repolarization

49. A 34-year-old woman is the restrained driver in a motor vehicle collision. She arrives complaining of chest pain. She has normal vital signs and has a negative radiographic workup as well as a normal ECG. What is the MOST APPROPRIATE NEXT course of action?
    (A) Admit to a monitored bed for serial troponins
    (B) Discharge to home, no further monitoring or testing is indicated
    (C) Monitor for 4 to 6 hours, discharge if no new complaints and EKG remains normal
    (D) Obtain STAT transthoracic echocardiogram

50. A 60-year-old man is involved in a high-speed motor vehicle crash. Vital signs are stable. As a primary survey adjunct, an AP chest x-ray is obtained. The mediastinum measures 10 cm and the trachea appears laterally displaced. What is the MOST APPROPRIATE NEXT course of action?
    (A) Administer sodium nitroprusside to maintain systolic blood pressure <120
    (B) Obtain immediate aortography
    (C) Obtain immediate CT angiography
    (D) Obtain immediate transesophageal echocardiography

51. What is the commonly injured intra-abdominal organ associated with sports-related injuries?
    (A) Duodenum
    (B) Liver
    (C) Pancreas
    (D) Spleen

52. Regarding diaphragmatic injuries, which of the following statements is CORRECT?
    (A) Diaphragmatic rupture is commonly seen in penetrating trauma but not in blunt trauma.
    (B) Diaphragmatic rupture usually occurs on the right side.
    (C) Signs and symptoms of diaphragmatic rupture are usually nonspecific and easily attributed to other associated injuries.
    (E) Undiagnosed diaphragmatic rupture is not associated with any clinically significant complications.

53. A 28-year-old man involved in a motor vehicle crash arrives with a HR 120 and BP 88. Primary survey with adjunct chest and pelvis x-rays is significant for multiple rib fractures. Secondary survey is significant for a soft but diffusely tender abdomen. Intravenous crystalloid resuscitation is initiated. What is the MOST APPROPRIATE NEXT step in the management of this patient?
    (A) CT scan of the head, cervical spine, chest, abdomen, and pelvis
    (B) Diagnostic peritoneal aspiration or lavage
    (C) FAST (focused assessment with sonography for trauma)
    (D) Institute massive transfusion protocol

54. A 32-year-old man involved in a motor vehicle crash arrives to the emergency department with a HR 120 and BP 88. Primary survey with adjunct chest and pelvis x-rays and secondary survey were performed. Multiple rib fractures were seen on chest x-ray. After 1000 cc IV crystalloid, the BP remained 88, and the HR remained 118. FAST (focused assessment with sonography for trauma) was negative, and on diagnostic peritoneal aspiration (DPA), 15 cc blood was aspirated. What is the MOST APPROPRIATE NEXT step in the management of this patient?
    (A) Administer tranexamic acid and admit to the surgical intensive care unit
    (B) Begin transfusing blood products, administer tranexamic acid (TXA), and page the surgeon to take the patient emergently for exploratory laparotomy
    (C) Immediately obtain CT of the head, cervical spine, chest, abdomen, and pelvis
    (D) Transfuse blood products in a 1:1:1 ratio and admit to the surgical intensive care unit

55. A 24-year-old woman presents with an anterior abdominal stab wound. Her HR is 98, and BP is 118/72. Primary survey with adjunct chest and pelvis x-rays as well as a secondary survey are performed. X-rays are negative for obvious intraperitoneal air. Physical examination is remarkable only for an anterior penetrating abdominal wound with localized tenderness. IV crystalloid is administered. What is the MOST APPROPRIATE STEP in the management of this patient?
    (A) Diagnostic peritoneal aspiration or lavage
    (B) Immediate CT scan of the abdomen and pelvis
    (C) Local wound exploration
    (D) The patient should be taken to the operating room for exploratory laparotomy

56. Regarding duodenal injuries, which of the following statements is TRUE?
    (A) Because the duodenum ruptures into the retroperitoneum, patients most often have early presentation of sepsis
    (B) Duodenal hematomas can lead to gastric outlet obstruction
    (C) Duodenal injuries are most often symptomatic on initial presentation
    (D) The duodenum can rupture and the contents generally spill into the peritoneal cavity leading to peritonitis

57. A 50-year-old man presents with a penetrating wound to the left flank, reportedly from a 6-inch knife. Vital signs are stable. After primary and secondary surveys are complete, what would be the MOST APPROPRIATE NEXT step in the management of this patient?
    (A) CT scan abdomen and pelvis with triple contrast
    (B) FAST (Focused assessment with sonography for trauma)
    (C) Immediately surgical consultation for exploratory laparotomy
    (D) Local wound exploration to determine depth of injury

58. A 26-year-old man presents after being stabbed in the right flank. Which of the following statements is TRUE?
    (A) A CT scan with IV contrast provides both anatomic and functional information in the evaluation of potential renal injury.
    (B) If the patient does not have gross or microscopic hematuria, renal injury can be excluded.
    (C) In patients with penetrating trauma to the flank, IV pyelography is sensitive in the detection of renal injury.
    (D) The amount of hematuria correlates with the extent and severity of renal injury.

59. A 60-year-old woman was kicked in the flank by her horse. Her HR is 72 and BP is 132/68. She has minimal pain on examination. Urinalysis shows 20 red blood cells/high power field. What is the MOST APPROPRIATE NEXT step to evaluate for potential renal injury in this patient?
    (A) Immediate CT scan of the abdomen and pelvis with IV contrast
    (B) Immediate IV pyelography
    (C) Immediate renal ultrasound
    (D) No further testing is indicated

60. Regarding penetrating trauma to the buttock, which of the following statements is TRUE?
    (A) Guaiac negative stool excludes rectal injury.
    (B) Penetrating trauma to the upper gluteal zone has lower incidence of major injury than trauma to the lower gluteal zone.
    (C) Sciatic nerve injury is common.
    (D) Vascular injury due to stab wounds to the buttock most commonly involves the superior gluteal artery.

61. What is MOST COMMONLY MISSED injury in penetrating flank trauma?
    (A) Occult colon injury
    (B) Occult duodenal injury
    (C) Occult pancreatic injury
    (D) Occult vascular injury

62. Which of the following statements is TRUE regarding traumatic ureteral injuries?
    (A) In stable patients with suspected ureteral injury, IV pyelography is the initial diagnostic study of choice.
    (B) Isolated ureteral injury is relatively rare in trauma patients.
    (C) The absence of hematuria excludes ureteral injury.
    (D) The majority of ureteral injuries are due to blunt trauma.

63. A 45-year-old unrestrained driver in a motor vehicle collision presents with the findings shown in Figure 19.6. Which of the following statements about this condition is MOST ACCURATE?

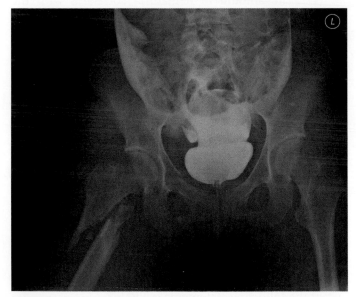

FIGURE 19.6 J.E. Tintinalli, J.S. Stapczynski, O.J. Ma, D. Yearly, G.D. Meckler, D.M. Cline: Tintinalli's Emergency Medicine: A Comprehensive Study Guide, 9th Edition: Copyright © McGraw Hill Education. All rights reserved.

    (A) Common physical findings include lower abdominal pain, tenderness, and perineal or scrotal edema.
    (B) Retrograde cystogram is no longer the gold standard diagnostic modality.

    (C) This injury is seen in approximately 20% of blunt abdominal trauma cases.
    (D) This injury can be excluded with a negative ultrasound.

64. Which of the following findings is NOT part of the classic triad associated with posterior urethral injury?
    (A) Blood at the urethral meatus
    (B) High riding prostate
    (C) Perineal hematoma
    (D) Urinary retention

65. A 25-year-old man presents after experiencing an acute onset of pain and penile deformity during sexual intercourse. He presents with an ecchymotic, deformed penis. The MOST APPROPRIATE NEXT course of action would be:
    (A) Color Doppler ultrasound
    (B) CT scan of the abdomen and pelvis
    (C) Immediate retrograde urethrogram
    (D) Immediate urologic consultation

66. A 43-year-old woman presents with flank pain after falling off a horse. She is hemodynamically stable. On physical examination, a right flank contusion is noted. What is the NEXT MOST APPROPRIATE NEXT course of action?
    (A) Immediate CT scan of the abdomen and pelvis with IV contrast
    (B) Immediate renal ultrasound
    (C) No further action unless there is gross hematuria
    (D) Urinalysis with basic and microscopic examination

67. A patient presents with a stab wound to the forearm. He has weakness on abduction of his fingers and reports decreased sensation of the little finger. His examination raises concern for injury to which nerve?
    (A) Median nerve
    (B) Musculocutaneous nerve
    (C) Radial nerve
    (D) Ulnar nerve

68. A patient presents with penetrating trauma to the lower extremity. EMS reported large blood loss at the scene, but there is no active hemorrhage on presentation to the emergency department. There is a small hematoma that does not appear pulsatile or expanding. What is the MOST APPROPRIATE NEXT step in the evaluation of the injury?
    (A) Emergent vascular surgery consultation
    (B) Immediate ankle-brachial index
    (C) Immediate CT angiography
    (D) No further evaluation is needed

69. Which of the following is NOT an advantage of CT angiography over conventional catheter angiography in the evaluation of vascular injuries of the extremities?
    (A) CT angiography allows for evaluation of extravascular injuries.
    (B) CT angiography allows for superior visualization of the tibial vessels.
    (C) CT angiography is less expensive than conventional catheter angiography.
    (D) CT angiography provides higher resolution images.

70. Which of the following statements regarding wound management in extremity trauma is TRUE?
    (A) Antibiotic administration is indicated in the management of gunshot and stab wounds to the extremities because the rate of infection is high.
    (B) Extremity wounds with major tissue destruction should be closed immediately.
    (C) Irrigation of wounds with antiseptic solutions decreases the rate of wound infection.
    (D) The most important factor in preventing wound infection in penetrating extremity trauma is copious irrigation.

ANSWERS

1. The answer is A. (Chapter 254) It is important to understand the resources that are available at a level 1 trauma center including 24-hour availability of all surgical specialists, coronary bypass, neuroradiology, and hemodialysis. The level 1 trauma center is also required to have organized research and a program that establishes injury prevention and education efforts.

2. The answer is D. (Chapter 254) This patient presents with a significant physiological derangement based on his Glasgow coma scale (GCS) of 12 and his anticoagulated status. While the trauma center is further away, the patient will likely benefit from having neurosurgery available and the other resources of the level 1 trauma center. From the question stem there is no concern for airway compromise imminently.

3. The answer is B. (Chapter 254) This patient is severely injured with evidence of diminished mental status, hypoxia, hypotension, and tachycardia. There are multiple priorities including establishing IV access, resuscitation of the patient with crystalloid and blood. However, in advanced trauma life support (ATLS) airway takes priority, so with a Glasgow coma scale (GCS) of 3, poor respiratory drive with RR of 6, and saturation of 89% on nonrebreather, the patient needs a definitive airway.

4. The answer is C. (Chapter 254) This patient has an unknown wound to the left antecubital fossa with evidence of reduced perfusion based on his physical examination. The most prudent choice would be able to establish a tourniquet proximal to the wound to evaluate the wound bed. Removing the clothing immediately is incorrect because if there is an underlying venous or arterial injury you will expose the patient to unnecessary blood loss and visualization of the wound bed will not be accomplished. Consultation with general surgery or transfer for vascular surgery is reasonable once the wound bed has been visualized and the injury has been established.

5. The answer is D. (Chapter 254) The patient has a positive FAST (focused assessment with sonography for trauma) examination in the setting of trauma. This is consistent with hemoperitoneum, most likely from a solid organ injury. This patient should be taken to the OR due to her hypotension. She should be concomitantly resuscitated with blood products. CT scan should be omitted given the patient is in class III shock and has an operative source of bleeding. CT scanning would be appropriate if this patient was hemodynamically stable.

TABLE 19.1	Classification of Hemorrhage Based on Estimated Blood Loss at Initial Presentation			
	Class I	Class II	Class III	Class IV
Blood loss (mL)*	Up to 750	750–1500	1500–2000	>2000
Blood loss (% blood volume)	Up to 15	15–30	30–40	40
Pulse rate (beats/min)	<100	100–120	120–140	>140
Blood pressure	Normal	Normal	Decreased	Decreased
Pulse pressure	Normal or increased	Decreased	Decreased	Decreased

*Assumes a 70-kg patient with a preinjury circulating blood volume of 5 L.

Reproduced with permission from J.E. Tintinalli, J.S. Stapczynski, O.J. Ma, D. Yealy, G.D. Meckler, D.M. Cline: Tintinalli's Emergency Medicine: A Comprehensive Study Guide, 9th Edition. McGraw-Hill Education; 2020.

6. The answer is B. (Chapter 254) The patient is in class II shock based on the classification of hemorrhage used by the American College of Surgeons (Table 19.1). She has experience between 750 and 1500 mL of blood loss, is tachycardic, and has a decreased pulse pressure with a normal blood pressure.

7. The answer is B. (Chapter 255) The patient presents after a fall with continued hip pain. The concern with persistent pain is an occult hip fracture. While CT scan imaging is fast, it can miss some occult fractures. Nuclear medicine scintigraphy is sensitive but less specific. Stress views are not typically performed in the emergency department. MRI is the best choice due to its sensitivity and specificity.

8. The answer is D. (Chapter 255) Geriatric patients have more difficulty tolerating large fluid boluses than younger patients due to their decreased myocytes and other cardiovascular aging. They are at increased risk of mortality and have decreased ability to compensate for hypoperfusion. They have a lower rate of epidurals and higher rate of subdural hematomas.

9. The answer is D. (Chapter 255) Elderly anticoagulated patients are known to have a low rate of delayed hemorrhage. Current practice patterns vary, but generally patients with a negative head CT scan and stable home situation without a supratherapeutic international normalized ratio (INR) may be discharged home with outpatient follow-up and return precautions.

10. The answer is B. (Chapter 255) Rib fractures are a serious cause of morbidity and mortality in the elderly patient population. Multiple rib fractures in an elderly patient will require aggressive pain control and close monitoring in an intensive care setting. The other options don't allow for sufficient monitoring for this patient.

11. **The answer is C.** (Chapter 255) Hip fractures are the most common injury that leads to hospitalizations. A recent study reports decreased morbidity and mortality, the sooner the hip is repaired. Traumatic brain and cervical spine fracture often lead to hospitalization but are less common. Rarely do arm fractures require hospitalization unless there is neurovascular compromise or concomitant medical or social issues.

12. **The answer is C.** (Chapter 256) Motor vehicle collisions are the most common source of blunt abdominal trauma for pregnant women, followed by falls and direct assaults. These patients can have concomitant multisystem injuries, but the abdomen is at particular risk due to seat belts, steering wheels, and airbags.

13. **The answer is D.** (Chapter 256) Due to the mechanism of injury, this patient has been placed on a backboard in the supine position. At her gestational age this causes significant compression of the inferior vena cava and uterus and can lead to up to a 1/3 loss in her circulating blood volume, leading to severe hypotension unresponsive to other maneuvers. This initial step must be done as other sources of hypotension are investigated. She has bilateral breath sounds with an acceptable respiratory status and Glasgow coma scale (GCS), so immediate airway interventions or chest tubes are not indicated at this point.

14. **The answer is C.** (Chapter 256) Twenty-four weeks is generally considered the age at which the fetus is viable, although some institutions lower that to 22. Ideally a multidisciplinary discussion between emergency medicine, neonatology, obstetrics, and trauma surgery based on the institution's unique resources should occur to determine the gestational age cutoff.

15. **The answer is B.** (Chapter 256) The next best step for this patient is to monitor for uterine irritability (3 or more contractions per hour). Uterine irritability is the most sensitive clinical finding for placental abruption. A negative ultrasound does not rule out placental abruption.

16. **The answer is C.** (Chapter 256) This patient was involved in a trauma and incidentally noted to have an early intrauterine pregnancy. The Rh status of this patient must be established. If she is Rh negative, Rhogam should be administered. She may then be discharged given the negative traumatic workup.

17. **The answer is D.** (Chapter 256) This question involves a severely injured woman who happens to be pregnant with unknown gestational age. The mother's management priorities include surgical control of bleeding and resuscitation. She should be treated as any other hemodynamically unstable patient with free fluid in the abdomen and taken to the operating room. Treat the mother first, consult with obstetrics for the fetus, and keep the patient tilted 30 degrees to minimize the chance of the supine hypotension syndrome. CT scanning would be more appropriate if the patient was hemodynamically stable, but given her unstable vital signs and positive FAST (focused assessment with sonography for trauma) examination, emergent operative exploration for hemorrhage control is indicated.

18. **The answer is C.** (Chapter 257) This patient is severely brain injured and likely has a loss of normal autoregulation. Therefore, mean arterial pressures (MAPs) should be maintained greater than or equal to 80 mm Hg, but not greater than 120 mm Hg, to promote cerebral perfusion despite impaired ability of the cerebral vasculature to autoregulate.

19. **The answer is C.** (Chapter 257) An epidural hematoma is most likely to need emergent neurosurgical intervention. On CT scan it appears as a biconcave hyperdensity that doesn't cross suture lines. Epidural hematoma is more likely to occur in younger patients. Immediate decompression is often required for this neurosurgical emergency. Subdural, diffuse axonal injury, and diffuse cerebral edema are also neurosurgical emergencies but are less likely to need immediate surgical intervention.

20. **The answer is C.** (Chapter 257) This patient presents after a severe head injury and has had a seizure. She now has a fixed, dilated right pupil most consistent with uncal herniation. The other herniation syndromes listed usually demonstrate pinpoint pupils, with more severe cases progressing to fixed and dilated bilateral pupils.

21. **The answer is C.** (Chapter 257) This patient has a Glasgow coma scale (GCS) of 8. He gets 2 points for opening his eyes to pain, 2 points for incomprehensible sounds, and 4 points for his ability to withdraw to pain.

22. **The answer is A.** (Chapter 257) This patient has a CT scan demonstrating delayed intraparenchymal hemorrhages from a traumatic contusion. Early CT for diffuse axonal injury may appear normal, or small hemorrhages may be seen at grey-white junction. Subdural hematoma crosses suture lines and are hyperdense if acute and hypodense if chronic. Diffuse swelling leads to

compressed, slit-like ventricles and can be seen in severe traumatic brain injury.

23. **The answer is B.** (Chapter 257) This patient has suffered a concussion and needs brain rest. Avoiding repeat head trauma is a key part of concussion treatment. He should not be allowed to return to sports until he is cleared by a physician who is able to follow him longitudinally and can provide definitive return-to-activity directions. This is an area of growing research and practice variation.

24. **The answer is B.** (Chapter 258) A bilateral facet dislocation occurs when the articular masses of one vertebra dislocate anteriorly and superiorly from the articular surfaces of the adjacent vertebrae below. This is highly unstable and requires immediate neurosurgical consultation and intervention. All the other choices are stable injuries.

25. **The answer is B.** (Chapter 258) Chance fractures are often associated with seatbelt injuries from a lap belt alone. There is anterior compression and associated transverse compression fracture through the vertebral body with displacement of the middle and posterior ligamentous structures. This can lead to cord compression. A burst fracture is more common with axial loading. Unilateral facet injuries are associated with rotational energy. Lateral mass fracture are rare and from axial loading and rotation of the cervical spine.

26. **The answer is D.** (Chapter 258) This patient has clinical evidence of a complete spinal cord transection at the level of the lower thoracic spine at approximately T10. He has no motor function or sensory function, which is inconsistent with the other incomplete spinal cord syndromes, and he has no evidence of sacral sparing. Patients with anterior cord syndrome present with loss of motor function and pain and temperature sensation distal to the injury with vibration, position, and tactile sense preserved. Brown-Seguard syndrome is characterized by ipsilateral loss of motor function, proprioception and vibratory sense and contralateral loss of pain and temperature sensation. Central cord syndrome with decreased strength and to a lesser extent decreased pain and temperature sensation more in the upper than lower extremities.

27. **The answer is C.** (Chapters 258 and 279) This patient's history is consistent with an axial load mechanism leading to a possible burst fracture with retropulsion of a fracture fragment into the spinal canal, leading to a progressive cauda equina syndrome. His examination demonstrates decreased perineal sensation, poor rectal tone, and lower extremity weakness suggestive of cauda equina syndrome. Consultation for emergent neurosurgical evaluation and concomitant MRI imaging of the spinal cord is warranted. His presentation is not consistent with anterior cord syndrome, complete transection of the spinal cord, or acute ischemic infarction of the spinal cord.

28. **The answer is D.** (Chapter 258) This patient has evidence of sacral sparing despite evidence of a spinal cord injury, likely from a burst fracture. Neurogenic shock is a form of hypotension in patients with higher spinal cord lesions leading to loss of sympathetic tone. Central cord syndrome leads to weakness in all four extremities as well as loss of pain and temperature sensation. Brown-Sequard syndrome is due to a transverse hemisection of the spinal cord and leads to ipsilateral spastic paresis, loss of proprioception and vibratory sensation and contralateral loss of pain and temperature sensation.

29. **The answer is D.** (Chapter 258) This patient has evidence of neurogenic shock related to loss of his sympathetic tone. Hemorrhagic shock has been excluded with his CT scans, which do not reveal any other injuries, so blood transfusion is not indicated. He has already received an adequate fluid challenge and has not responded to a 2-L bolus of saline. There is no mention of significant bradycardia, so atropine isn't warranted. Phenylephrine is the preferred pressor due to its alpha-1 agonism. Dopamine can be used if there is concomitant bradycardia.

30. **The answer is A.** (Chapter 259) The patient presents with maxillofacial trauma and he should have a maxillofacial CT to get thin cuts through the face to assess for facial fractures. However, before this is done his visual acuity should be assessed to determine whether he has a vision-threatening injury such as a retrobulbar hematoma that requires emergent intervention. Plain films of the face are less sensitive than a CT.

31. **The answer is B.** (Chapter 259) This patient has a suspected retrobulbar hematoma, which appears to be creating an ocular compartment syndrome. This can lead to acute ischemic optic neuropathy and vision loss. This is an emergent condition, which requires the patient undergo a lateral canthotomy as soon as possible to reduce ocular pressure and ischemia to the nerve. His anticoagulation status makes the retrobulbar hematoma more likely. The other choices listed should not delay performance of a lateral canthotomy.

32. **The answer is B.** (Chapter 259) This patient has clinical evidence of entrapment of the inferior rectus muscle of the eye leading to a gaze palsy. This requires emergent consultation to ear, nose and throat (ENT), maxillofacial surgery, or plastic surgery depending on the local practice.

The CT should be done, but the clinical picture alone warrants consultation since decompression is time-sensitive. Lateral canthotomy is indicated for retrobulbar hematoma leading to orbital compartment syndrome and is not appropriate in this case.

33. **The answer is D.** (Chapter 259) This photograph shows a septal hematoma. It can be seen in the right nare as a boggy, pale area of swelling. The hematoma must be incised to prevent pressure necrosis of the cartilage and an eventual saddle nose deformity.

34. **The answer is B.** (Chapter 259) This patient has an open mandible fracture. Typically, treatment requires consultation with an oral and maxillofacial surgeon for operative management and jaw wiring. IV antibiotics are also given due to this being an open fracture as well. The tongue-blade test can be used to assess for mandible fracture. The patient bites on to the tongue depressor and the examiner attempts to break it by twisting. If the patient is able to keep the tongue depressor compressed, it is unlikely that a fracture is present. A buccal laceration, maxilla fracture, or single tooth fracture are less likely to prevent the patient from being able to bite down adequately on a tongue depressor.

35. **The answer is C.** (Chapter 259) This image shows a retrobulbar hematoma with orbital emphysema. Depending on the clinical examination, the patient may require emergent lateral canthotomy for the treatment of a developing orbital compartment syndrome.

36. **The answer is D.** (Chapter 260) Hard signs of laryngotracheal injury include stridor, hemoptysis, dysphonia, air or bubbling in wound, and airway obstruction. Soft signs of laryngotracheal injury include hoarseness, neck tenderness, subcutaneous emphysema, cervical ecchymosis or hematoma, tracheal deviation or cartilaginous step-off, laryngeal edema or hematoma, and restricted vocal cord mobility.

37. **The answer is B.** (Chapter 260) Exsanguination from vascular injury is the leading cause of proximate death in penetrating neck trauma. Patients die from major vascular hemorrhage faster than even an unstable airway. Direct pressure should be used to control hemorrhage, taking care not to compress the airway or bilateral carotid arteries. Hemostatic dressings may be used and may decrease blood loss when used in combination with direct pressure. Uncontrolled hemorrhage is an indication for emergent surgery.

38. **The answer is B.** (Chapter 260) This patient has signs consistent with an acute Horner's syndrome, raising concern for an acute internal carotid artery dissection. The gold standard diagnostic study is four-vessel angiography; however, this modality may not be easily accessible and has potential associated complications. MRI and US have lower sensitivities in the detection of blunt cerebral vascular injury. MDCTA has a negative predictive value close to 100% making it a reasonable option as a screening test for blunt cerebral vascular injury in addition to the fact that is readily available in most the emergency departments. It is important to note that MDCTA has a false positive rate of approximately 45% so any positive study should be confirmed with angiography.

39. **The answer is B.** (Chapter 260) In strangulation, death is most commonly a result of the bilateral compression of the internal and external carotid arteries. Bilateral compression of these vessels causes cerebral vascular congestion, and ultimately cerebral edema and loss of consciousness. With the resultant loss of muscle tone, arterial compression and cerebral anoxia ensue.

40. **The answer is B.** (Chapter 261) The NEXUS Rules for Chest Radiography exclusion criteria are:

Age >60
Rapid deceleration: fall >20 ft (>6 m) or motor vehicle crash >40 mph (>64 km/h)
Chest pain
Intoxication
Abnormal alertness or abnormal mental status
Distracting painful injury
Tenderness to chest wall palpation

41. **The answer is A.** (Chapter 261) Tension pneumothorax must be considered in any patient who has bradycardia or cardiac arrest after intubation. This should be a clinical and not radiographic diagnosis. Needle decompression in the second intercostal space, mid-clavicular line should be performed immediately.

42. **The answer is B.** (Chapter 261) Indications for surgical exploration after tube thoracostomy placement include drainage of 1500 cc blood immediately following insertion, if blood continues to drain at 150 to 200 cc/h for 2 to 4 hours, or hemodynamic instability persists requiring ongoing blood produced administration.

43. **The answer is C.** (Chapter 261) While the sensitivity of CT scan and ultrasound is better than that of plain chest radiography, the incidence of delayed pneumothorax in the setting of penetrating chest trauma is estimated to be as high as 12%. Even if the initial study is negative, the current recommendation in asymptomatic patients is for

repeat imaging in 4 to 6 hours. Common practice remains to obtain a repeat chest x-ray. Repeat bedside ultrasound would also be an option.

44. **The answer is B.** (Chapter 261) Bedside ultrasound has 92% sensitivity and specificity approaching 100% in the diagnosis of pneumothorax compared to AP chest x-ray. It also has superior sensitivity and specificity in the diagnosis of hemothorax. This patient is hemodynamically stable with no signs of tension physiology, and therefore needle decompression or tube thoracostomy is not indicated.

45. **The answer is D.** (Chapter 262) The incidence of injury in penetrating cardiac injury is as follows: right ventricle 40%, left ventricle 35%, right atrium 20%, and left atrium 5%. The right ventricle has a large area of anterior exposure in the chest and is therefore most vulnerable to injury. The right and left atria are less frequently injured simply because of their smaller surface area.

46. **The answer is C.** (Chapter 262) This patient is presenting with penetrating chest trauma, distended neck veins, and a narrow pulse pressure. Concern is for acute pericardial tamponade. The fastest, most accessible imaging modality is bedside transthoracic ultrasound, which has 100% sensitivity in the detection of pericardial effusion. If a pericardial effusion is seen on ultrasound, immediate pericardiocentesis can be performed. CT scan would take more time, and chest x-ray will not provide a definitive diagnosis. Although, transfer to a trauma center is indicated, awaiting EMS arrival without acting emergently would lead to an unacceptable delay in diagnosis and treatment of this patient who is exhibiting signs of tamponade physiology.

47. **The answer is D.** (Chapter 262) Rapid deceleration can cause a shearing or tearing of the heart at points of fixation. Direct precordial impact is the second most common mechanism of blunt cardiac injury. Rapid change in intrathoracic pressure, crush injury due to compression between the sternum and spine, injury due to rib fracture fragments, and blast injuries are all less common causes of blunt cardiac injury.

48. **The answer is D.** (Chapter 262) Commotio cordis is a primary electrical event usually caused by a low velocity blunt impact to the chest wall and is most commonly seen in young athletes with structurally normal hearts. When the impact occurs 10 to 30 ms prior to the peak of the T wave during ventricular repolarization, ventricular fibrillation can be induced. Ventricular fibrillation is the

rhythm disturbance seen with this phenomenon, not asystole. Overall mortality is greater than 85%.

49. **The answer is C.** (Chapter 262) Patients who are suspected to have blunt cardiac injury with normal vital signs, negative imaging, and a normal ECG may be safely discharged after 4 to 6 hours of observation provided they have no new symptoms, and no EKG changes.

50. **The answer is C.** (Chapter 262) Ninety percent of patients with blunt traumatic aortic injury (BTAI) will die at the scene. The proximal descending aorta is the most commonly injured of the great vessels. Abnormalities on the AP chest x-ray associated with BTAI include widening of the mediastinum >8 cm, loss of the aortic knob contour, depression of the left mainstem bronchus, lateral displacement of the trachea, loss of paravertebral pleural stripe, apical pleural hematoma, and deviation of nasogastric tube to the right at the level of T4. The most appropriate imaging study to obtain is CT angiography. The study is faster and noninvasive compared to traditional aortography. Transesophageal echocardiography can be used to diagnose aortic injury, but it is contraindicated in patients with potential airway compromise or cervical spine injury. Sodium nitroprusside alone is not recommended for blood pressure control due to associated reflex tachycardia. Beta-blockers are most commonly recommended to control heart rate and blood pressure to reduce shearing forces. Sodium nitroprusside may be added to further assist with blood pressure control once the heart rate is controlled at about 60.

51. **The answer is D.** (Chapter 263) The most commonly injured intra-abdominal organ associated with sports-related injuries is the spleen. Otherwise, the liver is the most commonly injured intra-abdominal organ associated with blunt trauma. The pancreas and duodenum are injured much less commonly (4%), and these injuries are usually seen after highspeed deceleration events.

52. **The answer is C.** (Chapter 263) Diaphragmatic rupture is uncommon in patients with thoracoabdominal trauma (0.8% to 5%) regardless of whether the mechanism is penetrating or blunt. The diaphragm primarily ruptures on the left side and is associated with nonspecific signs or symptoms that are easily attributable to associated injuries. If undiagnosed, diaphragmatic rupture can be associated with herniation or strangulation of bowel through the defect.

53. **The answer is C.** (Chapter 263) In hemodynamically unstable patients, the benefit of the FAST

(focused assessment with sonography for trauma) examination is the ability to rapidly identify free intraperitoneal fluid in a noninvasive manner. The FAST examination can reliably detect about 200 cc of free infraperitoneal fluid. Sensitivity approaches 90%. In unstable patients who have negative FAST but index of suspicion is high for intraabdominal injury, diagnostic peritoneal aspiration (DPA) or diagnostic peritoneal lavage (DPL) is indicated. CT scan is not indicated in the hemodynamically unstable patient. Understanding that current literature supports permissive hypotension, particularly in the setting of penetrating trauma, current advanced trauma life support (ATLS) recommendations remain to initiate initial crystalloid resuscitation of 1 to 2 L, and then to start the administration of blood products in a 1:1:1 platelet:plasma:RBC ratio. Transfusing with this ratio of blood products offers potential mortality benefit and helps to mitigate transfusion coagulopathy.

54. **The answer is B.** (Chapter 263) This patient is unstable. In the case of the unstable patient with a negative FAST (focused assessment with sonography for trauma) and high index of suspicion for intra-abdominal injury DPA or DPL can be performed. More than 10 cc of blood on aspiration or >15,000 RBC/mm^3 in abdominal wounds or >25,000 RBC/mm^3 in lower chest wounds is the criteria for a positive aspirate/lavage. This patient has a positive DPA and hypotension after 1 L of crystalloid. CT is not indicated in the evaluation of the unstable trauma patient. Transfusion with a 1:1:1 ratio of platelets:plasma:RBCs offers potential mortality benefit and helps to mitigate transfusion coagulopathy. Tranexamic acid is an antifibrinolytic agent that when administered within 3 hours may favorably affect mortality. In this case, transfusion of blood products in a 1:1:1 platelet:plasma:RBC ratio, administration of tranexamic acid (TXA) and emergent exploratory laparotomy are indicated.

55. **The answer is C.** (Chapter 263) Mandatory exploratory laparotomy in the setting of anterior abdominal stab wounds without peritonitis is not recommended due to high rates of nontherapeutic laparotomies. Local wound exploration to determine if there has been violation of the fascia in the hemodynamically stable patient with an anterior abdominal stab wound and no signs of peritonitis or tenderness distant to the wound site are recommended. If the wound is found to be superficial and there is no evidence that the fascia has been violated, immediate surgical exploration may not be indicated, and the patient may be safely taken for CT scan. Persistent hypotension, peritonitis, or signs of fascial disruption are all indications for immediate surgical exploration.

56. **The answer is B.** (Chapter 263) Duodenal injuries can be difficult to diagnose and are often asymptomatic on initial presentation. Hematomas can be slow forming, but once they expand can lead to gastric outlet obstruction. Duodenal rupture can occur after a high velocity deceleration, with spilled contents generally retained in the retroperitoneum. For this reason, the symptoms of sepsis can be delayed.

57. **The answer is A.** (Chapter 264) CT with triple contrast (oral, intravenous, and rectal contrast) is the diagnostic study of choice in the hemodynamically stable patient with penetrating trauma to the flank. It provides the highest sensitivity for renal injury and also detects other coexisting abdominal injuries. Local wound exploration is not recommended in penetrating injuries of the flank. Hemodynamic instability is an indication for exploratory laparotomy: this patient is hemodynamically stable and can therefore undergo an imaging study. Ultrasound is not sensitive in the detection of retroperitoneal injuries.

58. **The answer is A.** (Chapter 264) The absence of hematuria does not exclude renal injury in the setting of penetrating trauma. Retrospective series have cited up to as high 45% of patients with significant renal injury with no hematuria on urinalysis. There has been no correlation between the amount of hematuria and severity of injury. The sensitivity of IV pyelography in the detection of penetrating renal injury is as low as 25%. CT with IV contrast is the most sensitive imaging modality and provides anatomical as well as functional information about the kidneys.

59. **The answer is D.** (Chapter 264) In the adult patient with blunt trauma to the flank, indications for further urologic imaging are gross hematuria (>50 red blood cells/high power field) or microscopic hematuria in the setting of hemodynamic instability. In hemodynamically stable patients with microscopic hematuria, no further imaging is indicated unless other intra-abdominal injury is suspected.

60. **The answer is D.** (Chapter 264) Stab wounds and gunshot wounds to the buttocks result in different patterns of injury. The upper and lower gluteal zones are divided at the level of the greater trochanters. Because the majority of the major pelvic vascular structures are in the upper gluteal zone, trauma of the upper zone is more likely to result in serious injury. The most commonly injured vascular structure seen with stab wounds to the buttocks is the superior gluteal artery. Gunshot wounds cause more widespread trauma but most commonly result in injuries

to the small bowel, colon, rectum, bladder, and pelvis. Guaiac testing is not sensitive enough to exclude bowel injury in the setting of penetrating trauma. Sciatic nerve injury is rare (<1%).

61. **The answer is A.** (Chapter 264) Penetrating trauma to the flank can cause injury to any of the retroperitoneal structures. The most common missed injury is an injury to the colon. Triple contrast CT can help in making the diagnosis of occult colon injury.

62. **The answer is B.** (Chapter 265) The majority (90%) of ureteral injuries are due to penetrating trauma. While approximately 70% of patients with ureteral injuries will have gross or microscopic hematuria, the absence of hematuria does not exclude ureteral injury. The initial study of choice in the evaluation of trauma patients with suspected ureteral injury is CT of the abdomen and pelvis with IV contrast and delayed phase images. IV pyelography is indicated if CT is negative and high index of suspicion exists.

63. **The answer is A.** (Chapter 265) Bladder rupture occurs in approximately 2% of blunt abdominal trauma cases and is commonly associated with pelvic fractures. Rupture can be intra or extraperitoneal. Extraperitoneal ruptures can often be managed nonoperatively with bladder catheter drainage, while intraperitoneal ruptures mandate surgical repair. Ultrasound is not sensitive in the diagnosis of bladder rupture, and retrograde cystography remains the gold standard for making the diagnosis.

64. **The answer is C.** (Chapter 265) The classic triad associated with posterior urethral injury is urinary retention, blood at the urethral meatus, and high riding prostate.

65. **The answer is D.** (Chapter 265) When the corpus callosum ruptures, usually due to vigorous sexual activity, patients typically experience an acute onset of pain, swelling, discoloration, and deformity of the penis. Penile fracture is an indication for emergent urologic consultation for surgical intervention.

66. **The answer is A.** (Chapter 265) Patients presenting with flank pain, ecchymosis, or lower rib fractures in the setting of blunt trauma require imaging to evaluate for renal injury. Renal injuries are present in up to 10% of patients with abdominal trauma. Urinalysis is commonly ordered in the evaluation of flank trauma, but there is no correlation of the presence or degree of hematuria with

the severity of renal injury. Clinically significant renal injuries can be present in the absence of hematuria. This patient has objective signs of trauma, and therefore warrants imaging.

67. **The answer is D.** (Chapter 266) Weakness of finger abduction would raise concern for an ulnar nerve injury. The radial nerve is responsible for forearm, wrist, and finger extension. The median nerve is responsible for wrist flexion and finger adduction. The musculocutaneous nerve is responsible for forearm flexion.

68. **The answer is B.** (Chapter 266) Hard signs of vascular injury include absent or diminished pulses, arterial hemorrhage, expanding or pulsatile hematoma, audible bruit, palpable thrill, and signs of distal ischemia. The presence of any hard sign of vascular injury is an indication for emergent vascular surgery consultation. In the absence of hard signs, the next most appropriate step in the evaluation of possible vascular injury would be calculation of the ankle-brachial index (ABI). An ABI measurement <0.9 is considered abnormal and suggests occlusive arterial injury requiring further evaluation with CT angiography. If the ABI is >0.9, the patient can be observed without further imaging provided no new signs or symptoms develop.

69. **The answer is B.** (Chapter 266) CT angiography is the diagnostic study of choice in the evaluation of potential vascular injuries of the extremities. It provides higher resolution images and involves less cost than conventional catheter angiography and is noninvasive. A limitation of CT angiography is that it does not provide good visualization of the tibial vessels. The sensitivity and specificity are comparable to conventional catheter angiography but can be limited due to scatter artifact if there are bullet fragments present.

70. **The answer is D.** (Chapter 266) Because the incidence of infection associated with simple gunshot and stab wounds is approximately 2%, the routine administration of antibiotics in the management of penetrating extremity trauma is not recommended unless the wound is grossly contaminated. The most important factor in the prevention of wound infection is copious irrigation. Irrigation with antiseptic solutions is not associated with decreased incidence of infection and may impair tissue healing. Wounds that are grossly contaminated, have suspected retained foreign body, or are associated with major tissue destruction should have delayed primary closure after 72 to 96 hours.

20
Injuries to Bones and Joints

QUESTIONS

1. A 21-year-old man with a history of mild intermittent asthma presents to the emergency department for left shoulder pain and difficulty swallowing for 1 day. Patient was playing in a football game last night and was struck hard in the left side of his chest. He had pain to left shoulder and left side of chest but did not seek treatment immediately. He noted this morning that it was hard to eat breakfast. He also states when he tried to lay back at night, it felt harder to breathe, so he slept upright in his chair. Physical examination demonstrates some decreased range of motion of the left arm. Vital signs are within normal limits, except for mild tachypnea when patient reclines. Which of the following would be the most appropriate imaging study to determine definitive management of this injury?
   (A) CT chest
   (B) MRI shoulder
   (C) X-ray chest
   (D) X-ray shoulder

2. Which of the following is TRUE regarding splinting a fracture in the emergency department?
   (A) A thumb spica splint is the treatment of choice for a typical scaphoid fracture.
   (B) The best way to immobilize a stable ankle sprain is with a posterior splint.

   (C) The colder the water temperature, the faster the plaster and fiberglass materials harden.
   (D) There is no need for sling or immobilizer after reduction of a dislocation.

3. Which of the following is a surgical emergency that requires an emergent orthopedic consult in the emergency department?
   (A) Clay Shoveler's fracture with intact neurologic examination
   (B) Mid-shaft radial fracture with an overlying, superficial laceration
   (C) Tibial fracture, complaining of severe pain, numbness, and tingling in the front part of the lower leg
   (D) Unstable ankle fracture that cannot bear weight

4. Which of the following maneuvers evaluates the ulnar nerve on a hand examination?
   (A) Abduction of the fingers
   (B) Flexion of the interphalangeal (IP) joint of the thumb against resistance
   (C) Hyperextension of the metacarpophalangeal (MCP) joints against resist
   (D) Making the "OK" sign

5. What is the name of the following fracture (Figure 20.1)?

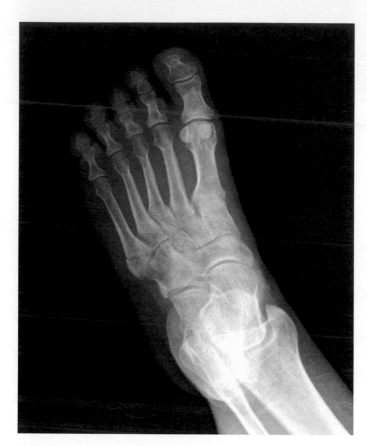

FIGURE 20.1 Image used with permission of Robert DeMayo, MD.

(A) Cuboid fracture
(B) Jones fracture
(C) Lisfranc injury
(D) Navicular fracture

6. A 26-year-old, right-hand dominant man presents with deformity and pain to left wrist after falling off of his bicycle earlier today. You obtain the following images on x-ray imaging (Figures 20.2A and B). What is the MOST APPROPRIATE emergency department treatment?
(A) Coaptation splint
(B) Forearm volar splint
(C) Radial gutter splint
(D) Sugar tong splint

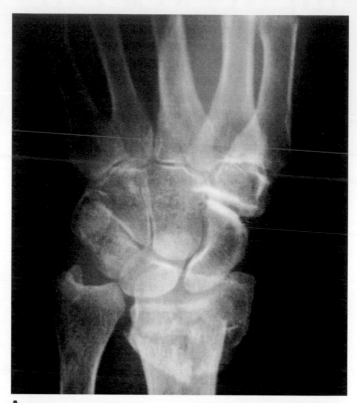

A

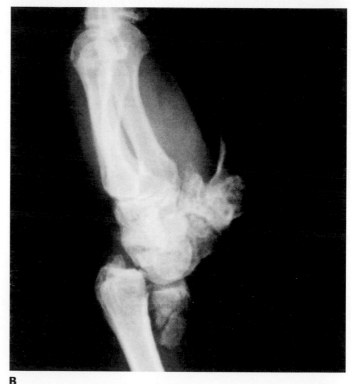

B

FIGURE 20.2 Reproduced with permission from J.E. Tintinalli, J.S. Stapczynski, O.J. Ma, D. Yealy, G.D. Meckler, D.M. Cline: Tintinalli's Emergency Medicine: A Comprehensive Study Guide, 9th Edition. Copyright © McGraw-Hill Education. All rights reserved.

7. A 47-year-old woman presents to the emergency department for evaluation of hand pain after a fall on her outstretched hand. On musculoskeletal examination, there are no neurological or vascular deficits, but there is tenderness to palpation between the patient's extensor pollicis brevis and longus tendons. You obtain imaging, which shows the abnormality noted on the x-ray shown in Figure 20.3. Which of the following is the treatment of choice for this injury?

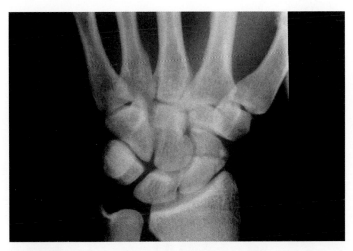

FIGURE 20.3 Reproduced with permission from J.E. Tintinalli, J.S. Stapczynski, O.J. Ma, D. Yealy, G.D. Meckler, D.M. Cline: Tintinalli's Emergency Medicine: A Comprehensive Study Guide, 9th Edition. Copyright © McGraw-Hill Education. All rights reserved.

(A) Forearm volar splint
(B) Long arm posterior splint
(C) Stat orthopedic surgery consult and admission for operative fixation
(D) Thumb spica splint

8. What is the name of the following injury (Figure 20.4)?
(A) Barton's fracture
(B) Colles' fracture
(C) Radial styloid fracture
(D) Smith's fracture

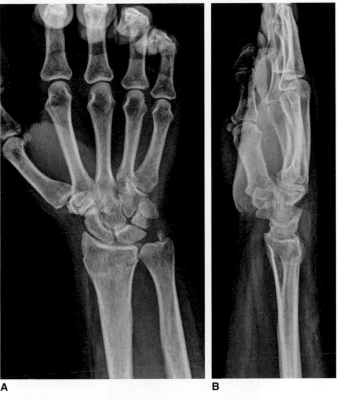

A   B

FIGURE 20.4 Photos contributed by Brooke Beckett, MD, Department of Radiology, Oregon Health & Science University, Portland, OR.

9. Fracture of the distal third of the radius in association with a dislocation of the distal radioulnar joint describes which of the following fractures?
(A) Galeazzi fracture
(B) Monteggia fracture
(C) Nightstick fracture
(D) Torus fracture

10. A 14-year-old man presents to the emergency department after falling onto his outstretched arm during a soccer game. He is crying, endorsing extreme pain at the elbow. On examination, his elbow demonstrates swelling, but patient is able to open the hand, can extend the wrist, and has a normal radial pulse. You obtain Figure 20.5 of the elbow. Which of the following is MOST COMMONLY associated with this injury?

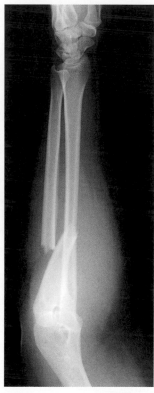

FIGURE 20.5 Reproduced with permission from J.E. Tintinalli, J.S. Stapczynski, O.J. Ma, D. Yealy, G.D. Meckler, D.M. Cline: Tintinalli's Emergency Medicine: A Comprehensive Study Guide, 9th Edition. Copyright © McGraw-Hill Education. All rights reserved.

(A) Radial head dislocation
(B) Scaphoid fracture
(C) Ulnar head dislocation
(D) Volkmann's contracture

11. A 14-year-old, right-hand dominant boy is brought in by his parents for an injury to his right third digit while fielding a groundball during a baseball game earlier today. He had immediate pain to the area, felt like his finger tip got jammed in, and has had trouble making a flat hand. You notice that the third digit's distal interphalangeal (DIP) is flexed compared to the other digits, and he is unable to extend the joint when examined. Imaging is negative for any fracture. What is the name of this injury?

(A) Bennett's finger
(B) Boutonniere deformity
(C) Jersey finger
(D) Mallet finger

12. Which of the following is not a risk factor for non-union of a middle clavicular fracture?
(A) Comminuted fracture
(B) Displaced fracture
(C) Female
(D) Initial shortening <2 cm

13. What is the mechanism for the following injury (Figure 20.6)?

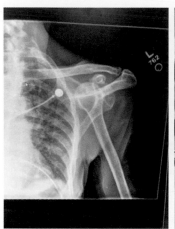 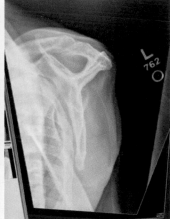

FIGURE 20.6

(A) Abduction, extension, and external rotation
(B) Abduction, flexion, and external rotation
(C) Adduction, extension, and internal rotation
(D) Adduction, flexion, and internal rotation

14. Which of the following is NOT a reduction method for an anterior glenohumeral dislocation?
(A) Cunningham technique
(B) Kocher's technique
(C) McMurray technique
(D) Stimson technique

15. Which one of the following tendons of the rotator cuff does NOT insert on the greater tuberosity of the proximal humerus?
(A) Infraspinatus
(B) Subscapularis
(C) Supraspinatus
(D) Teres minor

16. What is the MOST commonly injured nerve with proximal humeral fractures?
    (A) Axillary
    (B) Brachial
    (C) Radial
    (D) Suprascapular

17. A 67-year-old woman with early-onset dementia presents to your emergency department after being found down on the ground. She is unaccompanied and unable to tell you what happened but is repetitively saying "Ow" with any movement of the lower extremities. After your quick evaluation, the following is noticed on pelvic x-ray. What is the management of the following condition (Figure 20.7)?

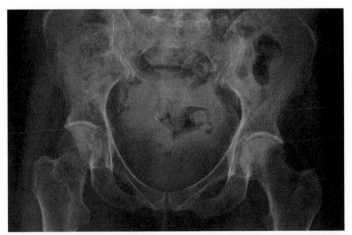

FIGURE 20.7 Reproduced with permission from J.E. Tintinalli, J.S. Stapczynski, O.J. Ma, D. Yealy, G.D. Meckler, D.M. Cline: Tintinalli's Emergency Medicine: A Comprehensive Study Guide, 9th Edition. Copyright © McGraw-Hill Education. All rights reserved.

   (A) Consult to orthopedic surgery for consideration of surgical repair
   (B) Consult to urology for operative evaluation for bladder rupture
   (C) Discharge with close outpatient follow-up with primary care physician
   (D) Pelvic binder, then retrograde urethrogram, then possibly Foley catheter

18. A 58-year-old man with a history of left hip replacement approximately 2 months ago presents to the emergency department by ambulance for left hip pain. The patient was stretching while playing golf and felt his left leg give out. He is unable to bear weight now. The extremity is shortened, internally rotated, and adducted. The patient is in significant pain. Which of the following is NOT a potential maneuver to fix this patient's condition?

   (A) Allis maneuver
   (B) Bigelow maneuver
   (C) Captain Morgan technique
   (D) Stimson technique

19. Which one of the following patients needs x-ray imaging just based on the following information?
    (A) A 24-year-old man who twisted his right knee playing soccer and is tender along the medial joint line
    (B) A 43-year-old man who had trauma to his left knee, but was able to bear weight for four steps both immediately after the injury and in the emergency department
    (C) A 53-year-old woman who is presenting with left knee stiffness without known trauma, worsening over the past 4 days, but it is able to flex her knee to 90 degrees
    (D) A 74-year-old woman with trauma to the right knee and isolated tenderness to the patella

20. A 34-year-old man is playing basketball when he twists his knee awkwardly, feels a pop, and immediately develops pain to his knee, and is having difficulty bearing weight due to instability. This occurred approximately 1.5 hours ago, and the patient's knee is already swollen. What is the MOST LIKELY injury?
    (A) Anterior cruciate ligament tear
    (B) Lateral meniscal tear
    (C) Medial meniscal tear
    (D) Posterior cruciate ligament tear

21. A 47-year-old man presents to the emergency department with severe, posterior, lower extremity/ankle pain, and difficulty with plantar flexion after running outside with his children. You perform a Thompson test, which does not move the foot at all. Which one of the following medications could have predisposed this patient to his injury?
    (A) Finasteride
    (B) Levothyroxine
    (C) Lisinopril
    (D) Moxifloxacin

22. The MOST SENSITIVE clinical finding for compartment syndrome is:
    (A) Color change in the extremity
    (B) Distal pulse deficit
    (C) Pain with passive stretch
    (D) Numbness

23. A 56-year-old patient presents to the emergency department with inability to bear weight on his right foot, and the pain worsens when putting pressure on his "tiptoes." He states he tripped over his dog earlier today and has had difficulty walking since that time. He has ecchymosis on the plantar aspect of his mid-foot with some tenderness over the dorsal midfoot. You obtain an x-ray and notice the following injury (Figure 20.8). The radiologist reports 2 mm of displacement. Which of the following is the treatment of choice?

(A) Emergent orthopedic surgery consultation for consideration of operative fixation

(B) Posterior short leg splinting with referral to orthopedic surgery

(C) Removable walking boot and weight bearing as tolerated

(D) Rest, ice, compression, and elevation

24. Which of the following is TRUE regarding the compartments of the extremities?

(A) The forearm of the upper extremity has four compartments: flexor, extensor, rotation, and mobile wad.

(B) The hand has one of the highest incidences of compartment syndrome.

(C) The lower leg has four compartments: anterior, lateral, superficial posterior, and deep posterior.

(D) The upper leg has four compartments: anterior, posterior, lateral, and medial.

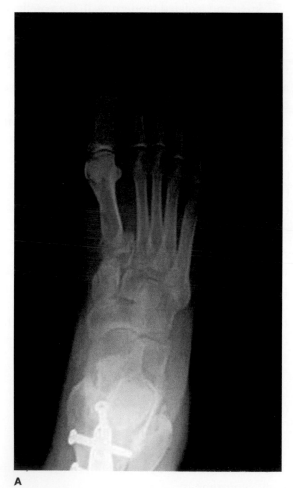

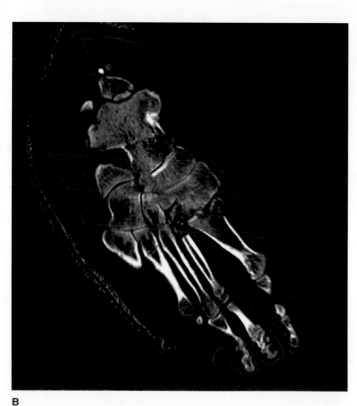

A   B

FIGURE 20.8 Image used with permission of Robert DeMayo, MD.

ANSWERS

1. **The answer is A.** (Chapter 271) This patient has a concerning history and physical for posterior sternoclavicular dislocation. This posterior dislocation can disrupt structures in the mediastinum and can impinge on the esophagus and trachea, leading to potential dysphagia and/or dyspnea. Examination findings often can demonstrate stridor when supine, concerning for compression of mediastinal structures. Patients can present with a decreased range of motion of ipsilateral arm, venous congestion, or decreased pulses. The imaging test of choice is CT scan, as plain radiographs frequently do not demonstrate sternoclavicular dislocation. Chest x-rays are helpful for ruling out acute problems such as pneumothorax, hemothorax, and/or pneumomediastinum. For acute posterior dislocations without evidence of mediastinal structure compromise, often these injuries can be managed with closed reduction under anesthesia, but for any concern for mediastinal compromise, these patients are taken to the operating room for open reduction with trauma or vascular available.

2. **The answer is A.** (Chapter 267) A thumb spica splint is a splint that immobilizes the wrist and the thumb. It is used for scaphoid fractures, as well as for fractures of the thumb metacarpal or proximal phalanx. It can be made with a wide splint that runs along the thumb and radial aspect of the wrist/forearm, but it is frequently improved by using two separate plaster splints and molding them together. In the latter case, the wrist/forearm piece runs along radial aspect, and the narrower thumb piece extends from the tip of the thumb down to the extensor aspect of the forearm, overlapping the wrist/forearm aspect of the splint. The higher the temperature of the water, the faster the splinting materials harden, both for plaster and fiberglass; however, room temperature water is safest. This is because the reaction of water interacting with plaster/fiberglass is an exothermic reaction, meaning the temperature of the skin is additive with the water and can cause burns if the water is too hot. All patients require a sling or other immobilizing contraption after reduction of a dislocation, as the stabilizing ligaments that normally keep joints in place need time to recover. The type of ankle injury determines the most suitable method of ankle splinting. A medial/lateral splint, or ankle stirrup, is useful for stable ankle sprains or stable lateral malleolus fractures as it allows for plantar and dorsiflexion at the joint. For ankle fractures that require non–weight-bearing status, a posterior splint is more suitable.

3. **The answer is C.** (Chapter 267) Severe pain and numbness with a tibial fracture is concerning for compartment syndrome, specifically of the anterior compartment of the lower leg, which is the most frequent site of compartment syndrome. Compartment syndrome is a surgical emergency due to an increase in pressure within a limb compartment leading to circulatory compromise, muscle necrosis, and neurologic damage. Other surgical emergencies necessitating urgent orthopedic surgery consultation include, but are not limited to, septic joints, open fractures, circulatory compromise due to musculoskeletal injury, irreducible dislocations, and flexor tenosynovitis. Although an open fracture is a surgical emergency, the example described is not a true open fracture, as it does not travel down to the bone. Of note, although musculoskeletal injuries that require surgery, such as an unstable fracture, need to have management with an orthopedic surgeon, they do not necessarily require emergency department consultation. An unstable fracture, may be splinted/immobilized, given crutches, and discharged with a prompt outpatient orthopedic follow-up. A clay-shoveler's fracture, also known as a spinous process fracture, is a stable fracture, and normally can be discharged with cervical collar in place, as there are high rates of union with conservative management.

4. **The answer is A.** (Chapter 268) The hand is supplied by three nerves: ulnar, radial, and median. The ulnar nerve innervates all seven interossei, the flexor digitorum profundus of the fourth and fifth digits, the flexor carpi ulnaris, the hypothenar muscles, the adductor pollicis, and the deep head of the flexor pollicus brevis. It can be tested by asking the patient to spread their fingers against resistance. It provides sensation to the medial aspect of the palm (both volar and dorsal aspects), the fifth digit, and the medial half of the fourth digit (refer to Figure 20.9 for cutaneous supply of the hand). Injury to the ulnar nerve can

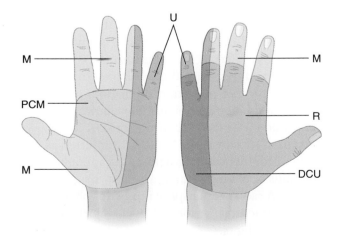

FIGURE 20.9 Reproduced with permission from J.E. Tintinalli, J.S. Stapczynski, O.J. Ma, D. Yearly, G.D. Meckler, D.M. Cline: Tintinalli's Emergency Medicine: A Comprehensive Study Guide, 9th ed, McGraw-Hill Education; 2020.

lead to a claw hand. The radial nerve provides innervation to the muscles that straighten the wrist and fingers. It travels along the humerus. When injured with a mid-shaft fracture, it can lead to a wrist drop. The radial nerve also supplies sensation to dorsal aspect of the thumb and majority of the dorsum of the palm (except what is supplied by the ulnar nerve). The median nerve supplies the thenar muscles and lumbricals to the second and third digits. The motor function may be tested by asking the patient to make the "OK" sign with their thumb and second phalanx. It also supplies almost all the flexor and pronator muscles of the forearm, except for the flexor carpi ulnaris and flexor digitorum profundus muscles to the fourth and fifth digits (which are done by the ulnar nerve). The median nerve provides sensation to the volar aspects of the thumb, second digit, and third digit, as well as half of the fourth digit; it also supplies the dorsal aspect of the distal second, third, and half the fourth digit (refer to Figure 20.9 for cutaneous supply of the hand). The median nerve is what is compressed during carpal tunnel syndrome.

5. **The answer is B.** (Chapter 277) This is an example of a Jones fracture, which is a fracture at the base of the fifth metatarsal. This usually presents with acute pain on the lateral foot, normally due to a sudden change in direction with the heel off the ground. Patients may or may not have edema, ecchymosis, and/or the inability to bear weight. A Lisfranc injury describes a midfoot injury, which affects the second metatarsal and the Lisfranc ligament. A typical mechanism for significant injury may involve plantar flexion with an axial load, such as in a car accident or sports-related injury. Navicular, cuboid, and cuneiform fracture diagnosis start with x-rays (weight-bearing AP, lateral, and oblique) but may require CT for better visualization.

6. **The answer is D.** (Chapter 269) The image shows a Barton's fracture. This is a fracture of the dorsal or volar rim of the distal radius. A sugar tong splint and orthopedic surgery referral are indicated for distal radius and ulnar fractures, including Barton's fractures. This splint helps prevent pronation/supination, wrist flexion/extension, and helps immobilize the elbow. A coaptation splint is used for humeral shaft fractures. A forearm volar splint is used for soft tissue hand/wrist injuries, as well as second to fifth metacarpal fractures. It cannot be used for distal radius or ulnar fractures, as it allows supination and pronation. A radial gutter splint is used for phalangeal and metacarpal fractures, or for soft tissue injuries of the second and third digits.

7. **The answer is D.** (Chapter 269) The scaphoid is the bone injured. The scaphoid is easily palpable in the anatomic snuffbox, which is formed by the bony radial styloid at its proximal base, the extensor pollicis brevis at radial aspect, and the extensor pollicis longus at ulnar aspect. Scaphoid fracture is also suspected if pain is elicited on supination or pronation of the hand or with axial pressure directed along the thumb's metacarpal. The scaphoid is the most common carpal bone fractured. Patients are at risk of developing avascular necrosis, as the vascular supply enters the distal portion of the scaphoid from the radial artery and palmar and superficial arteries. Delayed union, malunion, or nonunion of this joint can also develop after fracture, as 2/3 of the scaphoid is articular. All of these complications can lead to early, disabling arthritis. Nondisplaced fractures can be treated with short-arm thumb spica splint, though unstable fractures should be given a long-arm thumb spica splint and should be seen promptly by a hand surgeon or orthopedist for definitive operative treatment. A long-arm posterior splint is indicated for elbow and forearm injuries, such as distal humerus fractures, both bone forearm fractures, or sometimes unstable proximal radius or ulna fractures, though sugar-tone splints are normally preferred. Hospital admission is not normally required for these injuries. A forearm volar splint is the splint most frequently used for wrist fractures, second through fifth metacarpal fractures, wrist sprains, or even for night splints for carpal tunnel, but it does not provide enough stabilization for a scaphoid fracture.

8. **The answer is B.** (Chapter 269) The radiograph demonstrates a Colles' fracture, which is a distal radial metaphysis fracture that is dorsally angulated and displaced proximally and distally. This injury usually results from falling on an outstretched hand. On examination, the wrist commonly has a characteristic dorsiflexed appearance called a "dinner fork" deformity. It is important to obtain lateral imaging to evaluate angulation and comminution. It also helps differentiate from a Smith's fracture, which is also called a reverse Colles' fracture, as it is a volar angulated fracture of the distal radius. Barton's fractures are dorsal or volar rim fractures of the distal radius. Dorsal rim fractures are from dorsiflexion and pronation, whereas volar rim fractures are from a fall on an outstretched hand in supination. Radial styloid fractures, sometimes called Chauffeur's fractures, are fractures that extend from the scaphoid fossa to the metaphysis of the radius. These are often accompanied by lunate dislocations. Normally, these injuries are seen on PA radiographs as a thin, lucent line beneath the radial styloid.

9. **The answer is A.** (Chapter 270) Galeazzi fracture dislocation is the described fracture. It usually occurs with a fall on an outstretched hand or direct trauma. This is often called the "reverse" Monteggia's fracture. Monteggia's

fracture dislocation is a fracture of the proximal ulna with an associated dislocation of the radial head. The mechanism of injury is the same as the Galeazzi fracture. Nightstick fracture describes an ulna fracture that normally occurs after a direct blow. Torus fractures are cortical fractures secondary to compressive forces and show a bulging of the bony cortex.

10. **The answer is A.** (Chapter 270) The answer to this question is a radial head dislocation, which highlights the importance of imaging of the joint proximal and distal to the site of injury. The x-ray demonstrates a proximal ulnar fracture (Figure 20.10). A fracture of the proximal third of the ulna with a radial head dislocation is commonly referred to as Monteggia's fracture dislocation. In a Monteggia's fracture, the apex of the ulnar fracture points in the direction of the radial head dislocation. The most common direction is an anterior dislocation of the radial head (60%). It is very easy to miss the radial head dislocation due to the considerable pain and swelling of the elbow from the proximal ulnar fracture. A scaphoid fracture is also normally due to a fall on an outstretched hand but is not associated with a proximal ulnar fracture. A Galeazzi fracture is a distal third radial fracture with an associated distal radioulnar joint dislocation, rather than fracture. Volkmann's contracture is a term for compartment syndrome of the forearm. It is most commonly due to supracondylar fracture.

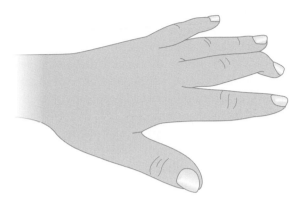

FIGURE 20.11 Reproduced with permission from J.E. Tintinalli, J.S. Stapczynski, O.J. Ma, D. Yearly, G.D. Meckler, D.M. Cline: Tintinalli's Emergency Medicine: A Comprehensive Study Guide, 9th ed, McGraw-Hill Education; 2020.

11. **The answer is D.** (Chapter 268) Mallet finger is a rupture of the extensor tendon of a digit and is normally caused by hyperflexion of the distal interphalangeal (DIP) joint (Figure 20.11). This results in the inability to extend the DIP joint. This injury is common in athletes, specifically baseball players, due to direct injury from a baseball striking the tip of a digit and forcing it into hyperflexion. Jersey finger is a flexor digitorum profundus rupture, which is also commonly seen in athletes who grab another athlete's jersey with the tip of a finger. Boutonniere deformity is an injury to the area over the proximal interphalangeal (PIP) joint. The central tendon is most commonly injured. Injury to this causes retraction of the extensor hood, which results in extension of the DIP and flexion at the PIP joint. Bennett's fracture is an intra-articular fracture of the thumb with associated subluxation or dislocation of the carpometacarpal (CMC) joint (Figure 20.12).

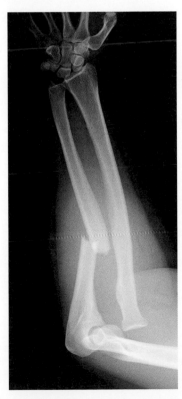

FIGURE 20.10 Reproduced with permission from J.E. Tintinalli, J.S. Stapczynski, O.J. Ma, D. Yealy, G.D. Meckler, D.M. Cline: Tintinalli's Emergency Medicine: A Comprehensive Study Guide, 9th Edition. Copyright © McGraw-Hill Education. All rights reserved.

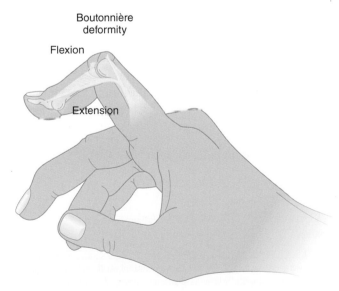

FIGURE 20.12 Reproduced with permission from J.E. Tintinalli, J.S. Stapczynski, O.J. Ma, D. Yearly, G.D. Meckler, D.M. Cline: Tintinalli's Emergency Medicine: A Comprehensive Study Guide, 9th ed, McGraw-Hill Education; 2020.

12. **The answer is D.** (Chapter 271) Initial shortening greater than 2 cm is not a risk factor for nonunion of middle third clavicle fractures. Fractures in the middle third of the clavicle are normally treated nonoperatively with immobilization by either sling or figure-of-eight brace. The length of immobilization is typically 4 to 8 weeks. However, if the above nonunion risk factors are present, the patient may benefit from an orthopedic surgery referral for possible intervention. The provider should also consider referral for athletes, impact on the patient's profession, or cosmetic concerns (Table 20.1).

13. **The answer is A.** (Chapter 271) Abduction, extension, and external rotation forces cause an anterior glenohumeral dislocation. Normally, prereduction radiographs are advisable especially for patients with first time dislocations or there those with have undergone significant trauma. It is entirely possible to have a fracture-dislocation and the methods to reduce them vary. Dislocations with a humeral fracture require orthopedic surgery consultation. Radiographs will also show if the patient has a Bankart lesion (glenoid labral defect) or a Hill-Sachs deformity (humeral head bony defect).

14. **The answer is C.** (Chapter 271) McMurray's test is a maneuver to test for meniscal injury of the knee. There are many reduction maneuvers for glenohumeral dislocation, but the major categories are traction, leverage, and scapular manipulation. The Stimson technique is a more prolonged technique, usually requiring approximately 30 minutes, where the patient is placed prone with the dislocated extremity hanging over the side of the stretcher and 10 lb attached to the wrist. Kocher's technique (Figure 20.13) is also known as the external rotation technique and involves the slow external rotation of the arm with the patient supine, arm against the body at 90 degrees of flexion. Often, this needs to be done slowly to allow resolution of the muscle spasms and may require the elbow to be brought anteriorly and internally rotated to the opposite shoulder. The Cunningham technique (Figure 20.14) is based on positioning

TABLE 20.1	Middle Clavicle Fracture Nonunion Risk Factors
• Initial shortening >2 cm	
• Comminuted fracture	
• Displaced fracture >100%	
• Significant trauma	
• Female	
• Elderly	

Reproduced with permission from J.E. Tintinalli, J.S. Stapczynski, O.J. Ma, D. Yearly, G.D. Meckler, D.M. Cline: Tintinalli's Emergency Medicine: A Comprehensive Study Guide, 9th ed, McGraw-Hill Education; 2020.

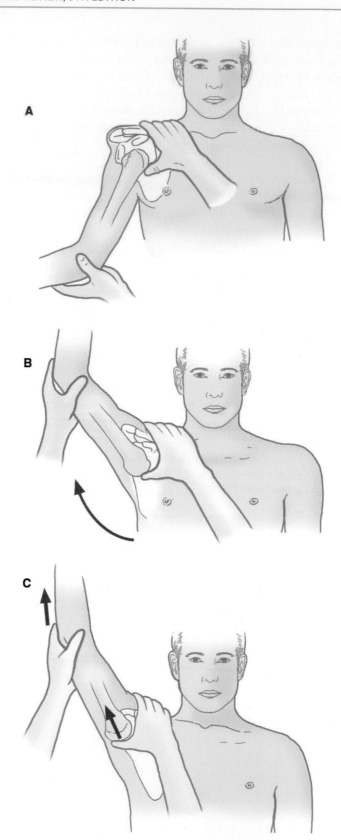

FIGURE 20.13 Reproduced with permission from Shoulder Joint Dislocation Reduction In Reichman EF: Emergency Medicine Procedures, 2nd ed. McGraw-Hill Inc., 2013.

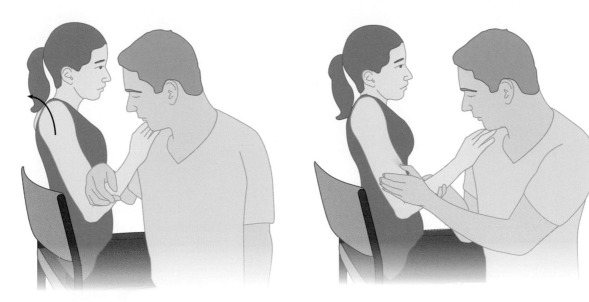

FIGURE 20.14 Reproduced with permission from J.E. Tintinalli, J.S. Stapczynski, O.J. Ma, D. Yearly, G.D. Meckler, D.M. Cline: Tintinalli's Emergency Medicine: A Comprehensive Study Guide, 9th ed, McGraw-Hill Education; 2020.

of the humerus and scapula and massaging the biceps muscle.

15. **The answer is B.** (Chapter 271) The supraspinatus, infraspinatus, and teres minor (SIT* of SITS) insert on the greater tuberosity, whereas the subscapularis (***S of SITS) inserts on the lesser tuberosity.

16. **The answer is A.** (Chapter 271) The most commonly injured nerve with a humeral fracture is the axillary nerve. Sensation over the deltoid should be tested to evaluate for the possibility of injury. Additionally, the most commonly injured vessel is the axillary artery. The second most commonly injured nerve is the suprascapular nerve, which innervates the supraspinatus and infraspinatus muscles of the rotator cuff. The most commonly injured nerve in humeral shaft fractures is the radial nerve, which will be manifested by wrist drop or altered sensation at the dorsum of the thumb. Distal humeral fractures are particularly prone to entrapment of the radial nerve. Distal humeral fractures typically require emergency orthopedic consultation, as they have a complex interaction with the neurovascular structures in the area, including the radial, median, ulnar, and anterior and posterior interosseous nerves.

17. **The answer is A.** (Chapter 273) The patient above has sustained a right femoral neck fracture, which requires an orthopedic consultation for further management depending on risk factors of the patient, management ranges from nonoperative to total hip arthroplasty. Because of the heavy vascular supply to this area, there is a high risk of avascular necrosis if this is not treated. This patient

does not have an open book pelvic fracture, as the pubic symphysis width is narrow. Plain x-ray imaging is not the study of choice for bladder trauma. Patients with this injury require orthopedic surgeon evaluation in the emergency department.

18. **The answer is B.** (Chapter 273). The Stimson technique is used for reduction of an anterior shoulder dislocation. The other technique/maneuvers are all well-documented ways to reduce a posterior hip dislocation, which is what this patient has in the vignette. Artificial hips are frequently much easier to reduce, and frequently native hip dislocations are emergencies, as they are more likely to damage the vascular supply. See Figures 20.15 through 20.18 for visual aids on how to proceed with the Allis maneuver, the Captain Morgan technique, and the Bigelow maneuver for posterior hip dislocation reductions.

19. **The answer is D.** (Chapter 274). This question assesses knowledge of the Ottawa knee x-ray imaging rules. Of the following, the only patient who definitely needs imaging is the 74-year-old patient who meets 2/5 criteria (Table 20.2).

20. **The answer is A.** (Chapter 274) Clues to this diagnosis include the pop and rapid development of swelling in the knee of the patient, which is likely a hemarthrosis and instability. The most common cause of hemarthrosis of the knee is ligamentous injury, most often of the anterior cruciate ligament. Anterior cruciate ligament tears can also be diagnosed by physical examination maneuvers,

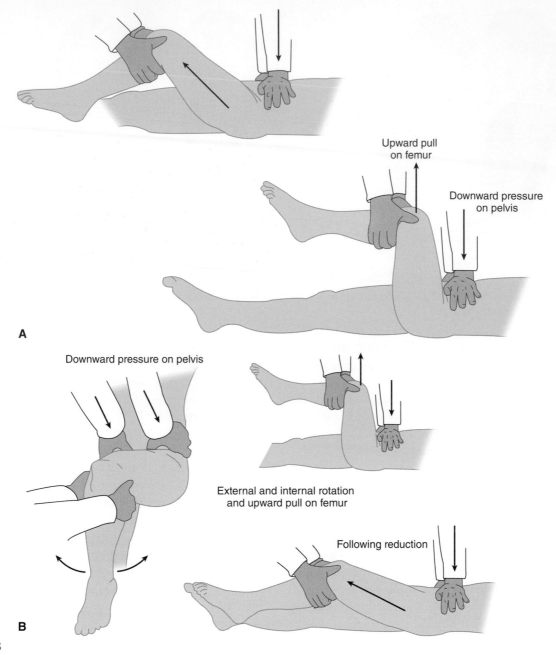

Upward pull
on femur

Downward pressure
on pelvis

A

Downward pressure on pelvis

External and internal rotation
and upward pull on femur

Following reduction

B

FIGURE 20.15

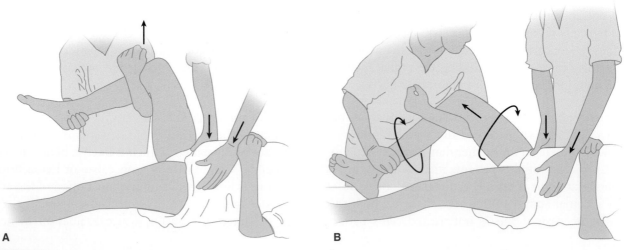

A

B

FIGURE 20.16

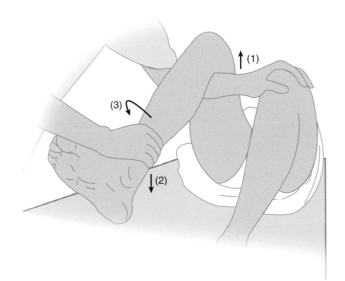

FIGURE 20.17

TABLE 20.2 Ottawa Knee Rules: Radiograph if One Criterion Is Met
• Patient age >55 y (rules have been validated for children 2–16 y of age)
• Tenderness at the head of the fibula
• Isolated tenderness of the patella
• Inability to flex knee to 90 degrees
• Inability to transfer weight for four steps both immediately after the injury and in the ED

Reproduced with permission from J.E. Tintinalli, J.S. Stapczynski, O.J. Ma, D. Yearly, G.D. Meckler, D.M. Cline: Tintinalli's Emergency Medicine: A Comprehensive Study Guide, 9th ed, McGraw-Hill Education; 2020.

including the Lachman test, anterior drawer test, lever sign, or pivot shift testing. Posterior cruciate ligament tears can be evaluated with a posterior drawer test or "sag sign," when the tibia seems to sag back on the femur at the joint. Meniscal tears can be diagnosed with McMurray testing, including varus/valgus stressing. They will often also have effusions, and patients may present with a joint "locked" in place. Patients will also have joint line tenderness on examination. For all instances, patients should be placed in a knee immobilizer and referred to either orthopedic surgery or sports medicine, the rapidity of which depends on that patient's functional status. If they are an athlete, they should be urgently referred for consideration of surgical repair.

21. **The answer is D.** (Chapter 276) The patient has suffered an Achilles tendon rupture. The Thompson test is a

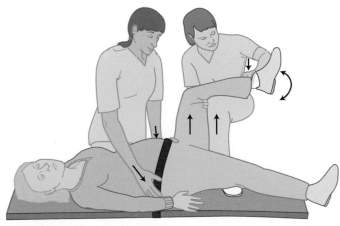

FIGURE 20.18

bedside maneuver to evaluate the Achilles tendon, where the patient lays prone with the knee bent at 90 degrees, and the examiner squeezes the patient's calf to see if the foot plantarflexes. If it does not, the Achilles is likely ruptured. There are several risk factors for Achilles tendon rupture, including prior steroid injections, prior quinolone use, and older age. Achilles tendon ruptures are often seen in the "weekend warrior," who engages in occasional strenuous activities. In these patients, management includes rest, ice, elevation, non–weight-bearing, and a short-leg posterior splint with the ankle in slight plantarflexion, with orthopedic surgery follow-up for consideration of surgery.

22. **The answer is C.** (Chapter 278) Patients with compartment syndrome will have pain in the extremity affected due to elevated pressures. The most sensitive finding initially is the pain with passive stretch of the area. When the nerve is affected, the patient will experience paresthesias. There will not be a change in distal pulses or skin color because the tissue pressure does not exceed the arterial pressure.

23. **The answer is A.** (Chapter 277) This patient has sustained a Lisfranc fracture, which is any fracture to the tarsometatarsal joint. Treatment of these injuries depends on displacement. A nondisplaced injury (<1 mm between the bases of the first and second metatarsals) should be treated with a non–weight-bearing splint, rest, ice, and elevation, with orthopedic follow-up within 2 weeks, and likely placement of a cast. A displaced Lisfranc is an unstable fracture and requires orthopedic consultation in the emergency department, and treatment ranges from open reduction, internal fixation, to primary arthrodesis. Compartment syndrome is a significant concern for these injuries.

24. **The answer is C.** (Chapter 278) The lower leg has four components: the anterior, lateral, superficial posterior, and deep posterior compartments. The most common site of compartment syndrome is at the level of the tibia and

fibula, where 40% of compartment syndromes occur. The upper leg has just three compartments: anterior, posterior, and medial compartments. Due to the larger size of these compartments, there is a lower incidence of compartment syndrome. The upper extremity forearm also has three compartments: the flexor, the extensor, and the mobile wad. The forearm is a high-risk area for compartment syndrome. The hand is less likely to develop compartment syndrome.

Musculoskeletal Disorders (Non-Traumatic) 21

QUESTIONS

1. A 68-year-old woman with a history of breast cancer treated with mastectomy 1 year ago presents with progressive neck pain for the past 2 months. She also notes paresthesias and slight weakness of her right hand for the past week. She denies fever, headache, vomiting, or dizziness. Her examination is notable for 4/5 grip strength in her right hand. Otherwise her neurological examination is unremarkable. Which of the following diagnostic studies is MOST APPROPRIATE?
   (A) CT of the cervical spine
   (B) CT myelogram
   (C) MRI of the cervical spine
   (D) Three-view cervical spine x-ray

2. What is the MOST COMMON location for metastatic epidural spinal cord compression?
   (A) Cervical spine
   (B) Cervical spine and thoracic spine equally
   (C) Lumbar spine
   (D) Thoracic spine

3. A 48-year-old man with a history of hypertension and chronic back pain presents with persistent low back pain for the past 3 days. The patient notes that the pain is worse with movement and radiates down his right leg. He denies trauma, fever, weight loss, IV drug use, difficulty walking, numbness, or weakness. His examination is notable for a normal neurologic examination and a positive right straight leg raise test. What is the NEXT BEST step in management?
   (A) CT of the lumbar spine with contrast
   (B) Ibuprofen and acetaminophen
   (C) MRI of the lumbar spine
   (D) X-ray of the lumbar spine

4. A 54-year-old woman with a history of intravenous drug use presents with progressive low back pain for the past 2 weeks. She notes that for the past 3 to 4 days she has had increasing difficulty ambulating and decreased sensation in her legs. She denies fever, urinary incontinence, nausea, or vomiting. Her examination is notable for 4/5 strength in lower extremities and decreased sensation to light touch in thighs bilaterally. Which of the following antibiotic regimens should you order?
   (A) Ceftriaxone plus metronidazole plus clindamycin
   (B) Imipenem
   (C) Nafcillin plus cefepime
   (D) Piperacillin-tazobactam plus vancomycin

5. A 39-year-old man presents with right-sided neck pain for the past 2 days. He reports a history of a car accident 1 year ago with initial neck pain that resolved after a few days, but no other prior similar episodes of pain. He denies new trauma, fever, headache, focal numbness, or weakness. On examination, he has no spinal tenderness, normal cranial nerve function, full range of motion of the neck, 5/5 strength in his upper and lower extremities, and a steady, narrow-based gait. Initial treatment with ibuprofen in the emergency department does not significantly improve his pain. What is the NEXT BEST step in management?
   (A) CT angiogram of the head and neck
   (B) Methocarbamol
   (C) Soft cervical collar
   (D) X-ray of the cervical spine

6. A 62-year-old woman presents with progressive right shoulder pain radiating to her chest. She started noticing tingling and pain in her right hand and forearm for the past month and feels like it is harder for her to hold objects with her right hand this week. She also endorses 15-lb weight loss but denies fever, neck pain, or trauma. On examination, you notice 4/5 grip strength of her right hand. What is the BEST diagnostic imaging study to order?
   (A) CT of the chest
   (B) CT of the right shoulder
   (C) X-ray of the cervical spine
   (D) X-ray of the right shoulder

7. Which of the following factors increases a patient's risk of developing adhesive capsulitis (frozen shoulder)?
   (A) Age <40 years
   (B) Coronary artery disease
   (C) Diabetes mellitus
   (D) Male sex

8. What is the MOST APPROPRIATE maneuver to evaluate for shoulder impingement?
   (A) Apley scratch test
   (B) Hawkins test
   (C) Spurling's test
   (D) Sulcus sign

9. A 42-year-old man presents with left knee pain for the past week which is worse with walking. He denies fever, swelling or trauma. On examination, you note tenderness of the left inferior patella, no erythema, warmth or swelling, and no joint laxity on valgus or varus stress testing. What is the NEXT BEST step in management?
   (A) Nonsteroidal anti-inflammatory drugs (NSAIDs) and a knee immobilizer
   (B) NSAIDs and increased exercise intensity
   (C) NSAIDs and rest
   (D) Steroid injection

10. A 58-year-old man with a history of chronic obstructive pulmonary disease (COPD) presents with 4 days of increasing left knee pain, which is worse after walking. He recently completed a course of antibiotics for pneumonia 1 week ago. He denies current fever, rash, swelling, numbness, or weakness. On examination, the patient has tenderness of the left inferior patella and slightly limited range of motion at the knee, but no joint laxity, swelling, or erythema. What is the MOST LIKELY cause of the patient's knee pain?
    (A) Azithromycin
    (B) Budesonide
    (C) Ipratropium bromide
    (D) Levofloxacin

11. A 13-year-old boy presents with persistent left hip and knee pain for the past 5 days. His mother states that he is having trouble walking today. The patient and his mother deny any recent fever, rash, or travel. He is well-appearing, lying on the stretcher with his left hip slightly externally rotated. On examination, he has mild tenderness of his left hip, no erythema or swelling, and full range of motion at the knee and ankle with 2+ peripheral lower extremity pulses. What is the MOST dangerous complication of this condition?
    (A) Avascular necrosis of the femoral head
    (B) Chondrolysis of the femoral head
    (C) Femoroacetabular impingement
    (D) Osteomyelitis of the femoral head

12. A 34-year-old woman with a history of type I diabetes presents with left flank and hip pain for the past week. The pain initially was intermittent but now has become constant with associated subjective fever, nausea, and anorexia. She denies diarrhea, constipation, vomiting, dysuria or hematuria, trauma, focal numbness, or weakness. On examination, you notice left lower abdominal tenderness plus limited active range of motion of the left hip. There is mild tenderness of the left hip but no swelling, erythema, or warmth. Her pelvic examination and urinalysis are unremarkable, and a urine pregnancy test is negative. What is the MOST COMMON pathogen associated with this condition?
    (A) *Proteus mirabilis*
    (B) *Pseudomonas aeruginosa*
    (C) *Staphylococcus aureus*
    (D) *Streptococcus pneumoniae*

13. A 38-year-old woman presents with fatigue, subjective fever, myalgias, and intermittent chest pain for the past 3 weeks. Today she felt light-headed and noticed more severe pain in her chest radiating down her right arm with associated numbness and tingling. Her vitals are notable for a BP 160/110, HR 112, SpO_2 96% on RA, and RR 22. On examination, she is fully oriented, and CN II–XII are intact. She has 5/5 strength in her upper and lower extremities, clear lungs, and a diminished right radial pulse. What is the MOST APPROPRIATE diagnostic imaging study?
    (A) Chest x-ray
    (B) CT angiogram of the aorta
    (C) CT angiogram of the head and neck with contrast
    (D) CT head without contrast

14. What is the MOST COMMON cause of death in systemic sclerosis?
    (A) Myocardial infarction
    (B) Pulmonary arterial hypertension
    (C) Pulmonary embolism
    (D) Renal failure

15. A 68-year-old woman with hypertension and type 2 diabetes mellitus presents with worsening vision in her right eye as well as a dull, right-sided headache for the past 2 days. On examination, her pupils are equal, round, and reactive to light, she has no conjunctival injection, and extraocular movements are normal. Her visual acuity is 20/100 in the right eye and 20/30 in the left eye. Her intraocular pressure is 18 bilaterally. There is no uptake on fluorescein stain of both eyes. You order a noncontrast head CT which is unremarkable. What is the NEXT BEST step in management?
    (A) Check erythrocyte sedimentation rate (ESR) and start high-dose steroids
    (B) Consult neurology and order an MRI brain without contrast
    (C) Discharge with ophthalmology follow-up
    (D) Discharge with prednisolone eye drops and ophthalmology follow-up

16. A 46-year-old man with systemic lupus erythematosus (SLE) presents with 3 days of worsening dyspnea, multiple episodes of hemoptysis, and subjective fevers. He notes chest pain bilaterally which is worse with inspiration. He denies sick contacts, recent travel, leg pain, leg swelling, or weight loss. Vitals in the emergency department are notable for RR 28, SpO_2 82% on RA, HR 122, and BP 138/72. After starting oxygen via non-rebreather mask, his SpO_2 is 94%. A portable chest x-ray shows diffuse patchy opacities. What is the NEXT BEST step in management?
    (A) Intubate and obtain a CT angiogram of the chest
    (B) Intubate and start a heparin drip
    (C) Obtain a CT angiogram of the chest and start a heparin drip
    (D) Start noninvasive ventilation and give broad-spectrum antibiotics

17. Why is endotracheal intubation potentially more dangerous in patients with rheumatoid arthritis?
    (A) Atlantoaxial instability
    (B) Immunosuppression
    (C) Interstitial lung disease
    (D) Laryngomalacia

18. A 32-year-old woman with systemic lupus erythematosus (SLE) presents with 1 day of urinary retention, lower back pain, and paresthesias of her legs. On examination, she has 5/5 strength in her upper and lower extremities, no spinal tenderness, and slightly diminished sensation to light touch in her medial thighs. What is the MOST APPROPRIATE diagnostic test?
    (A) CT of the abdomen and pelvis with IV contrast
    (B) MRI of the thoracic and lumbar spine with IV contrast
    (C) Renal ultrasound
    (D) Urinalysis

19. A 52-year-old woman with rheumatoid arthritis currently on prednisone and naproxen presents with nausea, fatigue, and body aches for the past 4 days. She has been visiting family for the past 2 weeks but accidently forgots to bring her medications. She notes a dry cough but denies fever, chest pain, or dyspnea. Her vitals are notable for HR 112, BP 80/52, SpO_2 96% on RA, RR 21, and T 37.1°C. Which of the following lab abnormalities would you expect based on her suspected condition?
    (A) Hyperkalemia
    (B) Hyperglycemia
    (C) Hypocalcemia
    (D) Hypoglycemia

20. A 54-year-old woman with diabetes and end-stage renal disease on hemodialysis presents with painful swelling of her right index finger for the past 4 days. She noticed a scratch on her finger about 1 week ago but then developed worsening redness and swelling and today feels like it is hard to move the finger. She denies fever or other injury to the hand. On examination, you note that the patient holds her right index finger slightly flexed, has significant swelling of the entire finger, and experiences severe pain with passive extension of the finger. Her vitals are notable for HR 94, BP 142/98, SpO$_2$ 97% on RA, RR 18, and point of care blood glucose of 221. What is the NEXT BEST step in management?
    (A) Consult hand surgery and give piperacillin-tazobactam plus vancomycin
    (B) Discharge with amoxicillin-clavulanate plus trimethoprim-sulfamethoxazole
    (C) Give piperacillin-tazobactam plus vancomycin and place in the observation unit
    (D) Incision and drainage and discharge with amoxicillin-clavulanate

21. A 22-year-old man is brought to the emergency department by ambulance after he was found outside of a bar intoxicated. He notes right hand pain but does not remember injuring his hand. On examination he is awake and oriented to person, place, and time and has no signs of facial trauma. The only notable examination finding is a cut on his right hand as shown in Figure 21.1:

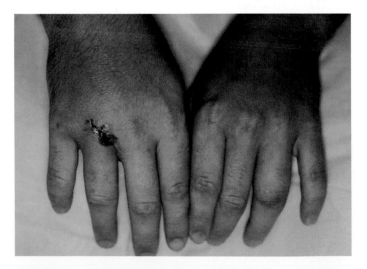

FIGURE 21.1 Photo contributor: Lawrence B. Stack, MD. Reproduced with permission from Knoop KJ, Stack LB, Storrow AB, Thurman RJ (eds): The Atlas of Emergency Medicine, 3rd ed. New York, NY: McGraw-Hill, Inc, 2010.

What is the BEST treatment for the patient's condition?
    (A) Amoxicillin-clavulanate
    (B) Cephalexin plus doxycycline
    (C) Piperacillin-tazobactam
    (D) Trimethoprim-sulfamethoxazole

22. How should the following hand infection be treated (Figure 21.2)?

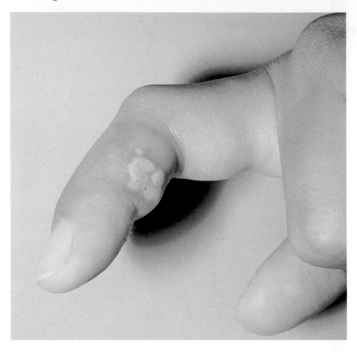

FIGURE 21.2 Photo contributor: Lawrence B. Stack, MD. Reproduced with permission from Knoop K, Stack L, Storrow A, Thurman RJ (eds): Atlas of Emergency Medicine, 3rd ed. New York, NY: McGraw-Hill, Inc.; 2010.

    (A) Amoxicillin-clavulanate only
    (B) Ibuprofen
    (C) Incision and drainage only
    (D) Incision and drainage plus amoxicillin-clavulanate

23. A 52-year-old woman presents with right arm and hand pain for the past 2 weeks. She notes that the pain seems to radiate up her arm and also feels tingling in her thumb, index, and middle fingers, worse at night. She denies trauma, weakness, swelling, or fever. On examination, sensation is intact throughout her right arm. She has 2+ radial and brachial pulses, and full range of motion at the digits, wrist, elbow, and shoulder. What test would be MOST HELPFUL in supporting your diagnosis?
    (A) Have patient hold her wrists fully flexed for 1 minute
    (B) Have patient hold her thumb in palm of her hand and then ulnar deviate her hand
    (C) Hold patient's arm at 90 degrees and forcibly internally rotate her shoulder
    (D) Obtain x-rays of the wrist and forearm

24. A 72-year-old man with a history of hypertension and coronary artery disease presents with a painful tender swollen "lump" over the dorsum of his left wrist for the past 2 weeks. He denies any recent trauma or fevers and does not think the lump has grown any bigger. On examination, he has a 3-cm firm nodule over the dorsum of his wrist without any surrounding erythema or warmth. What is the NEXT BEST step in management?
    (A) Incision and drainage and cephalexin
    (B) Incision and drainage and outpatient hand surgery follow-up
    (C) Nonsteroidal anti-inflammatory drugs (NSAIDs) and outpatient hand surgery follow-up
    (D) X-rays of the hand and wrist

25. What is the BEST method for draining a felon?
    (A) Cruciate incision
    (B) "Hockey stick" incision
    (C) Needle aspiration
    (D) Unilateral longitudinal incision

26. A 38-year-old woman presents with pain and swelling of her left thumb for the past 2 days. She denies any specific trauma, fever, numbness, or weakness. Her examination is shown in Figure 21.3:

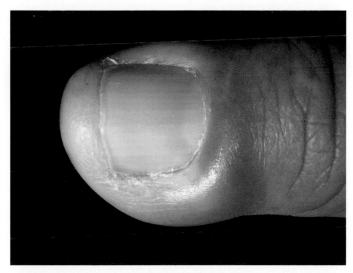

FIGURE 21.3 Courtesy of Richard P. Usatine, MD.

What is the BEST STEP in management?
(A) Incision and drainage
(B) Incision and drainage plus cephalexin
(C) Incision and drainage plus partial nail avulsion
(D) Warm soaks and elevation plus cephalexin

27. A 26-year-old woman presents with 2 days of right ankle pain. She also reports swelling and pain of her right index finger, subjective fevers, and fatigue for the past 5 days. On examination, you note a few small painless lesions on her hands and feet as well as moderate swelling and tenderness of her right ankle. What is the BEST STEP in management?
    (A) Check rapid human immunodeficiency virus (HIV) and syphilis tests, and give acetaminophen and ibuprofen
    (B) Obtain blood and synovial cultures, and give ceftriaxone plus vancomycin
    (C) Obtain blood, urogenital, and synovial cultures, and give ceftriaxone plus azithromycin
    (D) Obtain x-rays of the right ankle, and give acetaminophen and ibuprofen

28. A 62-year-old man with a history of diabetes, hypertension, and human immunodeficiency virus not currently on antiretroviral medications presents with right knee swelling and pain for the past week. He does not remember any specific fall or injury to the knee but notes that the pain has progressed and today he had difficulty walking. His vitals are notable for T 38.1°C, HR 98, BP of 137/62, SpO_2 96% on RA, and RR 18. He has erythema, diffuse swelling, and tenderness of the right knee and pain with passive and active range of motion. He refuses to ambulate in the emergency department. X-rays show a moderate to large effusion of the right knee and no acute fracture. You perform an arthrocentesis that shows negatively birefringent crystals and a white blood cell count of 44,000 with 88% PMNs. What is the NEXT BEST step in management?
    (A) Administer colchicine and discharge with outpatient follow-up
    (B) Administer indomethacin and discharge with outpatient follow-up
    (C) Administer intravenous cefepime and vancomycin and consult orthopedic surgery
    (D) Administer intravenous ceftriaxone and vancomycin and consult orthopedic surgery

29. A 72-year-old man with hypertension and diabetes presents with worsening right hip pain for the past 2 days. It is worse with walking or movement. He denies fever, recent fall, rash, or swelling. On examination the patient is well appearing, with limited active range of motion and mild tenderness at the right hip, sensation intact throughout the right leg, and 2+ peripheral pulses. You obtain the following x-ray (Figure 21.4), which demonstrates which of the following conditions?

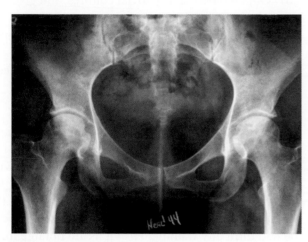

FIGURE 21.4 Imboden JB, Hellmann DB, Stone JH: Current Diagnosis & Treatment; Rheumatology, 3rd edition: www.accessmedicine.com

(A) Osteoarthritis of the right hip
(B) Right femoral neck fracture
(C) Right inferior pubic ramus fracture
(D) Right intertrochanteric fracture

30. A 32-year-old man presents with left knee swelling and pain for the past 4 days. He also notes low back pain and redness of his eyes for the past 3 days. Two weeks ago he had a few days of watery diarrhea and crampy abdominal pain, but this resolved without treatment. On examination you note bilateral conjunctival injection, no spinal tenderness, and left knee swelling with mild tenderness but no erythema or warmth. What is the BEST treatment for this patient's condition?
(A) Ciprofloxacin
(B) Methotrexate
(C) Naproxen
(D) Prednisone

31. A 24-year-old woman presents with 6 days of bilateral pain and swelling of the second to fourth proximal interphalangeal joints of her hands, followed by subsequent development of bilateral knee pain and swelling 4 days ago. She denies fever, redness, recent travel, or sick contacts. On examination she has full range of motion of her fingers and knees with tenderness and slight swelling of her bilateral knees, but no erythema or warmth. Her symptoms are MOST suggestive of which of the following conditions?
(A) Gout
(B) Lyme disease
(C) Rheumatic fever
(D) Systemic lupus erythematosus

32. A 45-year-old man with hypertension presents with pain of the right first digit of his foot for the past 2 weeks. He denies fever, rash or purulent drainage from the toe. On examination you note distal swelling and erythema of the right first digit and a significantly ingrown toenail without warmth or drainage. What is the NEXT BEST step in management?
(A) Perform partial toenail removal
(B) Perform partial toenail removal and chemical matricectomy
(C) Perform partial toenail removal and discharge with cephalexin
(D) Recommend daily foot soaks and comfortable shoes

33. A 42-year-old woman presents with progressive left foot pain for the past week. She has been training for a marathon for the past three weeks. She notes that the pain is located on the bottom of her foot and is worse with walking. She denies any swelling, redness, numbness or weakness of her foot or ankle. On examination you note full active range of motion of the left foot and ankle, 2+ dorsalis pedis pulses, and tenderness along the medial aspect of the calcaneus. What is the BEST initial strategy to manage this condition?
(A) Perform a corticosteroid injection
(B) Place posterior leg splint
(C) Recommend ibuprofen and dorsiflexion night splints
(D) Recommend tramadol and continued activity

34. A 36-year-old man presents with sudden severe right calf pain that developed after he was playing basketball with some friends 1 hour ago. He notes difficulty walking, with severe pain and weakness of his foot. On examination his sensation is intact to light touch throughout the right calf, ankle and foot, he has 2+ dorsalis pedis and posterior tibialis pulses, and difficulty plantar flexing the foot. What is the NEXT BEST step in management?
    (A) Consult orthopedic surgery
    (B) Give the patient crutches and discharge with orthopedic surgery follow-up
    (C) Place in a posterior leg splint in dorsiflexion and discharge with orthopedic surgery follow-up
    (D) Place in a posterior leg splint in plantar flexion and discharge with orthopedic surgery follow-up

35. A 35-year-old woman presents with lesions on the bottom of her feet for the past 2 weeks. She notes slight aching pain when walking but denies fever, rash elsewhere, or sick contacts. On examination you note two hard, circular lesions approximately 0.5 cm in size on the plantar surface of both feet. What is the BEST treatment option for this condition?
    (A) Cryotherapy
    (B) Duct tape
    (C) Ibuprofen
    (D) Valacyclovir

ANSWERS

1. **The answer is C.** (Chapter 279) An MRI of the cervical spine is the most appropriate diagnostic study to order given that the patient has several risk factors for a dangerous spinal cause of her neck pain, including pain for >6 weeks, age >50, history of cancer, and major motor weakness. Although a CT of the cervical spine or x-ray can show bony lesions, MRI is the best study to fully evaluate the spinal cord when there is significant concern for dangerous causes of neck pain, such as metastatic epidural spinal cord compression or spinal epidural abscess. A CT myelogram is only indicated if there are contraindications to MRI.

2. **The answer is D.** (Chapter 279) The majority of epidural cord compression cases occur in the thoracic spine. Compression at the cervical spine, multiple levels, or lumbar spine can occur, but they are less common.

3. **The answer is B.** (Chapter 279) The patient's presentation is most suggestive of sciatica. The initial best treatment option is ibuprofen and acetaminophen. The patient may need a nonemergent MRI of the lumbar spine to evaluate for a herniated disc, but without signs and symptoms of spinal cord compression, it is not indicated in the emergency department. A CT of the lumbar spine with contrast and an x-ray of the lumbar spine would not provide additional information that would change the patient's management.

4. **The answer is D.** (Chapter 279) The patient's presentation is concerning for a spinal epidural abscess. The best empiric antibiotic regimen provides coverage for *Staphylococcus aureus* including methicillin-resistant *S. aureus* (MRSA) (vancomycin) plus coverage of gram-negative bacteria and streptococci (piperacillin-tazobactam). Choice A provides coverage for gram-negative bacteria and streptococci (ceftriaxone), anaerobes (metronidazole), and some MRSA coverage (clindamycin), but given increasing resistance of MRSA to clindamycin, is not the best option. Nafcillin plus cefepime and imipenem do not provide MRSA coverage.

5. **The answer is B.** (Chapter 279) Despite minimal improvement after initial analgesia medication, imaging is not indicated for this patient given that he has no dangerous signs or symptoms suggestive of a more serious cause of neck pain. Additional treatment with a muscle relaxant such as methocarbamol, cyclobenzaprine, or diazepam may help with tension related neck pain or muscle spasm and is the bet next step. Soft cervical collars provide little actual neck support or significant benefit to patients with acute neck pain.

6. **The answer is A.** (Chapter 280) The patient's history of atypical shoulder pain with neurologic deficits is concerning for a Pancoast (superior pulmonary sulcus) tumor. The best imaging study to confirm the diagnosis in the emergency department is a CT of the chest, which will provide greater information about the tumor, its extension, and any additional pulmonary nodules, compared with an x-ray of the cervical spine or shoulder, which may not adequately visualize the tumor. Similarly, a CT of the right shoulder may not visualize the tumor.

7. **The answer is C.** (Chapter 280) Adhesive capsulitis is associated with a variety of conditions, including diabetes, thyroid disease, and autoimmune conditions, but not coronary artery disease. It is rare to see adhesive capsulitis in adults <40 years of age, and it is less common in men.

8. **The answer is B.** (Chapter 280) Impingement syndrome is a common condition where repetitive use of the arm can cause compression of the subacromial space by the humeral head, leading to rotator cuff edema, tendonitis, and eventually rotator cuff tears. The Hawkins test along with the maneuver of Neer specifically assess for impingement with fairly high sensitivity but lower specificity. The Apley scratch test evaluates shoulder range of motion, Spurling's test assesses cervical nerve root compression, and the Sulcus sign is a maneuver to evaluate glenohumeral instability.

9. **The answer is C.** (Chapter 281) The patient presents with nontraumatic knee pain suggestive of patellar tendinitis. The best initial management is nonsteroidal anti-inflammatory drugs (NSAIDs) and rest, but not complete immobilization which will delay the healing process. Increased exercise intensity, however, will exacerbate the condition further and put the patient at risk for potential patellar rupture. Steroid injection is not recommended for patellar tendinitis given risk for patellar rupture.

10. **The answer is D.** (Chapter 281) Medications can be an important cause of joint pain, tendinopathy, and tendon rupture. Fluoroquinolones such as levofloxacin have a black box warning for their increased risk of tendinopathy and tendon rupture. Azithromycin, inhaled steroids such as budesonide, and ipratropium do not significantly increase a patient's risk for tendinopathy.

11. **The answer is A.** (Chapters 141 and 281) The patient's presentation is concerning for slipped capital femoral epiphysis (SCFE). The most dangerous complication of this condition is avascular necrosis or osteonecrosis.

Chondrolysis, which is loss of cartilage and narrowing of the joint space, can also occur, but does not cause as much morbidity. Femoroacetabular impingement is associated with SCFE and increases risk of early osteoarthritis but not major damage to the hip. Osteomyelitis is not significantly associated with SCFE.

12. **The answer is C.** (Chapter 281) The patient's history of diabetes and left flank and hip pain with associated fever is concerning for a potential psoas abscess. The most common cause is *Staphylococcus aureus*, with *Proteus*, *Pseudomonas*, and *Streptococcus pneumoniae* seen much less frequently.

13. **The answer is B.** (Chapter 282) This patient's presentation of chest pain and neurologic symptoms with hypertension and a pulse deficit on examination is concerning for aortic pathology such as Takayasu arteritis, so a CT angiogram of the aorta is the most appropriate imaging study. This rare large vessel vasculitis is most often seen in women younger than 40 years of age and primarily involves the aorta and its main branches. A CT angiogram of the head and neck with contrast may or may not show evidence of vasculitis, but would not assess for the most immediately dangerous condition (aortic dissection) given the patient's presentation. A chest x-ray and a CT of the head without contrast would not evaluate the vasculature and so are not the most appropriate imaging studies.

14. **The answer is D.** (Chapter 282) The most common cause of death in systemic sclerosis is due to renal disease. Sudden renal failure, known as scleroderma renal crisis, can develop. Although myocardial infarction, pulmonary arterial hypertension, and pulmonary embolism can occur in patients with systemic sclerosis, these are not as commonly the cause of death.

15. **The answer is A.** (Chapters 241 and 282) The patient's history and examination are very concerning for temporal arteritis. The next best step is to check an erythrocyte sedimentation rate (ESR), as an elevated level (generally 70–110 mm/h) is seen in most cases, and give high dose intravenous steroids (A) to prevent progression to blindness. Treatment should not be delayed for a temporal artery biopsy. Patient discharge with ophthalmology follow-up without further diagnostic workup is not correct given that temporal arteritis is an ocular emergency. Although neurology consultation may be reasonable in certain cases of vision impairment, the patient's presentation is more suggestive of temporal arteritis than stroke.

16. **The answer is A.** (Chapter 282) This patient's presentation is most concerning for alveolar hemorrhage, an uncommon but serious complication of systemic lupus and other rheumatologic conditions, including antiphospholipid syndrome, dermatomyositis/polymyositis, and systemic sclerosis. Significant hemoptysis and pulmonary infiltrates on chest x-ray are suggestive of the condition, but it may often be mistaken for "atypical" pneumonia or pulmonary embolism early in the patient's presentation. Given the patient's significant dyspnea and persistent hypoxia, the best step is to intubate and obtain a CT angiogram of the chest for better characterization of the pulmonary infiltrates and to exclude potential pulmonary embolism. Initiation of an empiric heparin drip could be catastrophic without knowing if the patient has a pulmonary embolism or hemorrhage and thus is not advisable. Since the patient has had multiple episodes of hemoptysis and remains hypoxic despite oxygen, he is at high risk for aspiration and rapid deterioration, making non invasive ventilation an inappropriate option.

17. **The answer is A.** (Chapter 282) Patients with rheumatoid arthritis have an approximate 25% incidence of atlantoaxial instability, C1-C2 subluxation, or dislocation, putting patients requiring intubation at risk for spinal cord injury. It is thus of utmost importance to avoid hyperextending the neck during intubation of rheumatoid arthritis patients. Although patients with rheumatoid arthritis can develop interstitial lung disease and may have immunosuppression (B) from specific disease-directed therapies, these do not make the act of intubation more dangerous. Laryngomalacia is not a feature of rheumatoid arthritis.

18. **The answer is B.** (Chapter 282) Given the patient's history of SLE, she is at higher risk for transverse myelitis, a rare but very dangerous condition where acute inflammation of the spinal cord can lead quickly to irreversible paraplegia. This condition may initially present with only back pain and/or urinary retention, so physicians must have a higher index of suspicion for potential spinal cord pathology in patients with rheumatologic disease. The most appropriate diagnostic study to assess for transverse myelitis is an MRI of the thoracic and lumbar spine with IV contrast. CT of the abdomen and pelvis, renal ultrasound, and urinalysis will not provide information about spinal cord disease, so are not the best diagnostic tests.

19. **The answer is D.** (Chapters 230 and 282) Patients with rheumatologic conditions who are dependent on steroids are at risk for secondary adrenal insufficiency and acute adrenal crisis, either after abrupt withdrawal of steroids or due to an underlying stressful trigger (infection or other acute illness). Hypoglycemia is common in

secondary adrenal insufficiency, whereas hyperkalemia, hyperglycemia, and hypocalcemia are not likely to occur.

20. **The answer is A.** (Chapter 283) This patient's history and examination are concerning for flexor tenosynovitis, a surgical emergency. Three out of the four of Kanavel's cardinal signs of flexor tenosynovitis are present on examination, and the patient has additional risk factors for a serious infection (diabetes, hemodialysis). The best step is early consultation of hand surgery and broad-spectrum antibiotics. Discharge or placement in observation is not appropriate in cases of suspected flexor tenosynovitis given the potential for significant morbidity due to inadequate treatment. The patient's examination does not suggest a focal abscess, so bedside incision and drainage is not a reasonable option.

21. **The answer is A.** (Chapter 283) The patient's examination suggests that he was involved in a fight, likely sustaining a human bite after striking another person's teeth. Given this type of penetrating injury with exposure to human oral flora, he is at risk for infection and should receive antibiotic prophylaxis with amoxicillin-clavulanate. Cephalexin plus doxycycline or trimethoprim-sulfamethoxazole is not necessary as he has no community acquired MRSA risk factors. Piperacillin-tazobactam is an intravenous option if the patient were to have signs of infection from a human bite, but is not the correct option for antibiotic prophylaxis.

22. **The answer is B.** (Chapter 283) This picture shows herpetic whitlow. Of the options, ibuprofen is the most appropriate as most cases of herpetic whitlow resolve within 2 to 3 weeks without a need for acyclovir unless the patient is immunocompromised or has a protracted case. Antibiotics such as amoxicillin-clavulanate are only recommended if there is bacterial superinfection. Incision and drainage is not advisable and may increase risk of secondary bacterial infection.

23. **The answer is A.** (Chapter 283) The patient's history and examination are most suggestive of carpal tunnel syndrome. The presence of Phalen's sign, whereby flexing the wrist maximally reproduces tingling and numbness along a median nerve distribution, supporting a diagnosis of carpal tunnel syndrome. Choice B describes the Finkelstein test, which can be used to assess for De Quervain's tenosynovitis, and choice C demonstrates how to perform the Hawkins test for shoulder impingement. X-rays will not help support a diagnosis of carpal tunnel syndrome.

24. **The answer is C.** (Chapter 283) The patient most likely has a ganglion cyst, commonly located over the

dorsal and volar wrist. Initial treatment is with nonsteroidal anti-inflammatory drugs (NSAIDs) and outpatient hand surgery follow-up for future cyst aspiration or surgical excision as needed. It is not recommended to perform incision and drainage of these cysts in the emergency department and x-rays will provide no additional helpful information to manage this condition.

25. **The answer is D.** (Chapter 283) The best method for draining a felon is the unilateral longitudinal incision, which minimizes potential damage with the sensate areas of the finger pad. Cruciate and "hockey stick" (B) incisions are not indicated as they may damage sensation of the fingertip or affect vascularity. Although evidence for felon drainage techniques is limited, needle aspiration could lead to incomplete drainage of the felon, so is not currently recommended.

26. **The answer is A.** (Chapter 283) The patient has a paronychia, an infection of the lateral nail fold which can typically be treated with elevation of the eponychial fold using a #11 blade, or for larger infections, as shown in this picture, incision and drainage. Early paronychia without fluctuance can be treated with warm soaks, elevation, and antibiotics, but most paronychia will require drainage. The addition of antibiotics is not necessary in the absence of surrounding cellulitis or immunocompromise, as in this case. Partial nail avulsion is also not indicated for most paronychia.

27. **The answer is C.** (Chapter 284) The history of migratory arthritis as well as painless cutaneous lesions in a young adult is most suggestive of gonococcal septic arthritis. It is important to obtain blood, urogenital, and synovial cultures to aid in positive identification of Neisseria gonorrhoeae (since synovial fluid cultures are positive only in 25%–50% of cases) and give empiric treatment with ceftriaxone plus azithromycin to reduce emergence of resistance. Choice B is a reasonable option for the management of nongonococcal septic arthritis but is inadequate for cases of disseminated gonococcal infection. Checking for concomitant sexually transmitted infections and obtaining x-rays would not provide appropriate management for the most likely and dangerous condition.

28. **The answer is C.** (Chapter 284) The patient has risk factors (human immunodeficiency virus [HIV], diabetes) and physical examination findings concerning for septic arthritis. Although the synovial fluid white blood cell count is <50,000 and shows crystals, the cell count may be significantly diminished in immunocompromised patients, and crystal-induced arthritis can coexist with septic arthritis. The best management step is to consult

orthopedics and give intravenous cefepime and vancomycin for likely septic arthritis in an immunocompromised patient. Choice D would be a reasonable option for a patient with normal immune function. Choices A and B are management options for acute gout, but not for a patient with suspected septic arthritis.

29. **The answer is A.** (Chapter 284) The x-ray demonstrates significant osteoarthritis of the right hip, including severe joint space narrowing and sclerosis. There is no fracture.

30. **The answer is C.** (Chapter 284) The patient presents with arthritis, conjunctivitis, and a history of recent gastrointestinal illness suggestive of reactive arthritis. Reactive arthritis can develop after certain bacterial gastrointestinal infections (postdysentery reactive arthritis) or exposure to sexually transmitted disease (chlamydia, ureaplasma). Treatment for post-dysentery reactive arthritis is supportive, with nonsteroidal anti-inflammatory drugs (NSAIDs) such as naproxen. If the patient no longer has gastrointestinal symptoms such as diarrhea, there is no indication for antibiotics such as ciprofloxacin. Methotrexate and prednisone are treatment option for rheumatoid arthritis but are not indicated for treatment of reactive arthritis.

31. **The answer is D.** (Chapter 284) Of the conditions listed, only systemic lupus erythematosus presents most commonly as a symmetric polyarthritis (involving greater than three joints). Gout and Lyme disease typically present as a monoarthritis, while rheumatic fever tends to be an oligoarthritis involving two to three joints.

32. **The answer is A.** (Chapter 285) Ingrown toenails with swelling and inflammation of the toe but no evidence of infection typically require only partial toenail removal as opposed to supportive care. If there is no evidence of infection, antibiotics such as cephalexin are not indicated.

Chemical matricectomy may be considered if there is significant granulation tissue or infection present.

33. **The answer is C.** (Chapter 285) This patient presents with signs and symptoms suggestive of plantar fasciitis, the most common cause of heel pain. This condition typically resolves within 12 months but can be very painful, so initial treatment involves nonsteroidal anti-inflammatory drugs (NSAIDs) such as ibuprofen. Dorsiflexion night splints help to stretch the plantar fascia and Achilles tendon, reducing pain while sleeping. Placement of a posterior leg splint is not necessary, and corticosteroid injections increase risk of plantar fascia rupture, so are only considered in more severe cases under the care of an orthopedist. Tramadol, an opioid pain medication with no anti-inflammatory properties and abuse potential, is not the best analgesic option.

34. **The answer is D.** (Chapter 285) This patient's history and examination are concerning for an Achilles tendon rupture. Initial management involves placement of the patient in a posterior leg splint in plantar flexion with prompt orthopedic surgery follow-up. The posterior leg splint should not be in dorsiflexion, as this will impair proper healing of the tendon. Crutches alone without splinting puts the patient at risk for delayed healing and impaired ankle mobility, so is not advised. Orthopedic surgery consultation is not immediately necessary in the emergency department as long as the patient is able to see an orthopedist for follow-up within 5 to 7 days.

35. **The answer is A.** (Chapter 285) This patient's presentation is consistent with plantar warts, a common condition caused by human papillomavirus and typically found on the feet or hands. The main treatment options are salicylic acid or cryotherapy via liquid nitrogen. Ibuprofen, valacyclovir, and duct tape will not treat the actual underlying condition.

Psychosocial Disorders

22

QUESTIONS

1. Which of the following demographic groups have the greatest incidence of completion of suicide?
   (A) Females <20 years old and single
   (B) Women 21 to 40 years old and married
   (C) Men 21 to 40 years old and married
   (D) Men >59, widowed, separated or divorced

2. A family brings their 80-year-old patriarch with acute onset of confusion. The patient has no psychiatric history, has not started any recent medication, and has been declining in mental status for the past 2 days. Currently, the patient is easily distracted, has disorganized thinking, and appears to respond to visual stimuli. Which of the following is the MOST LIKELY diagnosis?
   (A) Delirium
   (B) Dementia
   (C) Normal-pressure hydrocephalus
   (D) Psychosis

3. An 76-year-old man is brought in by his family for acute onset of confusion over the last 2 days. He has no psychiatric history and normal vital signs. On arrival, the patient was easily distracted, had disorganized thinking, and appeared to respond to visual stimuli. He is now becoming more agitated, attempting to climb out of bed and pull out his IVs despite several attempts at verbal redirection. He does not have any history of alcohol or drug use. Which medication would you want to avoid with this patient?
   (A) Alpha 2 agonists
   (B) Atypical antipsychotics
   (C) Benzodiazepines
   (D) Typical antipsychotics

4. Which class of medications can exacerbate the hypotensive side effects of intramuscular olanzapine if given concurrently?
   (A) Alpha 2 agonists
   (B) Anticonvulsants
   (C) Antihistamines
   (D) Benzodiazepines

5. A patient is complaining of neck pain with the neck "twisted" to one side after receiving both haloperidol and lorazepam for agitation in the emergency department. What is the BEST agent to treat this condition?
   (A) Benztropine
   (B) Dantrolene
   (C) Diazepam
   (D) Flumazenil

6. A 35-year-old woman presents with chest pain that has been constant for the past 12 hours. She also has nausea, dizziness, and sweating. She has a history of panic attacks, migraines, and fibromyalgia. What element in her history is MOST CONCERNING for a more serious etiology of her symptoms than panic attack?
   (A) Duration of chest pain
   (B) Dizziness
   (C) Nausea
   (D) Sweating

7. Which of the following is NOT a benefit of atypical antipsychotics over typical antipsychotics?
   (A) Decreased extrapyramidal effects
   (B) Decreased incidence of hypotension
   (C) Increased efficacy of the negative symptoms in psychosis
   (D) No prolongation of the QTc interval on electrocardiogram

8. Which of the following is a symptom of opioid withdrawal?
   (A) Constipation
   (B) Delirium
   (C) Miosis
   (D) Piloerection

9. A patient in acute opioid and/or alcohol withdrawal is experiencing acute agitation. What is the BEST medication to use for this patient?
   (A) Antidepressants
   (B) Antipsychotics
   (C) Benzodiazepines
   (D) Selective serotonin reuptake inhibitors

10. What is the MOST common comorbid psychiatric disorder seen in patients with generalized anxiety disorder?
    (A) Conversion disorder
    (B) Depression
    (C) Obsessive-compulsive disorder
    (D) Panic disorder

11. A 35-year-old man who has been seen in the emergency department in the past for complaints of paralysis in his lower extremities presents again in the same fashion. The patient has an unrevealing repeat workup including MRI, blood work, and a neurology consultation. What is his MOST LIKELY diagnosis?
    (A) Conversion disorder
    (B) Dysthymic disorder
    (C) Hypochondriasis
    (D) Somatization disorder

12. Which of the following medications is NOT paired correctly with its major side effect?
    (A) Clozapine—agranulocytosis
    (B) Lamotrigine—Stevens-Johnson syndrome/toxic epidermal necrolysis

(C) Olanzapine—weight loss
(D) Ziprasidone—QTc prolongation

13. A 15-year-old very thin girl was brought to the emergency department by her parents for evaluation for generalized weakness. The patient has signs of dental erosion, callous formation to the dorsal hands, facial petechiae, and subconjunctival hemorrhages. What is her expected acid/base status?
    (A) Metabolic acidosis
    (B) Metabolic alkalosis
    (C) Respiratory acidosis
    (D) Respiratory alkalosis

14. A 15-year-old girl presents to the emergency department with her parents for generalized weakness and weight loss. She has a history of bulimia and admits to routinely purging after she eats. Which of the following abnormalities would you MOST expect to find on her electrocardiogram?
    (A) Flattened T waves
    (B) Peaked T waves
    (C) Prolonged QTc
    (D) Prolonged QTc and U waves

15. What is the MOST COMMON life-threatening problem for patients with significant eating disorders like bulemia?
    (A) Cardiac arrhythmias
    (B) Dehydration
    (C) Hyponatremia
    (D) Mallory Weiss tears

16. A combative 24-year-old man arrives in handcuffs, still fighting with police and staff when brought into your emergency department. What is the BEST medical treatment for him at this time?
    (A) Chlorpromazine and trazadone
    (B) Clozapine and diazepam
    (C) Haloperidol and lorazepam
    (D) Valproic acid and lorazepam

17. Which of the following is NOT an adverse effect of antipsychotics?
    (A) Bradycardia
    (B) Extrapyramidal symptoms
    (C) Neuroleptic malignant syndrome
    (D) QTc prolongation/torsades de pointes

18. Which of the following is NOT indicative of a substance use disorder?
    (A) Failed attempts to cut back or quit substance
    (B) Failure to fulfill responsibilities in work, school, and/or home because of recurrent use
    (C) Increased physical activity
    (D) Persistent use despite social or interpersonal problems

19. What kind of hallucinations are MOST COMMON in an acutely psychotic patient, as opposed to a delirious patient?
    (A) Auditory
    (B) Olfactory
    (C) Tactile
    (D) Visual

20. You are about to evaluate a patient with a history of psychotic schizophrenia who was brought in by police for increased agitation and aggressiveness. What should you AVOID when you approach this patient?
    (A) Have a nonthreatening attitude
    (B) Look the patient in the eye
    (C) Maintain a calm, controlled posture, and tone of voice
    (D) Stand in a location that neither threatens the patient nor blocks the exit of the healthcare worker in the room

ANSWERS

1. **The answer is D.** (Chapters 288 and 289) Patients who are single, separated, widowed, or recently unemployed are at higher risk than those who are married and employed. Recently widowed older white males with access to lethal means (e.g., a firearm) form the population at highest risk for completing suicide in the United States and thus should elicit a very careful evaluation. A useful aid to assessing suicide risk and appropriate treatment plan is provided by the acronym SAD PERSONS which is based on the first letters of 10 literature-identified suicide risk factors.

Modified SAD PERSONS scale

S—Sex: 1 if male; 0 if female; (more females attempt, more males succeed)

A—Age: 1 if 15-25 or ≥ 59

D—Depression or hopelessness: 2 if present

P—Previous suicide attempts or psychiatric care: 1 if present

E—Excessive ethanol or drug use: 1 if present

R—Rational thinking loss (psychotic or organic illness): 1 if present

S—Single, widowed or divorced: 1 if present

O—Organized plan or serious attempt: 2 if present

N—No social support: 1 if not present

S—Stated future intent: 2 if present

This score is then mapped onto a risk assessment scale as follows:

• 0–5: May be safe to discharge (depending upon circumstances)

• 6–8: Probably requires psychiatric consultation

• >8: Probably requires hospital admission

2. **The answer is A.** (Chapters 286 and 288) The rapid onset of this patient's acute confusion makes delirium more likely than dementia or normal pressure hydrocephalus. Delirium would be more common than a sudden acute onset of psychosis in an 80-year-old man with no prior history of mental illness (Table 22.1).

3. **The answer is C.** (Chapter 288) If an elderly patient becomes agitated, begin with a nonpharmacologic approach by addressing patient needs (such as using the restroom and, if possible, allowing the patient to eat or drink), providing comfortable surroundings, and having the family close by. Avoid benzodiazepines in the elderly, if at all possible, unless alcohol withdrawal is the cause of delirium. Benzodiazepines can cause paradoxical disinhibition and increased agitation in the elderly. If a benzodiazepine must be used, consider a short-acting, glucuronidated agent such as lorazepam, oxazepam, or temazepam to minimize prolonged benzodiazepine effects. Avoid antihistamines because this drug class has strong anticholinergic effects and can induce or worsen delirium in the elderly.

4. **The answer is D.** (Chapter 287) Hypotension is a serious adverse effect of intramuscular olanzapine and has led to fatalities in patients who were concurrently given benzodiazepines or chlorpromazine. The product information for olanzapine warns against coadministration with benzodiazepines, because life-threatening sedation and hypotension can occur. While recommendations differ, it is best to wait 1 to 2 hours between administering benzodiazepines with IM olanzapine, and if coadministering with oral olanzapine, monitor blood pressure frequently.

5. **The answer is A.** (Chapter 287) Treat acute dystonias with anticholinergic agents such as intramuscular or

TABLE 22.1	Features of Delirium, Dementia, and Psychiatric Disorder		
Characteristic	Delirium	Dementia	Psychiatric Disorder
Onset	Over days	Insidious	Varies
Course over 24 h	Fluctuating	Stable	Varies
Consciousness	Reduced or hyperalert	Alert	Alert or distracted
Attention	Disordered	Normal	May be disordered
Cognition	Disordered	Impaired	Rarely impaired
Orientation	Impaired	Often impaired	May be impaired
Hallucinations	Visual and/or auditory	Often absent	May be present
Delusions	Transient, poorly organized	Usually absent	Sustained
Movements	Asterixis, tremor may be present	Often absent	Varies

Reproduced with permission from J.E. Tintinalli, J.S. Stapczynski, O.J. Ma, D. Yearly, G.D. Meckler, D.M. Cline: Tintinalli's Emergency Medicine: A Comprehensive Study Guide, 9th ed, McGraw-Hill Education.

intravenous diphenhydramine (25–50 mg) or benztropine (2 mg). These agents are sometimes administered along with a typical intramuscular antipsychotic to prevent dystonia and other extrapyramidal symptoms. Be aware that diphenhydramine and benztropine carry their own risks of adverse reactions including sedation, constipation, and blurred vision.

6. **The answer is A.** (Chapter 289) Panic attacks are short-lived episodes of anxiety or intense fear accompanied by a range of somatic symptoms (commonly cardiac, gastrointestinal, or neurologic), usually peaking within 10 minutes and lasting up to 1 hour. The criteria for panic disorder also stipulate that the panic attack must be followed by 1 month of persistent concern about having additional attacks, or worry about the implications of the attack or its consequences, or a significant change in behavior related to the attacks. Twelve hours of constant symptoms would be unusual for a panic attack. Patients experiencing a panic attack may experience dizziness, nausea, and sweating.

7. **The answer is B.** (Chapter 290) The atypical antipsychotics are generally newer medications that more specifically target the dopamine receptors or inhibit the reuptake of serotonin. They also offer increased efficacy in the treatment of the negative symptoms of psychosis. Based on this improved receptor specificity, adverse effects such as sedation, extrapyramidal effects, QTc prolongation, and tardive dyskinesia are generally reduced but not completely eliminated. The incidence of hypotension does not appear to have been significantly altered.

8. **The answer is D.** (Chapter 292) Symptoms of opioid withdrawal include dilated pupils and tearing, sneezing and runny nose, nausea, vomiting, diarrhea and abdominal cramping, yawning, piloerection (goose bumps), and myalgias. Constipation and miosis are typically seen with opioid use. Delirium is not usually associated with opioid withdrawal and may be indicative of another pathological process.

9. **The answer is C.** (Chapter 287) Benzodiazepines are considered the preferred treatment of agitation for the patient with alcohol or substance abuse.

10. **The answer is B.** (Chapter 289) Comorbid psychiatric illnesses are common with anxiety; about half of the patients diagnosed with anxiety have comorbid depression.

11. **The answer is A.** (Chapter 286) This patient's presentation is most suspicious for a conversion disorder.

However, diagnosis of conversion disorder should be made with extreme caution, if at all, in the emergency department; studies indicate that many patients (up to 50%) diagnosed with conversion disorder eventually develop signs of a physical disorder that explains the symptoms.

12. **The answer is C.** (Chapter 289) Olanzapine is associated with weight gain, not weight loss. The other medications listed are correctly paired with possible adverse side effects (Table 22.2).

13. **The answer is B.** (Chapter 291) This patient's presentation is suspicious for bulimia. Purging from bulimia results in a metabolic alkalosis from hypokalemia and hypochloremia. Purging and binge eating both may cause elevation of liver and pancreatic enzymes.

14. **The answer is D.** (Chapter 291) This patient is likely to have hypokalemia from her poor oral intake and purging behavior. Prolonged QTc interval and U waves are ECG findings of hypokalemia.

15. **The answer is A.** (Chapter 291) Purging behavior leading to electrolyte abnormalities can cause cardiac arrhythmias. Although dehydration, hyponatremia, and Mallory-Weiss tears can also occur, cardiac arrhythmias are the most common problem to occur to a life-threatening degree of severity.

16. **The answer is C.** (Chapter 287) Haloperidol and lorazepam are both standard-of-care therapy for acute agitation in the emergency department as they have fairly rapid onset of action and can be safely administered intramuscularly in uncooperative patients who lack intravenous access. Trazadone is only available orally and would not rapidly treat acute agitation in an uncooperative patient. Clozapine has a significant side effect profile with a risk of agranulocytosis and is not given first line for this reason. Valproic acid would not be a first-line agent for acute agitation.

17. **The answer is A.** (Chapter 287) Bradycardia is not an adverse effect of the antipsychotics. The rest of the list are known side effects.

18. **The answer is C.** (Chapter 292) Everything except increased physical activity is characteristic of a person with a substance use disorder. The *Diagnostic and Statistical Manual of Mental Disorders, Fifth Edition* (DSM-5) diagnosis includes at least two or more of 11 criteria.

TABLE 22.2 Medications Used for Bipolar Disorder

Generic Name	Brand Name	Mechanism of Action	Side Effects (BLACK BOX WARNING IN CAPS)	Usual Starting Dose	Comments
Lithium carbonate	Eskalith®, Lithonate®, Lithotabs®	? increase NE function ? increase serotonin function	TOXICITY closely related to serum lithium levels: diarrhea, vomiting, tremor, mild ataxia, drowsiness or muscular weakness. Initially: nausea, dry mouth, excessive thirst, tremors, polyuria, peripheral edema, cognitive impairment Long-term: polyuria, diabetes insipidus, goiter, hypothyroidism, rashes, leukocytosis	300 mg 2 or 3 times a day	Effective for both acute and maintenance therapy Narrow therapeutic window; toxicity common; symptoms may be delayed up to 48 h in acute overdose Avoid giving with NSAIDs, ACE inhibitors, or diuretics to avoid toxicity. Dose is lower in elderly and patients with renal dysfunction
Valproic acid	Depakene®, Depakote® (12 h), Depakote Sprinkles® (12 h), Depacon® (IV)	Antiepileptic; enhances transmission of GABA	HEPATOTOXICITY, FETAL RISK, PANCREATITIS, weight gain, nausea, vomiting, hair loss, bruising, tremor, thrombocytopenia	250 mg 2 or 3 times a day	Effective for both acute and maintenance therapy Can monitor drug levels Monitor liver and platelet function May be used alone to treat BD, or in combination with antipsychotic or lithium
Carbamazepine	Tegretol®	Antiepileptic; stabilizes sodium channels, potentiates GABA receptors	AGRANULOCYTOSIS, STEVENS-JOHNSON SYNDROME/TOXIC EPIDERMAL NECROLYSIS, nausea, vomiting, hyponatremia, rash, leukopenia	100–200 mg 1 or 2 times a day	Effective for acute or maintenance therapy Can monitor drug levels Monitor LFTs May be better in rapid cycling disorder Do not use with antipsychotics Many drug interactions with similarly liver-metabolized medications OCP failure
Lamotrigine	Lamictal®	Antiepileptic; sodium channel blockade	STEVENS-JOHNSON SYNDROME/TOXIC EPIDERMAL NECROLYSIS—rare complications but potentially fatal; nausea, vomiting, fatigue, dizziness	25 mg once a day (unless on other antiepileptic medication)	Used with more severe depressive symptoms Dose adjustment required with other antiepileptic Progestin-only OCP failure Requires slower dose titration when used with valproic acid
Olanzapine	Zyprexa®	Antipsychotic; muscarinic; dopamine and serotonin antagonist	INCREASED MORTALITY IN ELDERLY PATIENTS WITH DEMENTIA-RELATED PSYCHOSIS, sedation, constipation, dry mouth, glucose intolerance, orthostatic hypotension, hyperlipidemia	2.5–5.0 mg 1 or 2 times a day	May be used in combination with lithium or valproic acid Injection cannot be given within 1 h of injectable benzodiazepine
Quetiapine	Seroquel®	Antipsychotic; dopamine, serotonin, and adrenergic antagonist	INCREASED MORTALITY IN ELDERLY PATIENTS WITH DEMENTIA-RELATED PSYCHOSIS, SUICIDAL THOUGHTS AND BEHAVIORS WITH ANTIDEPRESSANT DRUGS, headache, dry mouth, weight gain, sedation, dizziness, orthostatic hypotension	25–50 mg 1 or 2 times a day	May be used in combination with lithium or valproic acid
Risperidone	Risperdal®	Antipsychotic; serotonin and dopamine antagonist	INCREASED MORTALITY IN ELDERLY PATIENTS WITH DEMENTIA-RELATED PSYCHOSIS, extrapyramidal side effects, prolactin elevation, sedation, dyspepsia, nausea, weight gain	0.25–1 mg 1 or 2 times a day	May be used with lithium or valproic acid Use lower doses in elderly due to orthostasis risk
Aripiprazole	Abilify®	Antipsychotic; partial agonist of dopamine/serotonin receptors; antagonist of other serotonin receptors	INCREASED MORTALITY IN ELDERLY PATIENTS WITH DEMENTIA-RELATED PSYCHOSIS, SUICIDAL THOUGHTS AND BEHAVIORS WITH ANTIDEPRESSANT DRUGS, headache, nausea, vomiting, extrapyramidal symptoms, especially akathisia	2–10 mg once a day	May be used with lithium or valproic acid
Ziprasidone	Geodon®	Antipsychotic; serotonin and dopamine antagonist; adrenergic antagonist; agonist at other serotonin receptors	INCREASED RISK OF DEATH IN DEMENTIA-RELATED PSYCHOSIS; rash, weight gain, constipation, nausea, tremor, extrapyramidal side effects, sedation, vision changes	40 mg twice a day	May be used with lithium or valproic acid
Lurasidone	Latuda®	Antipsychotic; serotonin and dopamine antagonist; adrenergic antagonist; agonist at other serotonin receptors	INCREASED RISK OF DEATH IN DEMENTIA-RELATED PSYCHOSIS, nausea, vomiting, extrapyramidal side effects, sedation, anxiety	20 mg once a day	

Abbreviations: ACE = angiotensin-converting enzyme; BD = bipolar disorder; GABA = γ-aminobutyric acid; LFTs = liver function tests; NE = norepinephrine; OCP = oral contraceptive pill.

Reproduced with permission from J.E. Tintinalli, J.S. Stapczynski, O.J. Ma, D. Yearly, G.D. Meckler, D.M. Cline: Tintinalli's Emergency Medicine: A Comprehensive Study Guide, 9th ed, McGraw-Hill Education.

19. **The answer is A.** (Chapter 290) Although hallucinations may occur in any sensory modality, they are most commonly auditory in schizophrenia and other psychotic disorders. Typically, these are experienced as voices distinct from the individual's own thoughts.

20. **The answer is B.** (Chapter 286) Avoid excessive eye contact when dealing with a potentially dangerous patient, as this may cause them to escalate if they perceive it as aggressive. The other answers are correct in how to interact with this patient.

Abuse and Assault

23

QUESTIONS

1. Which initial emergency department presentation is MOST consistent with epidemiology of sexual assault in the United States?
   (A) Male or female sexually assaulted at gunpoint
   (B) Female sexually assaulted by multiple unknown perpetrators while walking home
   (C) Female with severe anogenital injuries who was raped greater than 48 hours ago
   (D) Female sexually assaulted by a known perpetrator

2. A 23-year-old woman presents to the emergency department with a chief complaint of being raped by a family friend greater than 96 hours ago. Which of the following is NOT recommended emergency department management at this time?
   (A) Testing for syphilis, hepatitis, and HIV
   (B) Full history and physical examination with thorough forensic evaluation and maintained chain of custody
   (C) Referral for follow-up medical care and rape crisis counseling
   (D) Pregnancy test, emergency contraception, and prophylaxis for sexually transmitted infections

3. Repeat human immunodeficiency virus (HIV) antibody testing after a sexual assault is recommended at what intervals after the baseline testing at emergency department presentation?

   (A) 3 months and 6 months
   (B) 3 months, 6 months, and 1 year
   (C) 6 weeks, 3 months, and 6 months
   (D) 6 weeks and 6 months

4. Which of the following is TRUE regarding the forensic examination for sexual assault?
   (A) When obtaining photographic evidence, begin with a photograph of the patient's face, photograph all injuries including all contusions, laceration and bite marks, and end the series with a photograph of the patient's hospital wrist band.
   (B) Document position of genital injuries using an upside-down clock face reference, where 12 o'clock is the perineum, 3 o'clock is the right hip, 6 o'clock is pubic symphysis, and 9 o'clock is the left hip.
   (C) Wood's lamp can detect traces of saliva from the assailant; therefore, any illuminated areas should be swabbed, dried, labeled, and added to forensic evidence.
   (D) A completed rape kit can be stored in an unlocked refrigerator in the emergency department clean utility room until law enforcement collects it, if the kit has been properly sealed and labeled.

5. Which of the following BEST describes the Centers for Disease Control and Prevention (CDC) guidelines for prophylaxis of sexually transmitted infections following sexual assault?
   (A) Human papilloma virus (HPV) vaccination is not recommended.
   (B) Postexposure hepatitis B vaccination including hepatitis B immune globulin (HBIG) is recommended if assailant is unknown and survivor is not previously vaccinated.
   (C) Human immunodeficiency virus (HIV) postexposure prophylaxis (PEP) should be given to all sexual assault victims in the ED.
   (D) Empiric antimicrobial regimen should include coverage for chlamydia, gonorrhea and trichomonas.

6. Which of the following BEST describes the typical cyclical pattern of intimate partner violence?
   (A) Tension building → Escalation → Honeymoon Phase
   (B) Tension building → Honeymoon Phase → Escalation
   (C) Tension building → Resolution → Honeymoon Phase → Explosion
   (D) Tension building → Escalation → 'Honeymoon' Phase → Explosion

7. Which of the presenting emergency department complaints would be MOST concerning for intimate partner violence and neglect?
   (A) Broken arm
   (B) Fractured clavicle from a fall down the basement steps 1 hour ago
   (C) Suicidal ideation without a plan and a history of multiple visits for chronic depression
   (D) Upper chest bruising in a pregnant female after a fall

8. A 29-year-old woman presents to the emergency department with a periorbital contusion and bilateral forearm bruising. After questioning by the triage nurse, she tearfully admits that she was beaten by her live-in boyfriend but feels she cannot leave him at this time for reasons she refuses to disclose. Which of the following would NOT be an appropriate approach by the emergency department provider?

(A) Using nonjudgmental language, tell the patient that violence, abuse, and intimidation are not part of normal, healthy relationships, but respect the individual's wishes about the future of the relationship and her decision to return home.
(B) Let the patient know the situation is taken seriously with voiced concern for her health and safety as well as anyone else living in the home.
(C) Inform the patient that trained social workers and intimate violence advocates can help her develop a plan for safety or ending the relationship if she would want their assistance.
(D) Request that an intimate personal violence advocate directly call the patient's home after the patient is discharged without direct permission from the patient.

9. Which of the following is NOT recommended for emergency department record documentation of intimate partner violence and abuse?
   (A) Voluntary descriptions quoted and described in the patient's own words whenever possible
   (B) Description of any stated violence or abuse as "alleged" since the actual details are not yet known
   (C) Description of the patient's injuries, appearance, and demeanor with annotated body maps and photographs
   (D) Documentation of relevant forensic evidence, emergency department testing, and treatment in the occurrence of sexual assault

10. Which of the following is CORRECT regarding the epidemiology of intimate partner violence and abuse?
    (A) Individuals who are married or divorced are at greater risk than those who are separated.
    (B) Individuals who were abused as children are at greater risk of intimate partner violence as adults.
    (C) Intimate partner violence and abuse are experienced most often by those older than 30 years.
    (D) Weapons in the home act as deterrents lowering the risk of intimate partner homicide.

11. Which of the following emergency department presentations would be LEAST concerning for elder abuse?
    (A) 75-year-old man who fell out of bed with contusions to inner thighs
    (B) 80-year-old woman with dementia with circumferential abrasions to the wrists and ankles

(C) 70-year-old man with advanced multiple sclerosis and open sacral pressure sore

(D) 75-year-old woman with early dementia and midshaft ulnar fracture

12. Which of the following is TRUE regarding elder abuse/maltreatment?
    (A) The perpetrator is most often the spouse of the primary caregiver.
    (B) Elder abuse is more prevalent in residential settings than in institutional settings.
    (C) Perpetrators of elder maltreatment are less likely to be dependent on the elder for financial security.
    (D) Female caregivers are more likely to engage in abuse than male caregivers.

13. Which of the following is NOT categorized as elder abuse?
    (A) Deliberate restricted nutrition of an elderly woman by the son she lives with
    (B) Armed robbery of an elderly woman who is subsequently beaten in her home
    (C) Forcible changing of an elderly parent's will by his three children
    (D) Demeaning remarks regularly made by a home health caregiver to an elderly man in her care

14. Which of the following is NOT a barrier to the detection of elder abuse?
    (A) Elderly parents may not want to admit vulnerabilities and are ashamed of the betrayal by adult children and afraid of retaliation.
    (B) Differing perceptions by cultural backgrounds as to what constitutes abuse.
    (C) Lack of established hospital protocols for identifying or addressing elder abuse.
    (D) Physicians are required by law to obtain permission from a mentally competent elderly patient before reporting suspected abuse.

15. Which of the following examples BEST illustrates the most common form of elder abuse reported annually to adult protective service agencies in the United States?
    (A) Elderly woman with early dementia being slapped or punched by her daughter's family whenever they become frustrated with her
    (B) Inadequate hygiene by the primary caretaker of an elderly man with dementia and incontinence resulting in open pressure ulcers in his anogenital area
    (C) Sexual assault of an elderly woman by a caregiver in a nursing home
    (D) Social security checks of an elderly man being regularly used by his daughter for her own personal vacations

ANSWERS

1. **The answer is D.** (Chapter 293) According to the National Electronic Injury Surveillance System (NEISS), women are likely to seek treatment earlier for more severe assaults and are more likely to delay seeking assistance if assaulted by a known perpetrator. In most cases of rape in the United States, a single assailant is involved, and most often the perpetrator is known to the victim. It is estimated that only 26% of assailants are strangers. Force or coercion is used in most assaults. More significant injuries are more often found in those who present within 24 hours of assault. Injuries are more often found in females <20 years old or >49 years old.

2. **The answer is B.** (Chapter 293) Any individual presenting to the emergency department with a complaint of sexual assault must have a pertinent medical history and thorough physical exam. Pregnancy testing and testing for sexually transmitted infections, including syphilis, hepatitis B, and HIV should be performed, followed by prophylaxis as appropriate. If individuals present <72 hours from the time of assault, forensic evidentiary examination should be performed. Consent must be obtained from the patient and collection according to directions on the forensic kit; however, collection of evidence should be tailored to specifics of the assault. Completed kits must be properly sealed, dated, and signed using provided chain of evidence form, and locked in a refrigerator or cabinet until collected by law enforcement. The chances of finding forensic evidence >72 hours after the assault are slim, so forensic examination and collection is NOT necessary in these cases. (It should be noted, however, that some states allow for evidence collection up to 96 hours post-assault.)

3. **The answer is C.** (Chapter 293) As per current Centers for Disease Control and Prevention (CDC) recommendations, HIV testing should be obtained at baseline presentation with repeated testing at 6 weeks, 3 months, and 6 months using methods to identify acute HIV infection.

4. **The answer is A.** (Chapter 293) Sexual assault forensic evaluation includes collection of head and pubic hair and swabs of bodily fluids for DNA comparison, photographs and full descriptions of all injuries, including documented vaginal and perineal injuries. The photographic series should begin with a photograph of the patient's face and end with a photograph of the patient's hospital wrist band. Document location, position of patient, and position of injury, using a clock face reference. In lithotomy position, the patient's pubic bone is at 12 o'clock, left hip is at 3 o'clock, and right hip is at 9 o'clock. If photography is not available, describe traumatic injuries in detail using a body

map. Traces of semen over the entire body surface can be detected using a Wood's lamp. When all forensic evidence has been collected, chain of custody must be maintained, with the completed collection kit that must be properly sealed and labeled, proper signing of the chain of custody form, and never left unattended. Unless law enforcement is immediately available to collect the completed kit, it should be temporarily stored in a locked cabinet or refrigerator in the emergency department designated for this purpose.

5. **The answer is D.** (Chapter 293) Survivors of sexual assault typically have poor compliance with follow-up visits; therefore, testing and appropriate prophylactic treatment are recommended in the emergency department setting. Centers for Disease Control and Prevention (CDC) guidelines recommend empiric antimicrobial treatment for chlamydia, gonorrhea, and trichomonas (Table 23.1).

6. **The answer is A.** (Chapter 294) Intimate partner violence is most often cyclical in nature. The cycle begins with a period of *tension building*, which may include arguing, controlling behaviors or jealousy. The following phase is *escalation* and may include verbal threats, physical and sexual abuse, or assault, including use of weapons. There may be a *honeymoon phase* in which the perpetrator apologizes or makes excuses for inappropriate behavior. With time, the cycle accelerates and the abusive behavior becomes more severe.

TABLE 23.1	Centers for Disease Control and Prevention Guidelines for Postassault Prophylaxis

- If assailant status unknown and survivor not previously vaccinated, give postexposure hepatitis B vaccination without HBIG, and inform survivor that subsequent doses must be given at 1–2 and 4–6 mo after first dose.
- If the assailant is known to be HBsAg positive, unvaccinated survivors should receive hepatitis B vaccine and HBIG at the time of initial examination.
- For survivors previously vaccinated but who have not had postvaccination testing, give a single hepatitis B vaccine booster.
- HPV vaccination is recommended for female survivors age 9–26 y and male survivors age 9–21 y at the time of initial examination. Inform survivor that subsequent doses must be given at 1–2 mo and 6 mo after the first dose.
- Empiric antibiotics for chlamydia, gonorrhea, and trichomoniasis.
- Tetanus prophylaxis if needed.
- Offer emergency contraception if the assault could result in pregnancy.
- Baseline testing for syphilis, hepatitis C, and HIV.
- Obtain serum chemistries and liver function studies if HIV postexposure prophylaxis given.
- Provide first follow-up at 1 week.

Abbreviations: HBIG = hepatitis B immune globulin; HBsAg = hepatitis B surface antigen; HIV = human immunodeficiency virus; HPV = human papillomavirus.

Source: Reproduced with permission from J.E. Tintinalli, J.S. Stapczynski, O.J. Ma, D. Yealy, G.D. Meckler, D.M. Cline: Tintinalli's Emergency Medicine: A Comprehensive Study Guide, 9th Edition. McGraw-Hill Education; 2020.

TABLE 23.2	Signs Suggestive of Intimate Partner Violence
Findings	**Comments**
Injuries characteristic of violence	Fingernail scratches, broken fingernails, bite marks, dental injuries, black eyes, broken bones, cigarette burns, bruises suggesting strangulation or restraint, and rope burns or ligature marks may be seen.
Injuries suggesting a defensive posture	Forearm bruises or fractures may be sustained when individuals try to fend off blows to the face or chest.
Injuries during pregnancy	Up to 45% of women report abuse or assault during pregnancy.[10]
	Preterm labor, placental abruption, direct fetal injury, and stillbirth can occur.
Central pattern of injury	Injuries to the head, neck, face, and thorax, abdominal and genital injuries.
Extent or type of injury inconsistent with the patient's explanation	Multiple injuries at different anatomic sites inconsistent with the described mechanism of injury.
	The most common explanation of injury is a "fall."
	Embarrassment, evasiveness, or lack of concern with the injuries may be noted.
Multiple injuries in various stages of healing	These may be reported as "accidents" or "clumsiness."
Delay between the time of injury and the presentation for treatment	Victims may wait several days before seeking medical care for injuries.
	Victims may seek care for minor or resolving injuries.
Visits for vague or minor complaints without evidence of physiologic abnormality	Frequent ED visits for a variety of injuries or illnesses, including chronic pelvic pain and other chronic pain syndromes.
Suicide attempts	Women who attempt or commit suicide often have a history of intimate partner violence.

Reproduced with permission from J.E. Tintinalli, J.S. Stapczynski, O.J. Ma, D. Yealy, G.D. Meckler, D.M. Cline: Tintinalli's Emergency Medicine: A Comprehensive Study Guide, 9th Edition. McGraw-Hill Education; 2020.

7. **The answer is D.** (Chapter 294) The overall features by which a person who has experienced intimate partner violence and abuse are not always typical. Careful screening and assessment for elements of the history and physical examination suggestive of abuse are necessary. Although any of these emergency department presentations could potentially be related to an incident of abuse, a central pattern of injury (head, neck, thorax, or abdomen) in a pregnant female are especially concerning for intimate partner violence and abuse. Signs suggestive of intimate partner violence are summarized in Table 23.2.

8. **The answer is D.** (Chapter 294) Ensuring the safety of the abused individual is the foremost goal. Ultimately the abused individual must make the determination of whether it is safe to return home. Let the patient know the situation is taken seriously with concern about the health and safety of her and anyone else living in the home, especially children. Patients must be told that violence, abuse, and intimidation are not a part of normal, healthy relationships, but respect the abused individual's wishes about the future of the relationship. By providing information about risks and options, the emergency department provider can help the patient decide what is the best decision at that time. Emphasize she has done nothing to warrant violence and abuse, and that trained social workers or intimate violence advocates can help develop logistical plans either for safety or for ending the relationship. Finally, if the patient is discharged home and direct contact with a social worker or advocate cannot be made prior to discharge, the patient is given up-to-date community services and resources. Intimate personal violence advocates should NOT be asked to call the patient directly unless the patient agrees, because direct calls to the home could potentially jeopardize the patient's safety.

9. **The answer is B.** (Chapter 294) Emergency department documentation of intimate partner violence and assault should be clearly stated, with voluntary descriptions quoted and described in the patient's own words. Do NOT use the word "alleged" because it implies that the person recording the incident does not believe the complaint. Record past and current abuse, with details of date, time, location, witnesses, and specific injury. Describe the patient's current health complaints, injuries, appearance, and demeanor, with annotated body maps and photographs whenever possible. If sexual assault has occurred, obtain relevant forensic evidence, document emergency department testing and treatment, and follow the appropriate chain of custody of evidence.

10. **The answer is B.** (Chapter 294). Intimate partner violence and abuse occur in every racial, ethnic, cultural, and religious group, and affect individuals of all socioeconomic and educational backgrounds worldwide. Risk factors include female sex, age between 18 and 24 years, low income level, and relationship status of separated rather than married or divorced. Sexual and/or physical abuse during childhood and adolescence is a frequent predictor of future victimization. Weapons in the home and threats of murder are associated with increased risk of homicide.

11. **The answer is C.** (Chapter 295) Elder abuse is often detected when physical examination triggers the need for additional history-taking with results suggesting maltreatment. Although not the most common form of elder abuse, physical abuse is most easily recognized. Patterns of abuse include injuries to normally protected areas of the body such as contusions or lacerations on the inner arms or thighs, rope or restraint marks on the wrists or ankles from inappropriate restraints, and isolated midshaft ulnar (nightstick) fractures from attempts to shield blows by raising the forearm. Findings resulting from caregiver neglect are less specific, with the most identifiable finding being multiple or deep pressure ulcer sores, especially those not in the lumbosacral areas.

Incapacitated patients with prolonged immobilization, like those with advanced neurological conditions such as multiple sclerosis, amyotrophic lateral sclerosis (ALS), or Parkinson's disease are at risk for pressure ulcers even with appropriate care.

12. **The answer is B.** (Chapter 295) Elder abuse is more common in residential than institutional settings, although institutionalization is a risk factor for elder neglect and abuse. Abusers are most often the primary caregiver, frequently an adult child. The adult child is more likely to abuse than the child's significant other and is more likely to be financially dependent on the elder for financial security. Males are more likely to be perpetrators of elder abuse than females, and although well intentioned, abusers may be simply overwhelmed by the amount of care required and may themselves be impaired by personal physical or mental health issues.

13. **The answer is B.** (Chapter 295) Elder abuse is defined as harm to an elderly individual by someone the older individual already knows, has an established relationship with, or who is relied upon for services. Many forms of elder abuse are committed by family members or by paid caregivers. Note that elder abuse does NOT include general criminal acts by persons not previously known, such as home invasion, burglaries, or physical or sexual assault. Table 23.3 summarizes the categories of elder abuse.

14. **The answer is D.** (Chapter 295) Elders who sustain abuse often blame themselves, may not want to admit vulnerabilities, feel disgraced for having raised a child who would betray them, and are often unwilling to press charges against a family member. Abused older adults are often afraid of retaliation, including further abuse or being removed from the home and placed in a nursing institution. There may also be differing perceptions as to what constitutes abuse based on cultural background. ED physicians may fail to report abuse because of time constraints, unfamiliarity with reporting laws or concern of offending patients or their families. In addition, physicians may have the misperception that the law requires them to obtain the patient's permission before reporting suspected abuse. Hospitals may also lack protocols for identifying or addressing elder abuse.

TABLE 23.3	Categories of Elder Abuse
Categories of Abuse	**Example**
Physical abuse	Pushing, slapping, burning, striking with objects, improper use of restraint (physical or chemical)
Caregiver neglect	Deprivation of food, clothing, hygiene, medical care, shelter, or supervision
Sexual abuse	Unwanted touching, indecent exposure, unwanted innuendo, rape
Financial or material exploitation	Forcible transfer of property or other assets, including changing elderly person's will
Emotional or psychological abuse	Verbal threats (such as threats of violence, institutionalization, or deprivation), humiliation, intimidation, harassment, social neglect, and isolation
Abandonment	Desertion of an elder in the home or a hospital, nursing facility, shopping mall, or other public location by a caregiver or caretaker
Self-neglect	Failure or unwillingness to provide adequate food, clothing, shelter, medical care, hygiene, or social stimulation to self in individuals with diminished capacity to perform essential self-care tasks

Source: Reproduced with permission from J.E. Tintinalli, J.S. Stapczynski, O.J. Ma, D. Yealy, G.D. Meckler, D.M. Cline: Tintinalli's Emergency Medicine: A Comprehensive Study Guide, 9th Edition. McGraw-Hill Education; 2020.

15. **The answer is B.** (Chapter 295) Elder neglect, defined as a caregiver's failure to provide basic patient care and provide goods and services necessary to prevent physical harm or emotional discomfort, is the most common form of elder abuse/maltreatment—accounting for >50% of all annual reported cases to adult protective service agencies. It also likely accounts for most unreported abuse cases. Examples of elder neglect include deprivation of food, clothing, hygiene, medical care, or supervision considered essential for a person's well-being. The second most common form of elder abuse is financial exploitation, accounting for 20% to 30% of reported cases. When family members or other caregivers assume control of the elder's financial resources, coercion or outright theft may occur, including savings accounts, pensions, or social security checks used for personal gain. Although physical abuse is more easily recognized, it is less common than other forms of elder abuse. Less common types of elder maltreatment also include sexual assault, emotional or psychological abuse, abandonment, and self-neglect.

QUESTIONS

1. A 35-year-old woman presents with cough and dyspnea. Vitals are T 38.9°C, P 109, BP 105/86, and RR 27. Examination reveals crackles over her right lung fields and track marks on her bilateral upper extremities and feet. Chest x-ray reveals a right upper lobe cavitary infiltrate. Documented purified protein derivative (PPD) 6 months ago is negative. Blood cultures are obtained, intravenous fluid resuscitation is initiated, and broad-spectrum antibiotics are given. Which of the following is the MOST APPROPRIATE NEXT step in management?
   (A) Admission for echocardiogram
   (B) Admission for bronchoscopy
   (C) Obtain computed tomography of the chest
   (D) Place the patient in negative pressure isolation

2. A 40-year-old man with a history of intravenous drug use presents to the emergency department with fever and pain in his groin. Vitals are T 38.8°C, HR 85, BP 126/83, and RR 16. There is a fluctuant, pulsatile mass in his left inguinal region that is tender to palpation with erythema extending over the thigh and groin, but no crepitus is appreciated. Which of the following is your NEXT STEP in management?
   (A) Admission to the floor for intravenous antibiotics for 48 hours
   (B) Doppler ultrasonography
   (C) Stat surgical consultation
   (D) Ultrasound-guided incision and drainage in the emergency department

3. A 63-year-old man received a cadaveric kidney transplant for end-stage renal disease due to a diabetic nephropathy approximately 8 weeks ago. The patient presents to the emergency department with 3 days of moderately decreased urine output, tenderness over the graft site, and a potassium level of 5.6 mEq/L (baseline, 4.8 mEq/L posttransplant). Vital signs include BP 185/98, HR 92, and T 100°F (37.8°C). Given this patient's presentation, which of the following should be at the forefront of the differential diagnosis?
   (A) Acute renal artery occlusion
   (B) Infection from cytomegalovirus (CMV)
   (C) Medication noncompliance
   (D) *Staphylococcus aureus* bacteremia

4. A 52-year-old man who underwent liver transplantation due to hepatitis C cirrhosis 1 year ago presents to the emergency department with fever, confusion, and ascites. His transplant medications include low-dose prednisone and tacrolimus. The patient's wife reports that he was doing well until approximately 2 weeks ago when their child came home from school with a fever and runny nose. The patient subsequently became ill with an upper respiratory infection and presented to his primary care physician, where he was given pseudoephedrine, azithromycin, and a cough suppressant. The patient improved over the next 3 to 5 days but became ill again with malaise, myalgias, and low-grade fevers and delirium. She brought him to the emergency department when she noticed that his symptoms were similar to "liver episodes" he experienced before the transplant. What is the MOST LIKELY etiology for this patient's presentation of hepatic encephalopathy?
   (A) Acute hepatitis C
   (B) Disappearing duct syndrome
   (C) Primary graft failure
   (D) Tacrolimus toxicity

5. A 70-year-old morbidly obese woman presents to the emergency department with a fever. Vital signs on presentation are T 39.1°C, HR 105, BP 128/75, RR 40, and SpO_2 92%. Labs are concerning for white blood cell count of $17 \times 10^3/\mu L$ with a neutrophilic predominance and a lactate of 3.5 mmol/L. On examination, she is tachypneic with a capillary refill of 4 seconds. Chest x-ray shows a right lower lobe infiltrate. Her weight is estimated to be 200 kg. As you are considering appropriate treatment and resuscitative efforts, you must recall which of the following will be TRUE for this patient?
(A) She is at risk for a falsely elevated blood pressure cuff measurement.
(B) She is not a candidate for rapid sequence intubation if she decompensates.
(C) She should receive a bolus of 3 L normal saline.
(D) She would benefit from femoral venous central catheter placement as opposed to the internal jugular central catheter.

6. A 50-year-old morbidly obese man with a history of atrial fibrillation on warfarin presents with altered mental status after being found by a family member in his bed. He was last seen normal 90 minutes prior to arrival. Vitals are T 36.1°C, P 120, BP 115/79, RR 23, and SpO_2 90% on a nonrebreather mask. He is making incomprehensible sounds, does not open his eyes, and withdraws from noxious stimuli. There is vomitus in his oropharynx. You have made the decision to intubate him. This patient's obesity places him at greatest risk for which of the following?
(A) Aspiration secondary to decreased intra-abdominal pressure
(B) Hypoxic arrest in the peri-intubation period
(C) Inadequate sedation post-intubation when fentanyl or benzodiazepines are administered as an infusion
(D) Increased Cormack-Lehane grade views in the ramping position as compared to the sniffing position

7. A 50-year-old man with a history of metastatic pancreatic cancer and recently diagnosed depression presents to the emergency department for abdominal pain. He has presented multiple times in the past 3 months for similar symptoms and has required admission for pain control. The patient lives with his daughter, who is his healthcare proxy, and is present at the bedside. He has documentation that reflects his wishes to not be resuscitated or intubated, although

he is agreeable to other indicated medical interventions. Which of the following is the BEST reason to obtain a palliative care consult in the emergency department for this patient?
(A) Age
(B) Code status
(C) Increased frequency of emergency department evaluations and admissions
(D) Mental health history

8. A 3-year-old boy was brought to the emergency department after being found unresponsive in a swimming pool. One hour of resuscitation efforts were unsuccessful. You are informed that the patient's family has arrived and would like to see their deceased child. Which of the following is TRUE?
(A) Organ donation is no longer possible.
(B) Removal of the endotracheal tube removal may occur at the physician or parents' request.
(C) The parents do not have the right to refuse an autopsy.
(D) The patient cannot be viewed by the family.

9. A 63-year-old man presents to the emergency department from a state prison with complaints of chest pain. He is handcuffed and there is a prison officer at bedside. You are informed that he has a history of violence toward others and has attempted to escape in the hospital in the past. He is currently calm, cooperative, and with no chest pain. His troponin is negative and an electrocardiogram shows T-wave inversions laterally. What must be considered when caring for this inmate?
(A) He should be sedated prophylactically before being examined.
(B) The Health Insurance Portability and Accountability Act (HIPPA) does not apply in this case.
(C) The patient may be observed in the prison infirmary.
(D) The patient should be handcuffed during your history taking and physical examination.

10. A patient presents from prison after sustaining an isolated open humeral fracture sustained in an assault. Vital signs on arrival are HR 110, BP 146/92, RR 21, and SpO_2 97% on RA. He informs you that he takes buprenorphine for his opiate use disorder. His pain is currently a 10/10. What is the MOST APPROPRIATE choice of intravenous analgesia for relief of this patient's acute pain?

(A) Fentanyl 1 mg/kg
(B) Ketamine 0.3 mg/kg
(C) Ketorolac 15 mg
(D) Morphine 0.1 mg/kg

11. When under fire, according to the Tactical Combat Casualty Protocol, which of the following interventions is indicated?
(A) Chest compressions in cardiac arrest
(B) Needle decompression for tension pneumothorax
(C) Rapid sequence intubation for airway protection
(D) Tourniquet application for massive hemorrhage

12. A member of the armed forces is shot in his left forearm during combat. A tourniquet is placed on the battlefield due to copious pulsatile bleeding from the wound. Which of the following is TRUE regarding tourniquet placement in this situation?
(A) An attempt to apply a pressure dressing should be made. If effective, the tourniquet should be removed from the extremity.
(B) Application pressure should equal the estimated diastolic blood pressure.
(C) The tourniquet should be placed approximately 2 in proximal to the wound.
(D) The tourniquet should be removed within 3 hours.

13. Which of the following is recommended for the initial resuscitation for a severe hypovolemic shock in the combat setting?
(A) Fresh whole blood
(B) Lactated ringers
(C) Packed red blood cells
(D) Packed red blood cells:plasma:platelets 1:1:1

14. A 50-year-old man presents to the emergency department with shortness of breath. He is alert and oriented and hemodynamically stable. You have decided the patient has decision-making capacity. In which of the following scenarios may informed consent be waived for further evaluation and treatment?
(A) Chest tube insertion for a pneumothorax
(B) Isolation and treatment for active pulmonary tuberculosis in a homeless man
(C) Observation for serial troponin testing in a prisoner with known coronary artery disease
(D) Transfusion of blood for anemia in a Jehovah's Witness

15. A pediatric patient presents to the emergency department without a legal guardian. Which situation requires consent by a legal guardian in order to provide them with treatment?
(A) A 13-year-old pregnant girl at 22 weeks gestation presenting with abdominal pain
(B) A 14-year-old sexually active girl with foul-smelling vaginal discharge
(C) A 16-year-old girl who suffered a deep self-inflicted laceration to her left flexor palmaris tendon after cutting it with a razor blade
(D) A 17-year-old boy presenting after motor vehicle collision whose systolic blood pressure is 70

ANSWERS

1. **The answer is D.** (Chapter 296) There is a broad differential of both infectious and noninfectious entities in the febrile IV drug user who presents with cough. Community-acquired pneumonia is most common, although other etiologies including aspiration, tuberculosis, human immunodeficiency virus complications. Additionally, septic pulmonary emboli secondary to right-sided endocarditis and hypersensitivity reactions should be considered. Although this patient had a recent negative purified protein derivative (PPD), injection drug use is associated with a high degree of immune dysregulation. The finding of a right upper lobe cavitary infiltrate in this individual warrants negative pressure isolation until tuberculosis can be excluded with further testing. Blood cultures and an echocardiogram to evaluate for bacteremia and endocarditis should be obtained in this patient, but the immediate priority is isolation to prevent spread of tuberculosis. While bronchoscopy and chest computed tomography can help to further evaluate the characteristics of this lesion, negative pressure isolation should not be delayed to obtain these tests.

2. **The answer is B.** (Chapter 296) Diagnosis is primarily clinical when evaluating cutaneous infections, except when pulsations are present. Pulsatile masses and masses in highly vascular regions should be imaged with Doppler ultrasound prior to incision and drainage. It is crucial to evaluate for the involvement of vascular structures and pseudoaneurysm formation, as incision and drainage of an infected pseudoaneurysm can result in severe hemorrhage. Antibiotics may give empirically, although definitive drainage will ultimately be needed for appropriate treatment of a fluid collection. Stat surgical consultation is appropriate when there is concern for necrotizing fasciitis due to findings of crepitus, rapid extension of infection, or pain out of proportion to examination. Bedside ultrasound is a useful adjunct to physical examination and can better define the margins of an underlying abscess for safe bedside incision and drainage, but Doppler ultrasonography is needed in this case to assess for vascular involvement first.

3. **The answer is B.** (Chapter 297) From 1 to 6 months posttransplant, cytomegalovirus (CMV) DNA virus is an important detrimental organism affecting the long-term viability of all transplants. CMV can precipitate rejection in every type of solid organ transplant. CMV can infect a transplanted organ at any time after transplantation; however, primary infection classically occurs approximately in the first 6 months of transplantation. Immunosuppression, which is typically maximized in the first 1.5 months

after transplantation, contributes to the early appearance of CMV. CMV is transmitted through the transplanted organ or infection in the donor's blood infections or through reactivation of latent infection. Diagnosis can be made either by blood titers or biopsy. In this patient's case, CMV has triggered rejection in the cadaveric kidney, which is identified by decreased urine output, pain over the transplant site, and an elevated potassium level. Given that infection is the most common cause of organ demise in all transplants, it is reasonable to consider *Staphylococcus aureus*; however, these nosocomial organisms generally cause infection in the first month after transplantation when immunosuppression is at its highest. Acute renal artery occurs more precipitously than as described in this patient's course, within 2 weeks after transplantation. Medication noncompliance is unlikely since transplant patients are under vigilant care of the transplant service during the first few weeks after transplantation and routinely receive blood tests to assess levels of transplant-related medications.

4. **The answer is D.** (Chapter 297) The most likely etiology is tacrolimus toxicity. Immunosuppressive agents are the cornerstone of posttransplant longevity. However, there is a delicate balance between immunosuppressive agents and the risk of infection. One of the most significant side effects of immunosuppressive agents is potential medication toxicity. Immunosuppressive medications such as cyclosporine and tacrolimus not only cause individual toxicities but also cause interactive toxicities. In this case, the patient was recently placed on a macrolide (azithromycin), which can increase serum concentrations immunosuppressive agents such as tacrolimus and cyclosporine. Inappropriate levels of these medications can precipitate graft rejection in an otherwise healthy transplanted organ. Although acute hepatitis C, disappearing duct syndrome, and primary graft failure can also lead to liver transplant rejection, the most likely culprit in this case is medication toxicity due to an interaction between the macrolide and immunosuppressive medications. Therefore, although medication toxicity is the most likely cause of this patient's hepatic encephalopathy, other potential causes must be carefully considered.

5. **The answer is A.** (Chapter 298) Improper blood pressure cuff width and circumference will artificially elevate blood pressure readings. Patients who are overweight require larger than 32 cm circumference cuff sizes. It is crucial to recognize this in this septic patient as her blood pressure may be falsely elevated. While obese patients are more difficult to mask ventilate and are at increased risks

for rapid desaturation, obesity is not a contraindication for rapid sequence intubation. Rapid sequence intubation in the obese patients decreases their risks of aspiration and improves intubating conditions as when compared to awake intubation. Emphasis on advanced preparation and backup techniques should be considered, including bougie and video laryngoscopy. Even if the patient is normotensive, she has an elevated lactate, poor perfusion, and multiple other signs of sepsis such as fever, tachypnea, and leukocytosis. Current sepsis guidelines recommend resuscitation with 30 cc/kg of crystalloid, which is significantly more than 3 L in this patient. In the morbidly obese, there is an increased incidence of infection and deep venous thrombosis when using the femoral approach and therefore should be avoided. The internal jugular vein can be accessed with equal success to the subclavian approach in patients who are obese.

6. **The answer is B.** (Chapter 298) Obese patients are known to desaturate more rapidly during preoxygenation when compared to those who are not obese and it is important to optimize rates of first pass success in this population. This patient has a high probability of suffering from hypoxia during intubation and is at increased risk for peri-intubation hypoxic cardiopulmonary arrest. Preoxygenation may be optimized by maintaining a 25-degree head-up position during preoxygenation and is appropriate as long as cervical spine injury is not a concern. Obese patients have increased intra-abdominal pressure and incidence of gastroesophageal reflux disease making them more prone to aspiration during airway management. Fentanyl and benzodiazepines are lipophilic and have a prolonged half-life in obese patients. Obese patients are actually at risk for oversedation after intubation and ideal body weight should be used for continuous dosing of sedatives and be titrated closely to clinical effect as ideal body weight doses may also be supratherapeutic. Initial dosing, however, may be based on total body weight in order to achieve clinically appropriate induction during intubation. The "sniffing" position results in suboptimal positioning for laryngoscopy as compared to the "ramping" position in obese patients. Ramping can be achieved by placing multiple folded blankets under the upper body, head, and neck in an attempt to horizontally align the external auditory meatus with the sternal notch and should result in improved laryngeal exposure.

7. **The answer is C.** (Chapter 300) Patients with chronic, progressive, and life-threatening diagnosis will almost always benefit from palliative care. Multiple visits to the emergency department for the same prognostically unfavorable disease state indicate that the care plan is failing and in many settings this patient would benefit from a palliative care consult while in the emergency department. Patients of any age may require a palliative care consult depending on their symptoms and prognosis, so his age is irrelevant in this case. Do not resuscitate or intubate status is not required or indicative of the need for palliative care involvement. Palliative care can be implemented even if the patient is full code, with an emphasis on comfort and maintenance of high quality of life during medical treatment. On the other hand, not all patients who have a do-not-resuscitate or intubate status mandate a need for palliative care. While addressing depression would certainly be a part of the patient's palliative care plan, it is a less acute reason to obtain palliative care consultation from the emergency department.

8. **The answer is C.** (Chapter 301) The majority of pediatric deaths will be subject to investigation by the medical examiner, especially in cases in which there is trauma, the possibility of child abuse, medical procedure complications, or when the death was unexpected. An autopsy may or may not be performed in these cases, but the family is not allowed to refuse an investigation or autopsy if the medical examiner deems it to be necessary. In this case, the family can see the patient in the emergency department, but they may not disturb the body. All lines and tubes must remain in place for verification by the medical examiner. Medical examiner investigation does not preclude the ability for a family to consider organ donation as an option for their child, but the consent of the medical examiner is needed before organ procurement.

9. **The answer is D.** (Chapter 303) Prisoners will be restrained when arriving at the emergency department. Physical mechanisms of restraint may vary. Although many physicians are uncomfortable to examine a patient with handcuffs, it may be necessary if the patient is considered a risk due to a past history of violent behavior. Providers should attempt to comply with the Health Insurance Portability and Accountability Act (HIPPA) regulations and protect medical confidentiality to the greatest degree possible. In the case of serious criminal offenses or a history of violence, however, safety needs take precedence over medical confidentiality. Regardless of the patient's history of violence, police custody is not a substitute for observation or administration of treatment of those who would otherwise be admitted to the hospital if they were not in custody. The use of sedatives should only be used if the patient becomes agitated to minimize harm to himself or others, not as a preventative measure.

10. **The answer is B.** (Chapters 35 and 301) Increasingly, inmates are being managed with medication-assisted treatment therapies such as buprenorphine for opiate use

disorder or chronic pain. Buprenorphine is a partial agonist at the mu receptor and has a higher affinity for the receptor than other opioids. In these cases, it is important to acknowledge that standard therapies of treatment for acute pain may be ineffective. Ketamine is a potent analgesic and may be administered at a dose of 0.1 to 0.3 mg/kg. Although more commonly used at higher doses for procedural sedation or induction for rapid-sequence intubation, subdissociative doses of ketamine are very effective for pain control. Ketamine maintains its effectiveness even when mu receptors are blocked, as in this case. Opiate therapy could be used in this patient, but much higher doses would be needed to achieve analgesia. It is important to keep in mind that respiratory depression may occur in these cases prior to achieving analgesia. Fentanyl at a dose of 1 mg/kg IV or morphine at 0.1 mg/kg IV would be ineffective. Nonnarcotic options such as ketorolac 15 mg IV may be used in appropriate settings but would be inadequate to address the severity of pain from a fracture and should be avoided in patients who are likely to need surgery in the next few hours due to their antiplatelet activity.

11. **The answer is D.** (Chapter 302) Tactical combat casualty care is a standardized, prehospital combat trauma guideline designed to address preventable causes of death. There are three phases of care: care under fire, tactical field care, and casualty evacuation. Medical actions during care under fire are extremely limited. Hemorrhage control with tourniquet application is one of the few measures shown to have benefit while under fire. Emphasis is otherwise placed on moving the wounded to safety and returning fire to secure the area. Even when no longer under fire, combat medics will often deviate from the traditional airway, breathing, and circulation algorithm, as massive hemorrhage is the most common correctable cause of death in the battlefield. Subsequent interventions for tactical field care after primary hemorrhage is controlled include performing needle decompressions for penetrating chest trauma. The threshold to perform this in the tactical setting is low given penetrating trauma will likely have some degree of hemo/pneumothorax and even in the absence of tension the decompression is unlikely to cause harm. Cardiopulmonary resuscitation on combat victims has failed to show any benefit, and apneic or pulseless victims of blast or penetrating trauma are not likely to survive and are not resuscitated per combat trauma guidelines.

12. **The answer is C.** (Chapter 302) Tourniquets have been shown to significantly reduce major hemorrhage from extremity wounds and they should be used when bleeding cannot be controlled with direct pressure alone.

Proper application is crucial to ensure effectiveness and to reduce complications. Windlass-equipped tourniquets with a width greater than 1.5 cm are recommended, and the device should be placed approximately 2 in proximal to the wound. The tourniquet should be tightened until pulsatile flow stops or distal pulses are no longer palpable in the affected extremity. Increased bleeding may result if the tourniquet pressure exceeds venous/diastolic pressure but is less than arterial/systolic pressure. It is important to note that every minute a tourniquet is in place increases the risk of permanent damage. Steps should be made to convert to a pressure dressing once homeostasis is achieved. Tourniquet tension may then be released. Even if a pressure dressing is effective; however, the tourniquet should be left in place on the extremity so that tension may be reapplied if bleeding recurs. Tourniquet application is a temporizing measure only and tourniquets should be removed within approximately 2 hours of placement.

13. **The answer is A.** (Chapter 302) The first-line resuscitation fluid for severe hypovolemic shock in trauma in the combat setting is fresh whole blood. It has all the blood components in a natural state and limits iatrogenic injury of resuscitation. While the use of whole blood is rare in the civilian world, on the battlefield whole blood is obtained from fellow soldiers who are the only blood source, these donors are often referred to as "walking blood banks." If fresh whole blood is not available, packed red blood cells, plasma, and platelets in a 1:1:1 ratio would be the next best resuscitation fluid. Packed red blood cells (PRBCs) alone could be used, but PRBCs lack clotting factors and are inferior to combined blood products. Lactated ringers and other crystalloids are inferior for resuscitation in major hemorrhage, as they lack oxygen-carrying capacity and clotting factors and may contribute to tissue damage and edema when administered in large quantities.

14. **The answer is B.** (Chapter 303) There are several scenarios under which informed consent may be waived in the emergency department. Consent is considered implied for the stabilization of critically ill patients, as long as this is not in conflict with a patient's previously stated wishes (such as those made in a do-not-resuscitate order or advance directive). Accordingly, providers may proceed directly with life-saving measures without first obtaining consent. Consent may also be waived when the patient is judged to lack capacity, is a risk to himself or others, or in instances of public health imperatives. Finally, patients suffering from high-risk communicable diseases such as tuberculosis may be required to undergo treatment in order to prevent transmission to other community members. A hemodynamically stable patient with capacity may refuse a procedure but should be offered

reasonable alternatives to that procedure such as admission for observation. Prisoners maintain decision-making capacity and have autonomy to make their own health care–related decisions. Patients' religious beliefs must be respected as long as the individual has capacity to understand the risks and alternatives to the recommended treatment plan.

15. **The answer is C.** (Chapter 303) Pediatric patients presenting to the emergency department are generally unable to consent to treatment. Exceptions to this rule are outlined in the mature minor doctrine, which is a guideline that stipulates minors may consent to medical treatment without parental consent if he or she is sufficiently mature to understand the nature and consequences of a proposed medical treatment. Although no exact is stipulated, it is generally accepted that patients need to be 14 years or older to consent on their own. The patient who sustains a serious self-inflicted wound will not qualify for the mature minor statute and her wounds will require surgical repair and therefore consent of a legal guardian should be obtained prior to treatment, although it is also important to consider she will need to be evaluated for suicidality regardless of the consent of the legal guardian. Minors may be treated for sexually transmitted infections without legal guardian consent. Most states also allow pregnant minors access to prenatal and other pregnancy-related care independently. Pregnant patients are often considered emancipated minors and may provide consent as adults independently of their legal guardian. Last, the need for consent is waived in patients with imminently life-threatening conditions. A patient's condition may be stabilized by the treating physician without obtaining consent first. The legal guardian should be contacted and consent obtained for further indicated treatments once his condition is stable.

Point-of-Care Ultrasound in the Emergency Department

QUESTIONS

1. A healthy 24-year-old G2P1 woman presents to the emergency department with small-volume vaginal bleeding. She had a positive pregnancy test at home last week. Vital signs are normal and her abdomen is non-tender. Urine pregnancy test is confirmed positive and additional labs are ordered. Pelvic examination shows closed cervical os without active bleeding. You perform a point-of-care transvaginal ultrasound and obtain the following midsagittal view of the uterus (Figure 25.1). Assuming this image is representative of the remainder of the examination, what is your diagnosis?

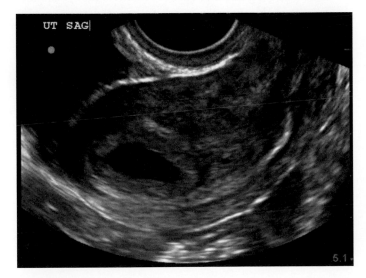

FIGURE 25.1

    (A) Early intrauterine pregnancy
    (B) Ectopic pregnancy
    (C) Incomplete abortion
    (D) Pregnancy of undetermined location

2. A 65-year-old man with history of chronic obstructive pulmonary disease and heart failure with reduced ejection fraction is brought to the emergency department for respiratory distress. Continuous positive airway pressure (CPAP) was initiated by EMS prior to arrival. He is tachycardic and hypertensive. Breath sounds are distant but with some scattered rales. You perform a point-of-care lung ultrasound and obtain the following image. Which of the following findings on point-of-care lung ultrasound suggests exacerbation of his obstructive lung disease as the etiology of his symptoms (Figure 25.2)?

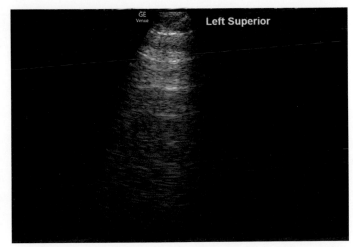

FIGURE 25.2

    (A) Bilateral A-lines
    (B) Bilateral B-lines
    (C) Small bilateral pleural effusions
    (D) Pleural irregularities

3. You are evaluating a patient with metastatic breast cancer for symptomatic pericardial effusion. You perform a point-of-care cardiac ultrasound and obtain the following image. Which of the following echocardiographic features suggests that cardiac tamponade is NOT present (Figure 25.3)?

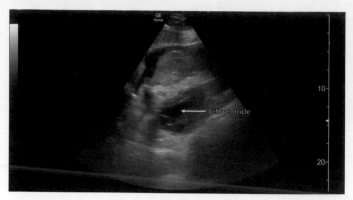

FIGURE 25.4

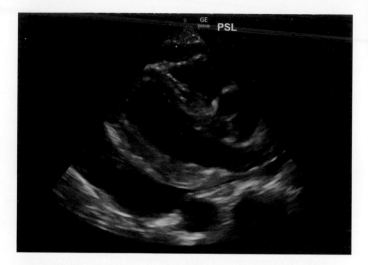

FIGURE 25.3

(A) Collapse of the right ventricle during diastole
(B) Swinging of the heart within the effusion
(C) Inferior vena cava diameter of 1.5 cm with respiratory variation greater than 50%
(D) Small size (<1 cm) of the effusion

4. You are working in an emergency department in a rural hospital when a 45-year-old man arrives via emergency medical services (EMS) after sustaining a stab wound to the chest. He is tachycardic, confused, and combative. You are unable to obtain a blood pressure due to combativeness. After successful endotracheal intubation, blood pressure is found to be 80/50. One unit of packed red blood cells is being given under pressure bag with normalization of blood pressure and improvement in heart rate. You proceed to FAST (focused assessment with sonography for

trauma) examination, which shows no pneumothorax but does reveal the following subxiphoid view. What is the BEST NEXT step (Figure 25.4)?
(A) Administer tranexamic acid
(B) Initiate transfer to trauma center
(C) Obtain computed tomography of the chest
(D) Perform bedside emergency pericardiocentesis

5. You are working overnight when a 42-year-old woman presents to the emergency department for recurrent episodes of epigastric abdominal pain. These episodes typically occur after eating and resolve without intervention. She is afebrile and vital signs are reassuring. Abdomen reveals mild right upper quadrant tenderness without guarding. Labs reveal no leukocytosis and unremarkable hepatic panel. Computed tomography of the abdomen reveals no acute findings. As no sonographer is available at your facility, you perform a point-of-care ultrasound of the gallbladder and obtain the following images. The remainder of your ultrasound examination is reassuring. Her pain is well controlled with oral medication (Figure 25.5). What is the BEST NEXT step?
(A) Consult general surgery
(B) Discharge home with general surgery follow-up
(C) Intravenous antibiotics and admission to internal medicine
(D) Transfer to tertiary care center for additional imaging

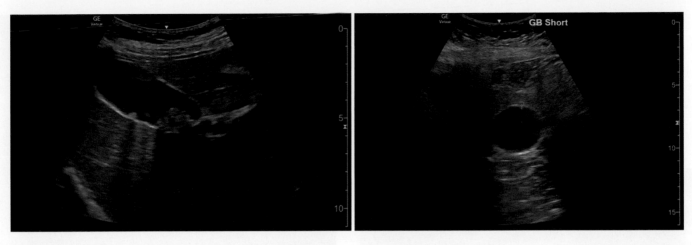

FIGURE 25.5

6. A 70-year-old man with pancreatic adenocarcinoma presents to the emergency department for abrupt onset of chest pain. His HR is 95, BP 100/75, and SpO$_2$ 93% on RA. Examination shows uncomfortable man without other significant abnormality. Electrocardiogram shows no ST-elevation. You perform a point-of-care cardiac ultrasound and obtain the following views (Figure 25.6). What finding suggests the MOST LIKELY etiology in this patient?

(A) Aortic root dilation
(B) Dilation of the right ventricle
(C) Pericardial effusion
(D) Reduced left ventricular ejection fraction

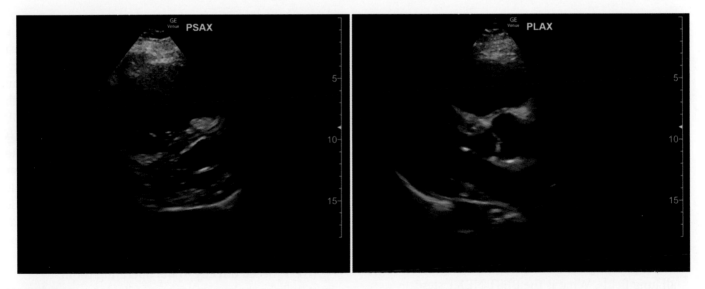

FIGURE 25.6

7. A 56-year-old man with history of end-stage renal disease on hemodialysis presents to the emergency department for acute shortness of breath. His HR is 118 and BP is 142/92. The patient's breathing is visibly labored. You perform a point-of-care limited echocardiogram and obtain the following subxiphoid view (Figure 25.7). What is the CORRECT interpretation of the provided image?

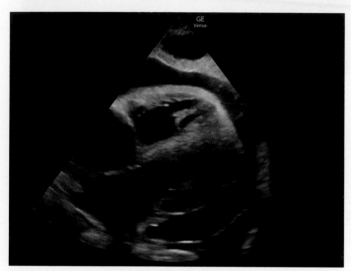

FIGURE 25.7

(A) No pericardial abnormality
(B) Pericardial effusion with features of tamponade
(C) Pericardial effusion without features of tamponade
(D) Pericardial fat

8. A 59-year-old man with history of chronic obstructive pulmonary disease, congestive heart failure, and obesity presents to the emergency department for shortness of breath which began abruptly. He arrives in respiratory distress. He is afebrile with BP 188/90, HR 98, and SpO$_2$ 85% on RA. Breath sounds are distant. You perform a point-of-care lung ultrasound and obtain Figure 25.8. Similar findings are seen in all lung fields. What is the BEST NEXT step?

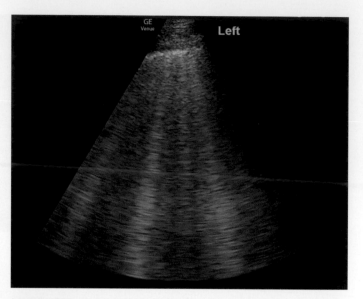

FIGURE 25.8

(A) Administer oxygen via nasal cannula and broad-spectrum antibiotics
(B) Initiate biphasic positive airway pressure (BiPAP) and nitroglycerin infusion
(C) Initiate BiPAP, steroids, and bronchodilators
(D) Needle decompression of the thorax

9. You are working in an emergency department at a tertiary care hospital and a trauma patient has just arrived. He is a 25-year-old man arriving after high-energy motor vehicle collision. His airway is intact but he is in respiratory distress on a nonrebreather. Breath sounds are diminished bilaterally. His HR is 135, BP 86/50, and Glasgow coma scale (GCS) 15. There is no obvious external hemorrhage. You proceed to extended focused assessment with sonography for trauma (eFAST) examination. Abdominal and cardiac views are negative. Figure 25.9 shows the M-mode tracing of the patient's bilateral upper anterior thoraces with a linear probe. What is the BEST NEXT step?
(A) Obtain portable chest x-ray
(B) Proceed directly to the operating room
(C) Tube thoracostomy or needle decompression
(D) Volume resuscitation with blood product

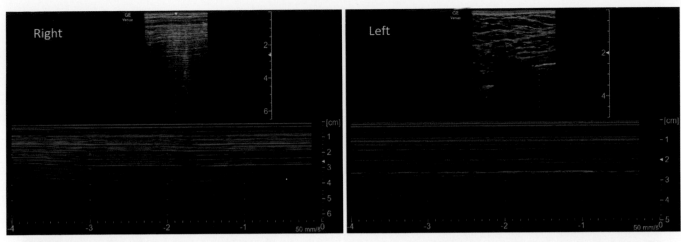

FIGURE 25.9

10. A 22-year-old woman with no significant past medical history presents to the emergency department for hand pain and swelling. Examination is concerning for a cutaneous abscess involving the dorsal aspect of the hand over the fourth to fifth metacarpal region. The patient is wary of incision and drainage, and you offer regional anesthesia via blockade of the ulnar nerve. You obtain the following ultrasound image in transverse plane along the ulnar-volar aspect of the distal third of the forearm (Figure 25.10). Which labeled structure represents the ulnar nerve?

11. A 33-year-old woman with history of infertility presents to the emergency department for vaginal bleeding. She is currently pregnant at approximately 6 weeks by intrauterine insemination. Her HR is 80 and BP is 116/78. Abdomen is soft with mild tenderness in the lower abdomen. Urine pregnancy test is positive. Labs reveal appropriately elevated human chorionic gonadotropin (hCG), Rh positive blood type, and normal complete blood count. Pelvic examination shows closed cervical os. You perform a point-of-care transvaginal ultrasound and obtain the following midsagittal view of the uterus (Figure 25.11). Ovaries are not well visualized and the remainder of the ultrasound examination is unremarkable. What is the BEST NEXT step?

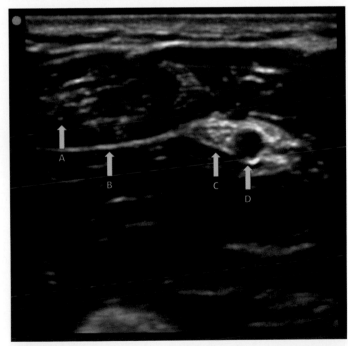

FIGURE 25.10

(A) A
(B) B
(C) C
(D) D

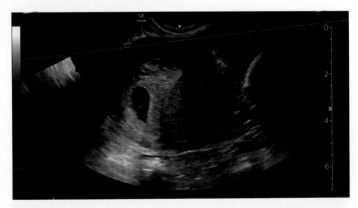

FIGURE 25.11

(A) Diagnostic laparoscopy
(B) Discharge home with obstetrics follow-up
(C) Radiology ("formal") pelvic ultrasound
(D) Magnetic resonance imaging (MRI) of the pelvis

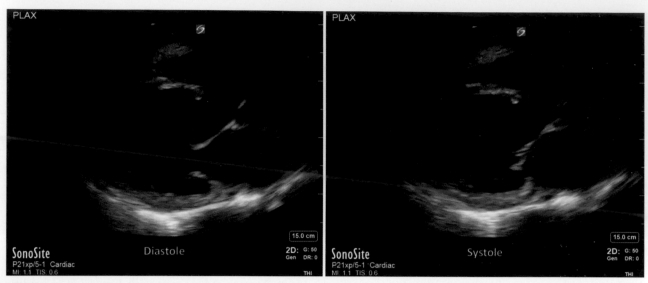

FIGURE 25.12

12. A 63-year-old woman with history of chronic obstructive pulmonary disease, coronary artery disease, and obesity presents to the emergency department with shortness of breath. She is dyspneic and uncomfortable. Lung examination is difficult due to obesity. Chart review shows prior transthoracic echocardiogram with normal left ventricle systolic function. You perform a point-of-care cardiac ultrasound and obtain the following parasternal long-axis view (Figure 25.12). Which of the following interpretations is CORRECT?
    (A) Depressed left ventricle ejection fraction
    (B) Left ventricular mass
    (C) Mitral valve vegetation
    (D) Pericardial effusion without tamponade

13. You are evaluating a 47-year-old man for upper abdominal pain. He is hemodynamically stable. Labs reveal mild leukocytosis with normal liver function tests. You perform the following point-of-care biliary ultrasound (Figure 25.13). What is the CORRECT interpretation of the provided image?

    (A) Choledocholithiasis
    (B) Cholelithiasis without cholecystitis
    (C) Findings concerning for acute cholecystitis
    (D) Intra-abdominal hemorrhage

14. A 72-year-old man with history of hypertension presents to the emergency department for back pain. Pain was abrupt in onset and severe in intensity. There was no associated trauma. On examination, the patient is in distress. Spine and neurologic examinations are normal. His BP is 88/54 and HR 105. Distal pulses are normal. You perform a point-of-care ultrasound of the abdominal aorta and obtain Figure 25.14. What is the BEST NEXT step?
    (A) Consult vascular surgery
    (B) Initiate blood product transfusion
    (C) Initiate norepinephrine infusion
    (D) Obtain computed tomography angiography (CTA) of the aorta

FIGURE 25.13

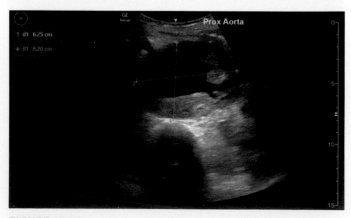

FIGURE 25.14

15. You are evaluating a 68-year-old man with history of hypertension for acute low back pain. The pain was abrupt in onset and is moderate in severity. There were no precipitating injuries. Vital signs and distal pulses are normal. His abdomen and back are non-tender to examination. You perform a point-of-care ultrasound examination of the abdominal aorta and find a maximum diameter of 3.3 cm. He has had no prior abdominal imaging. What additional imaging should this patient undergo for this finding?
    (A) Abdominal ultrasound by radiology ("formal" ultrasound)
    (B) Additional imaging to be determined at follow-up appointment
    (C) Computed tomography angiography (CTA) as an outpatient
    (D) CTA in the emergency department

16. A 65-year-old woman presents to the emergency department with abrupt-onset partial loss of vision in the left eye. There was no preceding trauma. Pupillary and extraocular muscular examination is unremarkable. You perform a point-of-care ultrasound of the affected eye and obtain the following image (Figure 25.15). Which of the following statements is TRUE regarding this diagnosis?

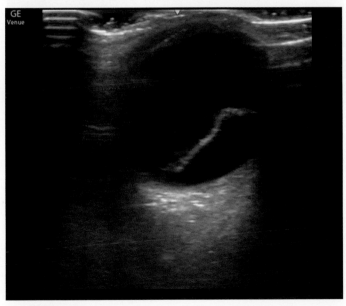

FIGURE 25.15

(A) Risk increases with age.
(B) The patient may be safely discharged to follow up with their ophthalmologist.
(C) The condition is typically painful.
(D) Treatment is generally limited to supportive care.

17. A 32-year-old woman arrives to the emergency department from the scene of a motor vehicle collision. Her airway is intact and bilateral breath sounds are present. Radial pulses are 2+. Glasgow coma scale (GCS) is 14. She has deformities of her left lower leg. Her HR is 128 and BP 84/50. You perform a focused assessment with sonography for trauma (FAST) examination and obtain the following image (Figure 25.16). Your trauma surgeon is expected to arrive at the hospital shortly. Which of the following is CORRECT regarding the FAST examination?

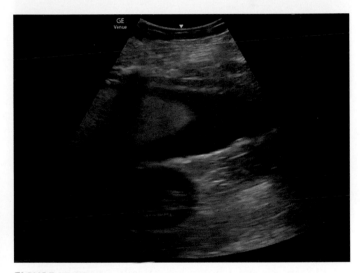

FIGURE 25.16

(A) FAST examination is reliable in excluding solid organ injury.
(B) Urinary catheter placement is helpful in facilitating image acquisition.
(C) Positive FAST examination findings should always be confirmed with additional imaging.
(D) Retroperitoneal hemorrhage is less likely to be detected on FAST than intraperitoneal hemorrhage.

18. A 43-year-old man presents for shortness of breath after fall from a single-story roof. He is awake and speaking in short sentences. He complains of pain in the right lower chest and right flank. His BP is 130/80, HR 95, and SpO$_2$ 92% on RA. You perform a focused assessment with sonography for trauma (FAST) examination and obtain the following image at the right flank (Figure 25.17). Lung sliding is present bilaterally and the remaining views show no free fluid. What is the BEST NEXT step?

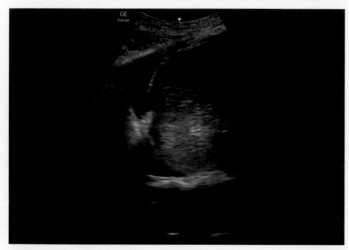

FIGURE 25.17

(A) Begin blood product transfusion
(B) Consult surgery for exploratory laparotomy
(C) Immediate needle decompression
(D) Proceed to computed tomography and prepare for tube thoracostomy

19. You are preparing to perform an emergency pericardiocentesis on a hemodynamically unstable patient after your point-of-care ultrasound revealed a large pericardial effusion evident on multiple views. You have gathered appropriate supplies and personnel. Which of the following is TRUE regarding pericardiocentesis in this case?

(A) Attempted ultrasound guidance results in unnecessary delay in intervention.
(B) Risk of damage to adjacent structures is decreased with ultrasound guidance.
(C) The apical approach should be avoided due to risk of pneumothorax.
(D) The traditional "blind" subxiphoid approach is preferred.

20. A 44-year-old woman with history of hypertension presents to the emergency department for acute upper and low back pain. She appears uncomfortable. Her BP is 192/104 and HR is 110. You perform a bedside ultrasound and obtain the following image of the abdominal aorta in cross section (Figure 25.18). Which of the following is TRUE regarding this scenario?

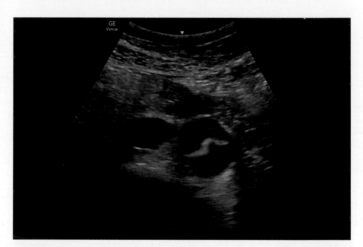

FIGURE 25.18

(A) Computed tomography angiography (CTA) is the imaging modality of choice for this condition.
(B) Negative inotropes should be avoided to prevent iatrogenic hypotension.
(C) Point-of-care ultrasound has excellent sensitivity for this condition.
(D) This finding should be confirmed with CTA as the next step in this patient's care.

ANSWERS

1. **The answer is D.** (Chapter 98) The provided image shows a sac in the uterus without visualized contents, representing an empty gestational sac. While the majority of gestational sacs proceed normally to an intrauterine gestation, a pseudogestational sac may appear in the setting of ectopic or heterotopic pregnancy. Diagnosis of an intrauterine pregnancy therefore requires visualization of a gestational sac with either a yolk sac or fetal pole. Ectopic pregnancy remains possible, but sonographic diagnosis requires visualization of an extrauterine gestational sac with yolk sac or fetal pole. Incomplete abortion may have this sonographic appearance but would require a previously known intrauterine pregnancy as well as an open cervical os (Figure 25.19).

2. **The answer is A.** (Chapter 53) The provided image shows a repeating pattern of horizontally oriented hyperechoic lines, which are termed A-lines. These are typically seen in normal or nonedematous lungs. B-lines are vertically oriented, hyperechoic, laser-like lines extending to the bottom of the field of view. The presence of three or more B-lines in any given field of view is considered abnormal and may be due to pulmonary edema, pneumonia, inflammation, or atelectasis. The presence of bilateral B-lines suggests pulmonary edema in the correct clinical context. The presence of A-lines and absence of B-lines suggest the lack of an infectious or edematous process. In this scenario, this leaves a chronic obstructive pulmonary disease exacerbation as the likely etiology. Pleural effusions are another indicator of hypervolemia. Pleural irregularities are typically seen with an inflammatory or infectious process such as pneumonia (viral or bacterial) (Figure 25.20).

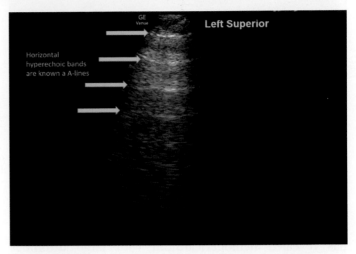

FIGURE 25.20

3. **The answer is C.** (Chapter 55) Determining the hemodynamic significance of an effusion can be challenging. It is therefore important to evaluate multiple markers for this condition. In tamponade, the obstruction begins at the level of the right atrium and/or right ventricle, resulting in buildup of venous pressure in the inferior vena cava. This manifests as a dilated (>2 cm) and plethoric (minimal respiratory variation) inferior vena cava. Collapse of the right ventricle during diastole suggests tamponade is present. Size of the pericardial effusion is not a reliable indicator of tamponade, as even a small effusion can cause hemodynamic instability if accumulated rapidly. Swinging of the heart is commonly seen in large effusions. Although swinging is often seen in tamponade, a large effusion may accumulate slowly and allow the pericardium to accommodate the fluid without hemodynamic consequence (Figure 25.21).

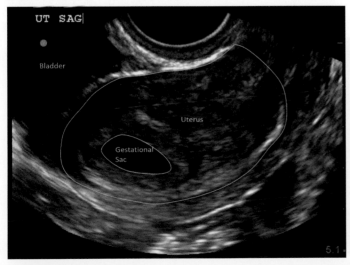

FIGURE 25.19

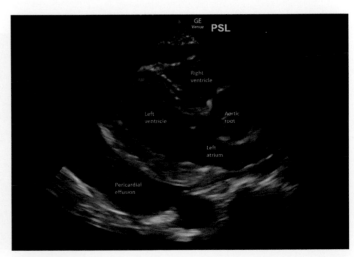

FIGURE 25.21

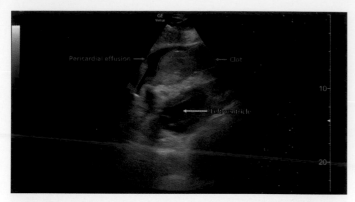

FIGURE 25.22

4. The answer is B. (Chapter 262) Your focused assessment with sonography for trauma (FAST) examination has revealed hemopericardium with large thrombus resulting in collapse of the right ventricle. Given the patient's hemodynamic instability, this is diagnostic of cardiac tamponade. This patient's condition is expected to rapidly deteriorate without definitive surgical management, and he should therefore be transferred as quickly as possible. Bedside emergency pericardiocentesis can be attempted as a temporizing measure and, if successful, can be accompanied by drain placement. However, with suspected hemopericardium and large thrombus visible on ultrasound, pericardiocentesis would likely be of limited utility. Tranexamic acid is indicated in this case if the injury occurred within 3 hours of evaluation, but definitive management of patient's cardiac tamponade takes precedence. Computerized tomography should not delay further resuscitative measures including transfer at this point (Figure 25.22).

5. The answer is B. (Chapter 79) The provided images show multiple shadowing stones within the gallbladder lumen with normal gallbladder wall thickness.

Her recurrent pain represents biliary colic due to uncomplicated cholelithiasis. With reassuring laboratory evaluation and adequate pain control, outpatient general surgery referral is appropriate. Consulting general surgery would be appropriate if she had evidence of acute cholecystitis. Sonographic features of cholecystitis are pericholecystic fluid, gallbladder wall thickening greater than 3 mm, and sonographic Murphy's sign. None of these sonographic features are present. Additionally, although CT has poor sensitivity for gallstones, it is a sensitive modality for acute cholecystitis. Intravenous antibiotics and admission to internal medicine would be appropriate for acute cholangitis. However, this patient has no fever, derangement in liver function tests, or concerning CT findings to suggest cholangitis. Transfer to tertiary care center for additional imaging is not necessary in this patient with a clear diagnosis of uncomplicated cholelithiasis with biliary colic (Figure 25.23).

6. The answer is B. (Chapter 50) This is an example of severe dilation of the right ventricle, suggesting right heart strain. The right ventricle is approximately two-thirds the size of the left ventricle in a healthy heart. Pancreatic cancer is a strong risk factor for pulmonary embolism and should raise suspicion for such in any patient with chest pain. The parasternal short axis also demonstrates septal bowing, wherein the septum is pushed into the cavity of the left ventricle. This is further evidence of right heart strain. Additional sonographic signs of right heart strain include McConnell's sign (apical hyperkinesis of the right ventricle), tricuspid regurgitation, or tricuspid annular plane systolic excursion (TAPSE) less than 2.0 cm. The aortic root is not dilated. The bulb appearance just distal to the aortic valve is due to the sinuses of Valsalva—a normal anatomic appearance. There is no pericardial effusion. The anterior leaflet of the mitral valve is approaching

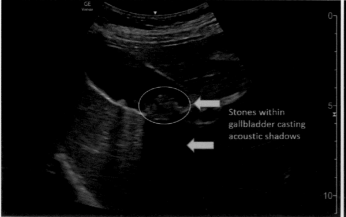

Stones within gallbladder casting acoustic shadows

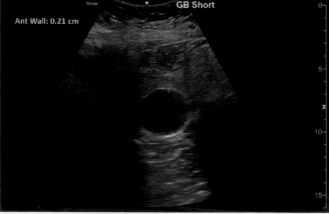

Ant Wall: 0.21 cm

GB Short

FIGURE 25.23

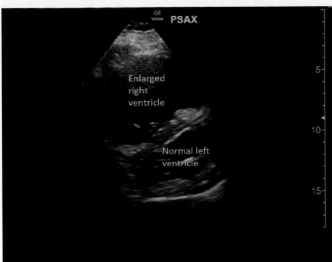

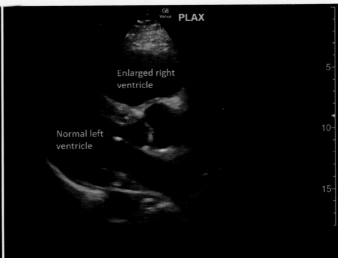

FIGURE 25.24

the interventricular septum, suggesting normal left ventricular ejection fraction (Figure 25.24).

7. **The answer is C.** (Chapter 55) While diagnosing cardiac tamponade remains ultimately a clinical endeavor, point-of-care ultrasound has been widely adopted to aid in this evaluation. In the provided image, there is seen simple anechoic fluid surrounding the heart representing a pericardial effusion. However, all four chambers of the heart are well-filled. In tamponade, we would expect to see collapse of the right atrium during systole and collapse of the right ventricle during diastole. Additional findings of cardiac tamponade include plethoric inferior vena cava, collapse of the left atrium and ventricle, and increased variation in atrioventricular valve inflow velocities. Pericardial or epicardial fat appears as a heteroechoic layer on ultrasound with limited mobility and is not present here (Figure 25.25).

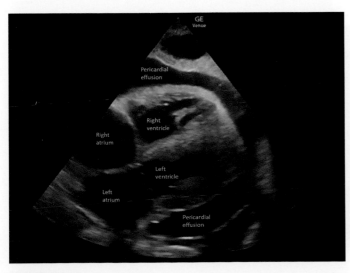

FIGURE 25.25

8. **The answer is B.** (Chapter 53) The provided image shows B-lines. B-lines are vertically oriented, hyperechoic, laser-like lines extending to the bottom of the field of view. They are a type of artifact that arises due to interstitial edema of the examined lung tissue. The presence of three or more B-lines in any given field of view is considered abnormal and may be due to pulmonary edema, pneumonia, inflammation, or atelectasis. With B-lines in all lung fields and significant hypertension, the diagnosis of pulmonary edema can be made. Acute hypertensive pulmonary edema (flash pulmonary edema, sympathetic crashing acute pulmonary edema) is best initially managed with a combination of positive airway pressure and a vasodilating agent such as nitroglycerin. Antibiotics may be needed if infection is suspected, but management of the patient's respiratory distress must be initiated first. Positive airway pressure with steroids and bronchodilators is appropriate management of obstructive lung disease. However, obstructive lung disease typically results in A-lines on lung ultrasound and would not be expected to show generalized B-lines. Needle decompression of the thorax is the treatment of choice for tension pneumothorax. Pneumothorax would be detected by the absence of lung sliding, which was not described in this scenario, nor is the patient hypotensive (Figure 25.26).

9. **The answer is C.** (Chapter 68) The provided images reveal evidence of a pneumothorax on the right. These are M-mode tracings of the chest wall, pleura, and lung. On the image labeled "Left," there is the typical "sandy beach" appearance showing horizontal lines of a static chest wall (the waves of the sea) and the speckled appearance of moving lung (the sand of the shore). On the image labeled "Right," there is an absence of the speckled appearance

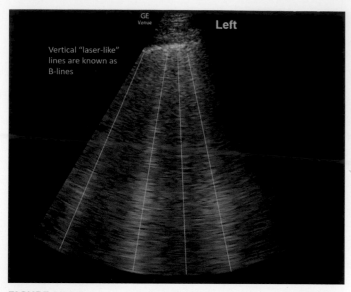

FIGURE 25.26

and instead we see horizontal lines extending throughout the depth of the image. This is sometimes referred to as the "Barcode" sign. This suggests a lack of lung sliding and, in the setting of trauma, pneumothorax. As this patient is hemodynamically unstable and in respiratory distress, an intervention is required in the primary survey. Moving sequentially through the primary survey results in a "breathing" intervention first. Decompressing the affected hemithorax is therefore the best next step. Chest x-ray would cause an unnecessary delay in treatment of this unstable patient, as lung ultrasound is sensitive and specific in this setting. There is no indication to proceed to the operating room at this point. Volume resuscitation with blood product is likely indicated, but a stepwise progression through the primary survey dictates treatment for suspected tension pneumothorax takes precedence (Figure 25.27).

10. **The answer is C.** (Chapter 36) It is important to be able to recognize all major structures on soft tissue point-of-care ultrasound in its applications in infection, vascular access, and regional anesthesia. Peripheral nerves are identified by their "honeycomb" structure with mixed hyperechoic and hypoechoic internal structure and predictable relationship to vascular and musculoskeletal structures. The brightness of a nerve is significantly dependent on the angle of probe relative to course of the nerve (termed anisotropy). Structure A is the typical speckled and striated appearance of muscle in cross section. Structure B is a linear and hyperechoic plane, representing fascia. Structure D is a blood vessel—the ulnar artery.

11. **The answer is C.** (Chapter 98) The provided image shows an intrauterine gestational sac with a yolk sac, diagnostic of an intrauterine pregnancy. Usually, confirmation of an intrauterine pregnancy is sufficient to exclude an ectopic pregnancy. However, this patient has received assisted reproductive technology (ART), which significantly increases their risk for heterotopic pregnancy. Heterotopic pregnancy is the simultaneous presence of both an intrauterine gestation and an ectopic gestation. In this patient with vaginal bleeding and abdominal tenderness, one must maintain a high suspicion for ectopic pregnancy. More comprehensive pelvic sonography performed by radiology will allow for better evaluation for adnexal masses and should be the next step. Depending on degree of clinical suspicion, consultation with an obstetrician may also be indicated. Diagnostic laparoscopy is not indicated at this point without additional imaging. Discharge home would be appropriate in the absence of ART. Magnetic resonance imaging does have a high sensitivity and specificity for ectopic pregnancy, but cost and availability limit its usage as first-line imaging in this case (Figure 25.28).

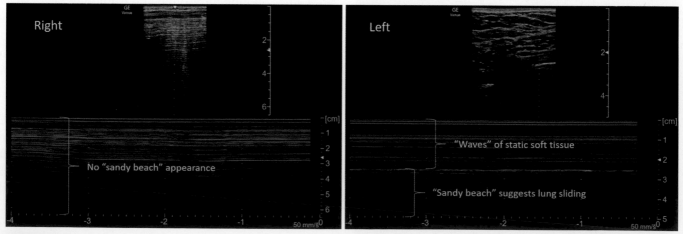

FIGURE 25.27

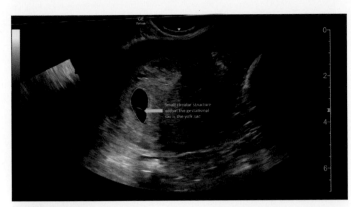

FIGURE 25.28

12. The answer is A. (Chapter 53) This is an example of typical sonographic features of left ventricular systolic dysfunction. The two key qualitative indicators of ejection fraction in a point-of-care cardiac ultrasound are mobility of the anterior leaflet of the mitral valve and motion of the left ventricular walls. The anterior leaflet of the mitral valve should closely approach the interventricular septum during diastole. In the provided images, the mitral valve shows little excursion in diastole, suggesting reduced systolic function. Subjectively, there is very little movement in the walls of the left ventricle between the two images, further suggesting reduced left ventricle ejection fraction. There is no pericardial effusion in these images. The fluid at the near field of the image has the typical triangular appearance of the right ventricle and there is no fluid at the posterior pericardial interface. There is no apparent left ventricular mass or mitral valve vegetation, although point-of-care ultrasound is insensitive for these entities (Figure 25.29).

13. The answer is C. (Chapter 79) The provided image demonstrates multiple sonographic features concerning for acute cholecystitis. Typical sonographic features of cholecystitis include pericholecystic fluid, gallbladder wall thickening greater than 0.3 cm, stones or sludge in the neck of the gallbladder, and sonographic Murphy's sign (maximal abdominal tenderness over the visualized gallbladder). In the provided image, we see multiple shadowing stones in the dependent portion of the gallbladder, gallbladder wall thickening, and pericholecystic fluid. Choledocholithiasis may be suggested by dilation of the common bile duct but requires visualization of a stone in the common bile duct for diagnosis. This is typically beyond the scope of point-of-care ultrasound in the emergency department. Cholelithiasis without cholecystitis is suggested when stones are visualized within the gallbladder without signs of inflammation (pericholecystic fluid, thickened gallbladder wall, sonographic Murphy's sign). Intra-abdominal hemorrhage is evidenced by free fluid in the correct clinical setting and may be seen in many places in the abdomen. However, it is most commonly seen in the focused assessment with sonography for trauma (FAST) examination views including the hepatorenal recess, the perisplenic area, and the rectovesical/rectouterine spaces (Figure 25.30).

14. The answer is A. (Chapter 60) The provided image shows a large aneurysm of the abdominal aorta. Aneurysm of the abdominal aorta is defined as diameter greater than 3 cm at any point. Aneurysms greater than 5 cm in diameter are at greater risk for rupture. This patient has an unstable aortic aneurysm as evidenced by his hypotension and distress. Ultrasound is sufficient

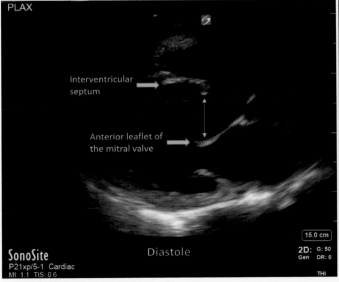

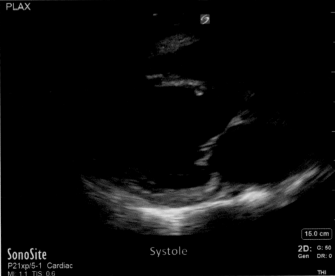

FIGURE 25.29

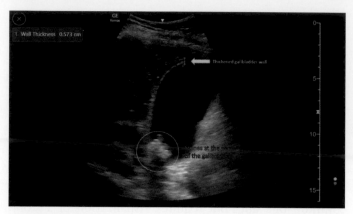

FIGURE 25.30

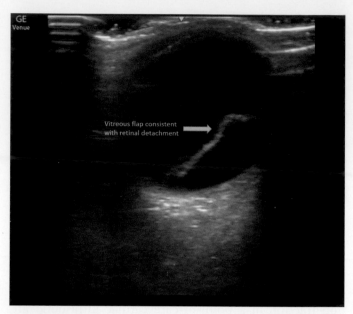

FIGURE 25.32

to make this diagnosis and vascular surgery should be immediately consulted for definitive management. Consulting vascular surgery should not be delayed by additional imaging in unstable patients. Although blood product or crystalloid administration may be used for resuscitation, the most important next step is rapid vascular intervention. Further, permissive hypotension with a goal systolic blood pressure of 80 to 90 is supported by current guidelines. Vasoactive medications are not the first-line agent in resuscitation of unstable aortic aneurysm (Figure 25.31).

15. **The answer is D.** (Chapter 60) This patient meets diagnostic criteria for abdominal aortic aneurysm. Aneurysm of the abdominal aorta is defined as diameter greater than 3 cm at any point. Aneurysms greater than 5 cm in diameter are at greater risk for rupture. This is a stable patient as evidenced by his reassuring examination and vital signs. Although aneurysms smaller than 5 cm are less likely to rupture, aneurysms may be symptomatic at any size and this is a new diagnosis for the patient. Computed

tomography angiography should therefore be performed in the emergency department if there is any suspicion this may a symptomatic aneurysm. Abdominal ultrasound in radiology is a good screening test for abdominal aortic aneurysm but is not the modality of choice for evaluating anatomic detail of an aneurysm. Additional imaging should not be deferred to the outpatient setting in this patient with a new diagnosis of abdominal aortic aneurysm and back pain.

16. **The answer is A.** (Chapter 241) The provided ultrasound image demonstrates a thin irregular echogenic line anterior to the retina consistent with a retinal detachment. Risk factors for retinal detachment include increasing age, myopia, and family history of retinal detachment. It is a time-sensitive condition, which requires prompt intervention to minimize vision loss. Ophthalmology should be consulted emergently. The condition is typically painless as opposed to painful monocular visual loss disorders such as acute glaucoma or optic neuritis. There are several vision-preserving interventions, which may be performed in a time-sensitive fashion. Treatment should be discussed with an ophthalmologist as soon as the diagnosis is suspected or confirmed (Figure 25.32).

17. **The answer is D.** (Chapter 263) The focused assessment with sonography for trauma (FAST) examination is a rapid tool to accurately detect the presence of intraperitoneal free fluid. The provided image demonstrates a large amount of fluid adjacent to the liver. Although FAST

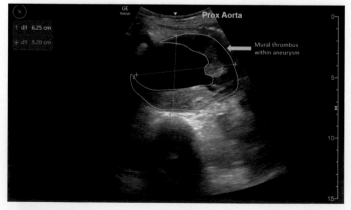

FIGURE 25.31

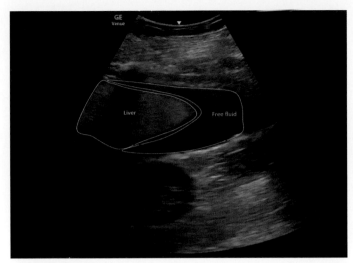

FIGURE 25.33

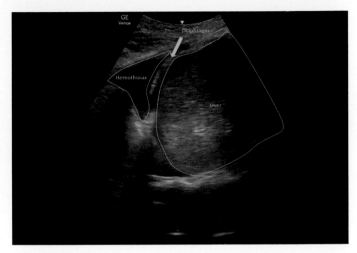

FIGURE 25.34

examination shows excellent specificity for peritoneal free fluid, there are important limitations of which operators must be mindful. Although the FAST examination performs well in detecting intraperitoneal hemorrhage, it is less reliable in the detection of retroperitoneal hemorrhage. FAST is not sensitive for solid organ injuries in isolation and computed tomography should be pursued if solid organ injury is suspected despite a negative FAST. A complete FAST examination requires a bladder, which is at least partially filled to visualize the rectovesicular or rectouterine space. Placement of a urinary catheter is therefore likely to render the pelvic view indeterminate. There are clinical situations in which confirmatory imaging is not necessary. The hemodynamically unstable patient described in this scenario is such a situation, as a positive FAST with hemodynamic instability is an absolute indication for exploratory laparotomy (Figure 25.33).

18. **The answer is D.** (Chapter 261) The provided image demonstrates free fluid near the liver. This fluid is intrapleural as evidenced by its location superior to the diaphragm and the typical triangular shape of the costophrenic recess. In the setting of blunt thoracic trauma, this likely represents acute hemothorax. Tube thoracostomy remains the treatment of choice for moderate-to-large sized hemothorax (greater than 200 mL). However, as this is a stable patient, it is appropriate to obtain cross-sectional imaging to further characterize the fluid collection prior to intervention. Blood product transfusion is not indicated in the initial management of this hemodynamically stable patient. There is no indication for exploratory laparotomy at this point given the patient's stability, and further radiographic evaluation should be pursued. A large pneumothorax was ruled out with bilateral lung sliding on

focused assessment with sonography for trauma (FAST) examination and needle decompression is therefore not indicated (Figure 25.34).

19. **The answer is B.** (Chapter 34) Emergency pericardiocentesis is a rarely performed but potentially life-saving procedure for the emergency physician. It has classically been performed via the traditional "blind" subxiphoid approach wherein a long needle is inserted percutaneously deep to the xiphoid process and directed toward the left shoulder. This approach remains preferred by many in the setting of cardiac arrest with chest compressions. In the nonarresting patient, ultrasound guidance decreases the risk of damage to adjacent structures such as the GI tract, liver, diaphragm, and lung. Using ultrasound guidance, one should identify the approach with the largest and most superficial pocket of pericardial fluid. As ultrasound is available in this scenario, the traditional "blind" subxiphoid approach is not preferred. Ultrasound guidance may result in small increases in preparation time, but the advantages of improved success rate and decreased iatrogenic injury generally outweigh the risk. The apical and parasternal approaches are often the safest approach when identified with ultrasound.

20. **The answer is A.** (Chapter 59) The provided image demonstrates an irregular echogenic line traversing the abdominal aorta representing a dissection flap. Point-of-care ultrasound has excellent specificity for the detection of dissection and, with appropriate clinical correlate, treatment should be initiated immediately. However, computed tomography angiography (CTA) remains the test of choice for aortic dissection in the emergency department given its excellent sensitivity and ability to

define extent of disease. Although CTA is likely to be obtained in the emergency department to determine the extent of disease and need for intervention, the next step in this patient's care is consulting vascular surgery and initiating blood pressure control for her likely unstable dissection. Negative inotropes such as esmolol or labetalol are first-line agents for blood pressure control. Point-of-care ultrasound has relatively poor sensitivity for aortic dissection and should therefore not be used in isolation as a rule-out test.